Oral Pathology for Dental Hygienists and Assistants

Adel M Abdel-Azim, MDSc, PhD

Professor and Former Chairman of

Oral Pathology Department,

Faculty of Dentistry, Ain Shams University, Egypt

Ahmed A Abdel-Azim, BDS, MD

Oral Medicine Consultant

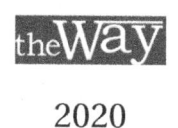

theWay

2020

Second Edition, 2020

theWay

Copyright 2020 by Adel M Abdel-Azim & Ahmed A Abdel-Azim

All rights reserved. No part of this publication may be reproduced, stored in a retrieval system, or transmitted in any form or by any means, electronic, mechanical, photocopying, recording or otherwise, without a written permission of the authors.

ISBN 978-1-7341882-3-3

Giza, Egypt, Zip Code 12555

https://dr-adel.site

E-mail: adelmam55@gmail.com

Medical knowledge is constantly changing. As new information becomes available, changes in treatment, procedures, equipment and the use of drugs become necessary. Readers are strongly recommended to follow up with recent medical information.

The use of registered names, trademarks, etc. in this book does not imply, even in the absence of a specific statement, that such names are exempt from the relevant protective laws and regulations and therefore free for general use.

Product liability: The publisher cannot guarantee the accuracy of any information about the dosage and application mentioned in this book. In every individual case, the reader must check such information by consulting the most recent literature.

PREFACE

This is a unique textbook of oral pathology. Although it is short and concise, it took a long time to write and evolve. Each sentence was fine-tuned for students studying for a degree in dental hygiene, dental assistants, and health professions. The aim of this book is to present the basic facts regarding oral pathology in a concise and clear short bullet. The normal anatomy, histology, physiology, and general pathological facts were sparingly touched to remind the students of what they studied in the past years. Although this caries some redundancy, we think that redundancy is not always a devil, and in many instances, it proves to be beneficial.

The book is also comprehensive covering almost all curricula currently required by many universities allover the world. Some of the microscopic and molecular details typically found in comparable textbooks have been eliminated. Each chapter focuses on the essential knowledge necessary to build a broad, fundamental understanding, with supporting detail where relevant.

In spite of best efforts, some mistakes may have sneaked in, which we request all our students and colleagues to kindly draw to our notification. Your recommendations, gratitude, and criticism will be appreciated.

Contents

1 **Developmental Disturbances: Back to Basics** 1
   1.1   Hereditary and Diseases 1
         1.1.1   Concept of expressivity 3
         1.1.2   Concept of penetrance 4
         1.1.3   Sex limited traits 4
         1.1.4   Classification of Hereditary diseases 4
   1.2   Environmental Factors and Diseases 10
         1.2.1   Teratogens 10
         1.2.2   Proven teratogenic agents in man 10

2 **Developmental Disturbances of Hard Dental Tissues** 13
   2.1   Normal Tooth Development 13
   2.2   Classification of Developmental Disturbances of Teeth 14
   2.3   Abnormalities in Number 16
         2.3.1   Increase in number (Hyperdontia) 16
         2.3.2   Decrease in Number (Hypodontia) 19
   2.4   Abnormalities in Size 21
         2.4.1   Macrodontia 21
         2.4.2   Microdontia 22
   2.5   Abnormalities in Shape 23
         2.5.1   Gemination (Schizodontia) 23
         2.5.2   Fusion 23
         2.5.3   Concrescence 24

Contents

- 2.5.4 Dilaceration 24
- 2.5.5 Taurodontism 24
- 2.5.6 Dens in dente (Dens Invaginatus) 25
- 2.5.7 Dens Evaginatus (Occlusal Enamel Drop) 25
- 2.5.8 Enamel Pearl 26
- 2.5.9 Talon Cusp 26
- 2.5.10 Supernumerary Roots 26
- 2.5.11 Supernumerary Cusps 26
- 2.5.12 Peg shaped laterals 27
- 2.5.13 Dental Abnormalities of Congenital Syphilis 27
- 2.6 Abnormalities in Structure 28
  - 2.6.1 Acquired Localized Enamel Hypoplasia 30
  - 2.6.2 Acquired Generalized Enamel Hypoplasia 30
  - 2.6.3 Dental Fluorosis (Mottled Enamel) 31
  - 2.6.4 Abnormal Tooth Discoloration 33
  - 2.6.5 Hereditary Defects of Enamel 35
- 2.7 Lyon Hypothesis 37
  - 2.7.1 Hereditary Defects of dentin 38
  - 2.7.2 Obscure Defects of dentin 45
- 2.8 Disturbances in Eruption 46
  - 2.8.1 Early Eruption 46
  - 2.8.2 Delayed Eruption 47
  - 2.8.3 Teething Problems 48
- 2.9 Multisystem Disorders Affecting Teeth 48

3 Developmental Disturbances of Oral & Para-Oral Tissues 53
- 3.1 Developmental Disturbances of Face 53
  - 3.1.1 Treacher Collins Syndrome 53
  - 3.1.2 Pierre Robin Syndrome 54
  - 3.1.3 Crouzon Syndrome 56

	3.1.4	Cleft Lip and Palate	57
	3.1.5	Oblique Facial Cleft	61
	3.1.6	Transverse Facial Cleft	61
	3.1.7	Macrostomia	62
	3.1.8	Microstomia	62
	3.1.9	Facial Hemihypertrophy (Hemifacial Hypertrophy)	62
	3.1.10	Facial Hemihypoplasia (Hemifacial Atrophy)	63
3.2	Developmental Disturbances of Jaws	64
	3.2.1	Agnathia (Aplasia of Mandible)	64
	3.2.2	Micrognathia (Mandibular Dysostosis)	64
	3.2.3	Macrognathia	65
3.3	Developmental Disturbances of Palate	65
	3.3.1	Cleft Palate	65
	3.3.2	Torus Palatinus	65
3.4	Developmental Disturbances of Lips	66
	3.4.1	Cleft Lip	66
	3.4.2	Double Lip	66
	3.4.3	Congenital Lip Pits and Fistulae	67
	3.4.4	Cheillits Glandularis	67
	3.4.5	Cheillitis Granulomatosa	68
	3.4.6	Melkersson - Rosenthal Syndrome	69
	3.4.7	Xeroderma Pigmentosa	70
	3.4.8	Peutz - Jeghers Syndrome	70
3.5	Developmental Disturbances of Oral Mucosa	72
	3.5.1	Fordyce's Granules (Spots)	72
	3.5.2	Leukoedema	72
	3.5.3	White Spongy Nevus	73
	3.5.4	Hereditary Benign Intraepithelial Dyskeratosis	74
	3.5.5	Darier's Disease	75
	3.5.6	Epidermolysis Bullosa	77

	3.5.7	Hereditary Hemorrhagic Telangiectasia	78
	3.5.8	Dyskeratosis Congenita	79
	3.5.9	Fanconi's Syndrome	79
	3.5.10	Pachyonychia Congenita	79
	3.5.11	Plumer-Vinson Syndrome	80
3.6	Developmental Disturbances of Tongue		80
	3.6.1	Aglossia	80
	3.6.2	Microglossia	81
	3.6.3	Macroglossia	81
	3.6.4	Ankyloglossia (Tongue Tie)	81
	3.6.5	Lingual Varicosities (Lingual Varices)	82
	3.6.6	Prominent Circumvallate Papillae	82
	3.6.7	Lingual Tonsils	83
	3.6.8	Cleft Tongue (Bifid Tongue)	84
	3.6.9	Fissured Tongue	84
	3.6.10	Median Rhomboidal Glossitis	85
	3.6.11	Glossitis Areata Exofoliativa	85
	3.6.12	Hairy Tongue (Black Hairy Tongue)	86
	3.6.13	Black Tongue	87
	3.6.14	Furred Tongue	87
	3.6.15	Thyroglossal Tract Cyst	88
	3.6.16	Lingual Thyroid Nodule	88
3.7	Developmental Disturbances of Salivary Glands		89
	3.7.1	Aplasia	89
	3.7.2	Atresia	89
	3.7.3	Aberrancy	89
	3.7.4	Latent Bone Cyst	90
3.8	Developmental Disturbances of Gingiva		90
	3.8.1	Fibromatosis Gingivae	90
	3.8.2	Gingival Cyst of Adult	91

		3.8.3	Gingival Cysts of Newborn (Bohn's Nodules)	91
		3.8.4	Epstein's Pearls	92
	3.9		Multisystem Disorders Affecting Oral and Para-Oral Tissues	92
		3.9.1	Cleidocranial Dysplasia	92
		3.9.2	Gardener's Syndrome (Polyposis Coli)	93
		3.9.3	Ehlers-Danlos Syndrome (Floppy Joint)	93
		3.9.4	Hypophosphatasia	93
		3.9.5	Hereditary Hypophosphatemia	94
		3.9.6	Early Onset Idiopathic Hypoparathyroidism	96
		3.9.7	Oral Facial Digital Syndrome *(OFDS)*	96
		3.9.8	Mongolism (Down's syndrome, Trisomy 21)	97
4	**Dental Caries**			**99**
	4.1		Definition	99
	4.2		Classification of dental caries	99
	4.3		Sequelae of caries	101
	4.4		Etiology of Dental Caries	102
		4.4.1	Contributing factors	102
		4.4.2	Theories of Dental Caries	115
	4.5		Pathology of enamel caries	116
		4.5.1	Macroscopic Picture	116
		4.5.2	Microscopic Picture	117
	4.6		Pathology of dentin Caries	119
		4.6.1	Macroscopic Picture	119
		4.6.2	Microscopic Picture	120
	4.7		Immunology of Dental Caries	122
5	**Periodontal Diseases**			**125**
	5.1		Back to Basics	125
	5.2		Periodontium in health	126
	5.3		Etiology of Periodontal Diseases	127

		5.3.1	Host-Bacterial Balance 127
		5.3.2	Dental Plaque: Formation and Mechanism of Action . 129
	5.4	Sequence of events leading to gingivitis 129
	5.5	Sequence of events leading to periodontitis 130
	5.6	Diagnosis of periodontal disease 131
		5.6.1	Chronic gingivitis 131
		5.6.2	Chronic periodontitis 132
	5.7	Non-surgical treatment of periodontal disease 132
		5.7.1	Supra-gingival calculus 134
		5.7.2	Subgingival calculus 135
	5.8	Surgical treatment of periodontal disease 136
		5.8.1	Gingivectomy 136
		5.8.2	Flap surgery 137
	5.9	Other periodontal conditions 138
		5.9.1	Acute necrotizing ulcerative gingivitis 138
		5.9.2	Lateral periodontal abscess 139
		5.9.3	Pericoronitis 139
6	**Diseases of Pulp and Periapical Tissues** **141**
	6.1	Characteristics of Pulp Inflammation 141
	6.2	Etiology of pulp inflammation 142
	6.3	Classification of Pulpitis 143
	6.4	Correlation Between Clinical Signs and Histological Features 144
	6.5	Pulp Diseases 146
		6.5.1	Focal Reversible Pulpitis (Pulp Hyperemia) 146
		6.5.2	Acute Pulpitis 149
		6.5.3	Pulp necrosis 150
		6.5.4	Chronic Pulpitis 151
		6.5.5	Chronic Hyperplastic Pulpitis (Pulp Polyp) 152
		6.5.6	Pulp Calcification 154

		6.5.7	Calcific Metamorphosis 156
		6.5.8	Internal Resorption 159
	6.6	Periapical Diseases 159
		6.6.1	Periapical Granuloma 159
		6.6.2	Periapical Abscess 162
		6.6.3	Acute Periapical Abscess 162
		6.6.4	Chronic Periapical Abscess 167
		6.6.5	Periapical Cemental Dysplasia and True Cementoma 168
		6.6.6	Hypercementosis 168

7 Cysts & Cyst-Like Lesions 169

	7.1	Introduction 169
		7.1.1	Definition 169
		7.1.2	Histogenesis of Epithelial Lining 169
		7.1.3	Pathogenesis of Cysts 170
		7.1.4	Mechanism of Cyst Enlargement 170
		7.1.5	Complications of Cysts 170
		7.1.6	Classification of Cysts 171
	7.2	Odontogenic cysts 173
		7.2.1	Inflammatory Odontogenic Cysts 173
		7.2.2	Developmental odontogenic cysts 179
	7.3	Non-odontogenic cysts 191
		7.3.1	Fissural cysts 191
		7.3.2	Cysts arising from embryonic vestiges (tracts) 195
		7.3.3	Cysts of salivary glands: 198
		7.3.4	Other soft tissue cysts 198
		7.3.5	Cysts of the Maxillary Antrum 200

8 Physical, Chemical & Idiopathic Pathology of Teeth 203

	8.1	Attrition 203
	8.2	Abrasion 205

8.3	Erosion	206
8.4	Abfraction	207
8.5	Dentinal Sclerosis	207
8.6	Secondary dentin and Tertiary dentin	208
8.7	Pulp Calcification	209
8.8	Resorption of Teeth	209
	8.8.1 External Resorption	211
	8.8.2 Internal Resorption	214
8.9	Hypercementosis (Cementum Hyperplasia)	217
8.10	Hypocementosis	218
8.11	Tooth Ankylosis	218
8.12	Tooth Concussion	221
8.13	Tooth Luxation	221
8.14	Tooth Avulsion	222

9 Spread of Dental Infection . . . 223

9.1	Basic Definitions	223
9.2	Introduction to Dental Infections	224
9.3	Methods of Spread of Odontogenic infections	224
9.4	Factors governing the spread of dental infection	225
	9.4.1 Microbial Factors:	226
	9.4.2 Host Factors:	226
9.5	Complications associated with the spread of dental infection	227
	9.5.1 Ludwig's Angina	228
	9.5.2 Cavernous Sinus Thrombosis	230
	9.5.3 Bacteremia	230
	9.5.4 Septicemia	231
	9.5.5 Septicemia and sepsis syndrome	231

10 Oral Tumors and Tumor-Like Lesions: Preamble . . . 233

10.1	Overview	233

		10.1.1	Definitions 233
		10.1.2	Structure of Tumors 234
		10.1.3	Differentiation 235
		10.1.4	Classification of Tumors 235
		10.1.5	Nomenclature of Tumors 236
		10.1.6	Biology of Tumor Cells 237
	10.2	Carcinogenesis 240	
	10.3	Basic Concepts of Carcinogenesis 240	
	10.4	Etiologic Factors of Malignancy 243	
		10.4.1	Essential factors in carcinogenesis 243
		10.4.2	Modifying factors in carcinogenesis 247

11 Benign Non-Odontogenic Tumors & Tumor-Like Lesions 251

	11.1	Benign Epithelial Tumors 251	
		11.1.1	Squamous Cell Papilloma 251
		11.1.2	Verruca Vulgaris (Common Wart) 252
		11.1.3	Focal Epithelial Hyperplasia (Heck's Disease) 253
		11.1.4	Keratoacanthoma 254
	11.2	Benign Connective Tissue Tumors 257	
		11.2.1	Fibroma 257
		11.2.2	Frenal Tag 259
		11.2.3	Retrocuspid Papilla 259
		11.2.4	Pyogenic Granuloma 259
		11.2.5	Epulis Granulomatosa 262
		11.2.6	Pregnancy Tumor 262
		11.2.7	Fibroepithelial Polyp 262
		11.2.8	Papillary Hyperplasia of the Palate 263
		11.2.9	Peripheral Giant Cell Granuloma 264
		11.2.10	Myxoma 265
		11.2.11	Lipoma 266

	11.2.12	Chondroma	266
	11.2.13	Benign Tumors of Bone	268
	11.2.14	Benign Tumors of Muscles	270
11.3	Nevi		272
	11.3.1	Pigmented Nevus	273
	11.3.2	Vascular Nevi	281
11.4	Benign Tumors of Nerve Tissue		283
	11.4.1	Neurofibroma	284
	11.4.2	Multiple neurofibromatosis	285
	11.4.3	NF-1 (Von Recklinghausen disease of skin):	285
	11.4.4	NF-2 (Bilateral acoustic neurofibromatosis)	286
	11.4.5	Neurolemmoma (Schwannoma)	286
	11.4.6	Traumatic Neuroma (Amputation Neuroma)	287

12 Premalignant Lesions of the Oral Cavity 289

12.1	Definitions		289
12.2	Epithelial Dysplasia		291
	12.2.1	Overview	291
	12.2.2	Criteria of epithelial dysplasia	291
	12.2.3	Grading of dysplasia	293
	12.2.4	Microbiology of Oral Dysplasia	295
	12.2.5	Oral premalignant lesions	297
12.3	Leukoplakia		297
12.4	Hairy leukoplakia		299
12.5	Carcinoma in Situ		303
12.6	Erythroplakia (Erythoplasia of Quirat)		303
12.7	Oral Submucous Fibrosis		304
12.8	Lichen Planus		305
12.9	Actinic Keratosis		306
12.10	Management of Oral Premalignancy		308

13 Malignant Non-Odontogenic Tumors 311
- 13.1 Classification of Malignancy 311
- 13.2 Malignant Epithelial Tumors (Carcinomas) 313
  - 13.2.1 Squamous Cell Carcinoma 313
  - 13.2.2 Variants of Squamous Cell Carcinoma 318
  - 13.2.3 Nasopharyngeal Carcinoma 322
  - 13.2.4 Basal Cell Carcinoma (Rodent Ulcer) 323
- 13.3 Malignant Mesenchymal Tumors (Sarcomas) 325
  - 13.3.1 Introduction 325
  - 13.3.2 Fibrosarcoma 326
  - 13.3.3 Osteosarcoma (Osteogenic Sarcoma) 327
  - 13.3.4 Chondrosarcoma 332
  - 13.3.5 Ewing's Sarcoma 333
  - 13.3.6 Kaposi's Sarcoma 334
  - 13.3.7 Lymphomas 336
  - 13.3.8 Burkitt's Lymphoma 336
  - 13.3.9 Plasma Cell Myeloma (Plasmacytoma) 338
  - 13.3.10 Vascular Tumors 342
- 13.4 Malignant Melanoma 345
  - 13.4.1 Cutaneous Melanomas 345
  - 13.4.2 Mucosal Melanomas 350
- 13.5 Metastatic tumors of the jaws 352

14 Benign Odontogenic Tumors 355
- 14.1 Benign Epithelial Odontogenic Tumors 357
  - 14.1.1 Ameloblastoma 357
  - 14.1.2 Calcifying Epithelial Odontogenic Tumor 366
  - 14.1.3 Adenomatoid Odontogenic Tumor 368
  - 14.1.4 Calcifying Odontogenic Cyst 369
  - 14.1.5 Squamous Odontogenic Tumor 371

		14.1.6	Enameloma	372
	14.2	Benign Ectomesenchymal Odontogenic Tumors		373
		14.2.1	Peripheral Odontogenic Fibroma	373
		14.2.2	Central Odontogenic Fibroma	374
		14.2.3	Odontogenic Myxoma	375
		14.2.4	Cementomas and Cemental dysplasias	376
	14.3	Benign Mixed Odontogenic Tumors		390
		14.3.1	Ameloblastic Fibroma	390
		14.3.2	Compound Composite Odontome	392
		14.3.3	Complex Composite Odontome	392
		14.3.4	Ameloblastic Fibro-Odontome	393
		14.3.5	Odonto-Ameloblastoma	393

15 Malignant Odontogenic Tumors 397

15.1	Malignant Ameloblastoma	397
15.2	Ameloblastic Carcinoma	398
15.3	Odontogenic Carcinoma	399
15.4	Primary Intraosseous Carcinoma of Jaw	399
	15.4.1 Solid primary intraosseous carcinoma	400
	15.4.2 Cystic primary intraosseous carcinoma	400
15.5	Ghost cell odontogenic carcinoma	400
15.6	Clear cell odontogenic carcinoma	401
15.7	Ameloblastic fibrosarcoma	401

16 Diseases of Salivary Glands 403

16.1	Classification of Salivary Gland Disorders	403
16.2	Functional Disorders of Salivary Glands	405
	16.2.1 Xerostomia	405
	16.2.2 Ptyalism	407
16.3	Infections of Salivary Glands	409
	16.3.1 Bacterial infections	409

	16.3.2	Viral Infections 412
16.4	Obstructive Diseases 414
	16.4.1	Sialolithiasis, (Sialolith, Salivary Calculus) 414
	16.4.2	Salivary Duct Stenosis 415
16.5	Cysts of Salivary Glands 416
	16.5.1	(Mucoceles) 416
16.6	Degenerative (Autoimmune Diseases) 418
	16.6.1	Sjogren's syndrome 418
	16.6.2	Mikulicz syndrome 422
	16.6.3	Hashimoto's thyroiditis 422
	16.6.4	IgG4-related diseases 422
16.7	Salivary Gland Neoplasms 422
	16.7.1	Benign Neoplasms 424
	16.7.2	Malignant Neoplasms 431
16.8	Tumor-Like Lesions 440
	16.8.1	Necrotizing Sialometaplasia 440
	16.8.2	Sialoadenosis *(Sialosis)* 441

17 Bone Diseases 443

17.1	Classification of bone diseases 443
17.2	Developmental Bone Diseases 446
	17.2.1	Fibrous dysplasia (Maccune-Albright Syndrome) ... 446
	17.2.2	Facial fibrous dysplasia 447
	17.2.3	Cherubism (Familial fibrous dysplasia) 450
	17.2.4	Marble bone disease 452
	17.2.5	Craniosynostosis 455
	17.2.6	Achondroplasia 456
	17.2.7	Osteogenesis Imperfecta 457
17.3	Bone Diseases of Unknown Etiology 459
	17.3.1	Paget's disease of bone (Osteitis Deformans) 459

17.4	Inflammatory Bone Diseases		464
	17.4.1	Dry socket (Alveolar Osteitis)	464
	17.4.2	Delayed Healing of tooth socket	468
	17.4.3	Acute Pyogenic Osteomyelitis	468
	17.4.4	Chronic Pyogenic Osteomyelitis	472
	17.4.5	Chronic Non-pyogenic Osteomyelitis	473
	17.4.6	Medication-related Osteonecrosis of the Jaw	476
	17.4.7	Irradiation Necrosis	479
17.5	Tumors of Bone		481
	17.5.1	Compact and Cancellous Osteoma	481
	17.5.2	Osteoid Osteoma	481
	17.5.3	Ossifying Fibroma	481
	17.5.4	Central Giant Cell Granuloma	481
	17.5.5	Giant Cell Tumor of Bone (Osteoclastoma)	483
	17.5.6	Tumors of Langerhans Cell Histiocytes	484
17.6	Hormonal bone diseases		488
	17.6.1	Hyperparathyroidism	488
17.7	Deficiency Diseases		490
	17.7.1	Rickets	490
	17.7.2	Osteomalacia	491
17.8	Metabolic Bone Diseases		492
	17.8.1	Osteoporosis	492

18 Infections of the Oral and Para-Oral Tissues 495

18.1	Classification of infectious agents		495
18.2	Bacterial Infections		499
	18.2.1	Acute Necrotizing Ulcerative Gingivitis, ANUG	500
	18.2.2	Vincent Angina	501
	18.2.3	Maxillofacial Gangrene (Noma, Cancrum Oris)	502
	18.2.4	Acute Streptococcal Gingivitis	503

	18.2.5	Pericoronitis	504
	18.2.6	Periodontal Abscess	508
	18.2.7	Scarlet Fever	510
	18.2.8	Diphtheria	511
	18.2.9	Anthrax	511
	18.2.10	Syphilis	512
	18.2.11	Leprosy (Hansen's disease)	514
	18.2.12	Tuberculosis of the Oral Cavity	517
	18.2.13	Actinomycosis	519
	18.2.14	Orofacial Granulomatosis	522
	18.2.15	Sarcoidosis	522
	18.2.16	Crohn's Disease (Regional ileitis)	525
18.3	Mycotic (Fungal) Infections		526
	18.3.1	Moniliasis (Candidiasis)	526
	18.3.2	Systemic Mycoses	534
18.4	Parasitic Diseases		535
	18.4.1	Leishmaniasis	535
18.5	Viral diseases		537
	18.5.1	Introduction	537
	18.5.2	Herpes Simplex I (Labialis)	539
	18.5.3	Varicella - Zoster Virus	543
	18.5.4	Hand-Foot and Mouth Disease	545
	18.5.5	Herpangina	546
	18.5.6	Measles (Rubeola)	546
	18.5.7	German Measles (Rubella)	550
	18.5.8	Infectious Mononucleosis	552
	18.5.9	AIDS	555

19 Diseases of the Maxillary Sinus 565
   19.1   Anatomy 565

Contents

- 19.2 Histology of the maxillary sinus 567
- 19.3 Dental Relevance 567
- 19.4 Sinus Diseases 569
  - 19.4.1 Infections 569
  - 19.4.2 Tumors 572
  - 19.4.3 Foreign Bodies 573
  - 19.4.4 Cysts 574
  - 19.4.5 Miscellaneous Conditions 574

20 Oral Manifestations of Skin Diseases 577
- 20.1 Back to Basics 577
  - 20.1.1 Skin Structure 577
- 20.2 Lichen Planus 579
- 20.3 Lichenoid Reactions 582
- 20.4 Pemphigus 582
  - 20.4.1 Pemphigus Vulgaris 585
  - 20.4.2 Pemphigus Vegetans 585
  - 20.4.3 Familial Benign Pemphigus 586
- 20.5 Pemphigoid 586
  - 20.5.1 Bullous Pemphigoid 587
  - 20.5.2 Benign Mucous Membrane Pemphigoid 587
- 20.6 Erythema Multiforme 588
- 20.7 Lupus Erythematosus 589
  - 20.7.1 Systemic Lupus Erythematosus 590
  - 20.7.2 Discoid Lupus Erythematosus 591
- 20.8 Psoriasis 591
- 20.9 Progressive systemic sclerosis 593
- 20.10 Rheumatoid Arthritis 594

21 White and Red Lesions of the Oral Cavity 599
- 21.1 Introduction 599

21.2	White Lesions		600
	21.2.1	Definition	600
	21.2.2	Classification of white lesions	600
	21.2.3	Oral Keratosis	603
21.3	Red Lesions		607
	21.3.1	Definition	607
	21.3.2	Classification of red lesions	608

22 Ulcers & Vesiculobullous Lesions of the Oral Cavity ... 611

22.1	Definitions		611
22.2	Classification		612
	22.2.1	Primary versus secondary ulcers	612
	22.2.2	Etiologic classification of ulcers	614
22.3	Ulcers due to Physical Injury		616
22.4	Ulcers due to Infectious Agents		618
22.5	Ulcers of Neoplastic Lesions		618
22.6	Ulcers due to Drugs		618
22.7	Ulcers of Immunological disorders:		619
	22.7.1	Recurrent Aphthous Stomatitis	619
	22.7.2	Behçet's Syndrome (Behçet's Disease)	625
	22.7.3	Reiter's Syndrome	627
22.8	Ulcers of Genodermatosis		628
	22.8.1	Epidermolysis bullosa	628
22.9	Ulcers due to Blood Disorders		628
22.10	Ulcers of Gastrointestinal Tract Diseases		629
	22.10.1	Celiac Disease	629
	22.10.2	Ulcerative Colitis	629
	22.10.3	Crohn's Disease	629
22.11	Ulcers of uncertain pathogenesis		629
	22.11.1	Eosinophilic Ulcer	629

	22.11.2	Lethal midline granuloma syndrome	630
	22.11.3	Wegener's granulomatosis	630
	22.11.4	Nasopharyngeal T-cell lymphomas	633
22.12		Guide Lines in the Diagnosis of Ulcers	634
22.13		Management of Oral Ulcers	636

23 Brown and Black Pigmented Lesions ... 639

23.1		Overview	639
23.2		Physiologic Pigmentation	640
	23.2.1	Racial Pigmentation (Oral Melanosis)	640
	23.2.2	Melasma (Mask of Pregnancy)	640
23.3		Developmental Pigmentation	640
	23.3.1	Incontinentia pigmenti	640
	23.3.2	Peutz-Jeghers syndrome	641
	23.3.3	Xeroderma Pigmentosa	641
	23.3.4	Polystotic fibrous dysplasia	641
23.4		Neoplastic	641
	23.4.1	Pigmented nevi	641
	23.4.2	Multiple neurofibromatosis	641
	23.4.3	Malignant melanomas	642
23.5		Hormonal Pigmentation	642
	23.5.1	Addison's disease (adrenal cortex insufficiency)	642
	23.5.2	Hyperpituitarism	642
23.6		Skin Diseases	642
	23.6.1	Lichen Planus	642
	23.6.2	Freckles (Ephelides)	643
23.7		Miscellaneous conditions	644
	23.7.1	Amalgam Tattoo	644
	23.7.2	Graphite Tattoo	644
	23.7.3	Drug-induced pigmentation	644

23.7.4	Heavy metal pigmentation	644
23.7.5	Black hairy tongue	645
23.7.6	Acanthosis nigricans	645
23.7.7	Oral Melanotic Macules	645

List of Figures

4.1	Contributing factors for dental caries	102
4.2	The metabolism of sucrose by cariogenic bacteria.	107
4.3	Acid production in the plaque	114
4.4	A diagram showing zones of initiation phase of enamel caries	119
4.5	A diagram showing zones of uninfected and infected dentin caries.	122
5.1	The Periodontium in Health	127
5.2	Chronic Gingivitis	130
5.3	Chronic Periodontitis	131
5.4	Types of periodontal probes	133
5.5	Hand Scalers	135
5.6	Subgingival Instruments	136
5.7	Gingivectomy	137
5.8	Flap Surgery	138
6.1	Classification of pulpitis.	145
6.2	Sequelae of pulp inflammation.	148
6.3	Various Types of Pulp Stones and Calcifications.	156
6.4	Diagrammatic illustration of periapical infections	163
6.5	Possible pathways for the spread of pus from an acute periapical abscess	167
6.6	Young female with a combined buccal and infraorbtial spaces infection	168

List of Figures

7.1	Types of Dentigerous Cysts	183
7.2	Proposed classification for cysts of the maxillary sinus.	202
8.1	Reactionary dentin vs reparative dentin	211
11.1	Diagrammatic representation of keratoacanthoma	256
11.2	Typical sites for the incidence of chondroma	267
11.3	Melanocytes and their function	275
11.4	Types of pigmented nevi	279
11.5	Diagrammatic structure of nerve trunk and nerve cell	284
12.1	Diagrammatic representation of stages of oral submucous fibrosis	306
13.1	Clinical characteristic features of squamous cell carcinoma ulcer	319
13.2	Clinical characteristic features of basal cell carcinoma ulcer	325
13.3	Diagrammatic representation of the radiographical feaures of osteosarcoma	330
13.4	Melanoma in radial and vertical growth phases.	347
13.5	Melanoma vs pigmented nevus and the warning signs of melanoma	348
14.1	Schema Showing Various Subtypes of Multicystic Ameloblastoma	362
14.2	Diagrammatic representation of unicystic ameloblastoma	364
16.1	Salivary gland acini and duct system	424
17.1	Diagrammatic representation of mosaic appearance	463
17.2	The 3 basic types of chronic non-pyogenic osteomyelitis	474
17.3	Diagrammatic representation of osteoporosis	494
18.1	Pericoronitis with the operculum	505
18.2	Natural History of Tuberculosis	561
18.3	Clinical Spectrum of Candidiasis	563

19.1 Diagrammatic representation of maxillary sinus 566
19.2 Anatomical relationship of the maxillary sinus with maxillary teeth. 568

20.1 Diagnostic criteria of lichen planus 581
20.2 Blistering conditions 596
20.3 The progress of the lesions from normal skin to psoriasis 598

21.1 White vs red lesions 600

List of Tables

1.1	The difference between some genetic terms	1
1.2	Useful Definitions for Some Genetic Concepts	5
1.3	Classification of Hereditary Diseases	5
1.4	Characteristics of Chromosomal Abnormalities	9
1.5	Characteristics of Single Gene Defects	9
1.6	Characteristics of Multifactorial Inheritance	10
2.1	Examples of craniofacial anomalies	49
2.2	Differences Between Hereditary and Acquired Defects of Enamel	50
2.3	Classification of Amelogenesis Imperfecta	50
2.4	Differences Between Coronal and Radicular Dentinal Dysplasia	51
6.1	Characteristics of pulpitis and periapical diseases	153
7.1	Aspiration Biopsy	177
8.1	Types of Dentin	209
8.2	Predentin	210
8.3	Principle Causes of External Resorption of Teeth	215
10.1	Main differences between benign and malignant tumors	237
10.2	Naming of Some Tumors	238
13.1	TNM of Oral Carcinomas	314
13.2	The ABCDE system of melanoma	349
14.1	Classification of Cementomas and Cemento-Osseous Dysplasias	377

14.2 Differential Diagnosis of Cemento-Osseous Dysplasias 395
14.3 Differential Diagnosis of Facial Fibrous Dysplasia from Ossifying Fibroma 396

16.1 Differential diagnosis of myoepitheloma and pleomorphic adenoma 428
16.2 Key features of Warthin's Tumor 432
16.3 Biologic classification of malignant salivary gland tumor 432
16.4 The problem of clear cells in salivary gland tumors 439

17.1 Classification of Fibro-osseous Lesions 448
17.2 Risk factors associated with dry socket 466
17.3 A summary of measures to prevent the risk of dry socket 469

18.1 Morphologic Classification of Medically Important Fungi 498
18.2 Classification of Streptococci 499
18.6 Summary of Viral Infections of the Oral Mucosa 539
18.7 Supportive Measures Used in Infections with Herpes Viruses. . 541
18.8 Diseases Associated with EBV 555
18.3 Principle Types of Virus Causing Human Disease 560
18.4 Clinical Features of Tuberuclous Lymphadenitis 562
18.5 Differential Diagnosis of Mucosal Leishmaniasis 562

20.1 Examples of drugs capable of causing lichenoid reactions ... 583
20.2 Features suggesting a lichenoid reaction 583
20.3 Classification of Vesiculo-bullous Lesions. 597

22.1 Key Features of Aphthae (Recurrent Aphthous Stomatitis (RAS)). 622

Chapter 1
Developmental Disturbances: Back to Basics

- Disturbance in normal development and growth of an individual result in developmental diseases.
- They may be manifested at birth (*congenital*) or appear later on life (*tarda*).
- The etiologic factors responsible for the causation of developmental diseases may be hereditary or environmental (acquired).
- See table (1.1) for the different terms used in the field of developmental diseases.

1.1 Hereditary and Diseases

- Each individual is different, and the difference is thought to lie in the coded information (or genetic material) that is passed down to that person from his or her parents.

Table 1.1: The difference between some genetic terms

> **Always Remember**
> - Not all congenital diseases are hereditary
> - All congenital diseases are developmental
> - Not all developmental diseases are congenital
>
> Note

Chapter 1. Developmental Disturbances: Back to Basics

- This information is very precise and is capable of exact analysis.
- Gregor Mendel noted that characteristics of any individual behave as if they were determined by units, which were passed unchanged from one generation to the next.
- To these units, the name *genes* were give, and it was postulated that a pair of them are situated at a specific site, or locus, on one of the pair of chromosomes, and the genes forming a pair are called alleles..
- If the two pairs are similar, the individual is called a homozygote for that particular gene, while if dissimilar the term heterozygote is used.
- The genetic makeup of an individual is called his *genotype*, and the effect which these genes produce is called *phenotype*.
- To explain Mendelian inheritance several assumptions have been made:
  - ★ Genes occur in pairs.
  - ★ Genes forming a pair are called alleles.
  - ★ One gene of each pair is received from each parent.
  - ★ Genes remain unchanged through many generations.
  - ★ Genes consist of DNA (deoxyribonucleic acid).
  - ★ The genome is the complete set of genes.
  - ★ The human genome consists of around 3 billion base pairs of DNA and includes 30,000 to 35,000 genes organized as 23 pairs of chromosomes.
  - ★ The genotype is the genetic makeup of an individual.
  - ★ Phenotype is the visible trait that results from a particular genotype.
  - ★ Many genes present in humans are also present in mice, fish, fruit flies, yeast, and bacteria and about 98% of human DNA sequences are shared with the chimpanzee.

- ★ If the two alleles are similar, the individual is called homozygous for that particular gene.
- ★ If the two alleles are dissimilar, the individual is called heterozygous for that particular gene.
- ★ Some genes may be considered as dominant and some as recessive. A dominant gene produces its effect both in heterozygote and in the homozygote while a recessive gene produces its effect only in the homozygous condition. However, it was shown that some genes occupy an intermediate position (described as being incompletely or partially dominant).
- ★ Some genes can express the phenomenon of codominance in which a gene and its allele will produce their effects in the same time as in the blood group genes A and B. An individual with a genotype AB will be phenotypically AB, this is because the gene A is dominant and the gene B is also dominant.

1.1.1 Concept of expressivity

- Genes have been considered as behaving either as dominant or recessive.
- In fact, the position is much more complex.
- Sometimes a dominant gene may produce severe disease in one individual but only a minor deformity in another. The concept of expressivity has been introduced to explain this phenomenon.
- If a gene that usually produces a severe effect is found to cause a minor one in a particular individual, it is said to show poor expressivity. See also table (1.2).

1.1.2 Concept of penetrance

- Sometimes a dominant gene fails to produce any detectable effect and a dominant trait may then miss a generation.
- This is an example of reduced penetrance, a term used when some individuals with the appropriate genotype fail to express it.
- In other words, penetrance could be defined as the ability of genes to penetrate (express) itself through every generation.

1.1.3 Sex limited traits

> **Remember !**
> Do not confuse sex-linked diseases with sex-limited diseases.

- Sometimes a dominant gene fails to produce its effect in one sex, although the gene is not carried on X or Y chromosomes.
- This is called sex limitation. Male pattern baldness behaves in this way and for the gene to become manifested; there must be a level of testosterone found naturally only in males.

1.1.4 Classification of Hereditary diseases

- Hereditary diseases by definition are diseases transmissible from parent to offspring through genetic abnormalities of genes.
- Genetic abnormalities, in general, may be inherited or they may be acquired.
- Inherited genetic abnormalities usually affect the developing germ cells and they will result in a developmental malformation.

Table 1.2: Useful Definitions for Some Genetic Concepts

> **Expressivity, Penetrance and Sex-Limited Traits**
>
> Expressivity — Is the ability of the gene to express its full features in every generation (some features of a gene are missing in some generations)
>
> Penetrance — Is the ability of the gene to express itself in every generation (some genes do skip some generations)
>
> Sex-Limited Traits — Is the ability of the gene to miss its feaures in certain gender although it is neither X nor Y linked e.g. male-type baldness.
>
> *Note*

Table 1.3: Classification of Hereditary Diseases

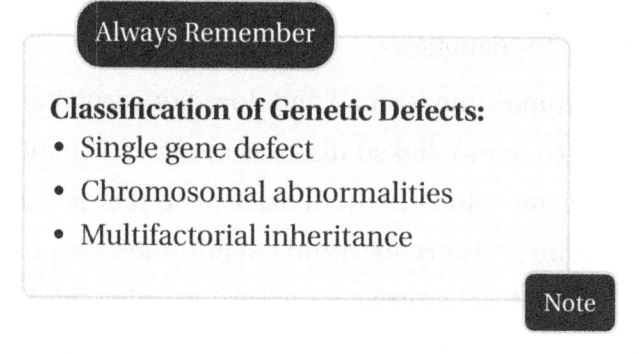

> **Always Remember**
>
> **Classification of Genetic Defects:**
> - Single gene defect
> - Chromosomal abnormalities
> - Multifactorial inheritance
>
> *Note*

- Acquired genetic abnormalities are not inherited and are not usually present at birth. They usually affect fully developed somatic cells and can result in cancer (refer to chapter "Oral Tumors and Tumor-Like Lesions: Preamble", page (233)).

- Inherited genetic abnormalities can be classified into (see also table (1.3)):

Single gene abnormalities

- Abnormalities may affect a single gene (single gene defect, unigenic, unifactorial). Diseases resulting from single gene defects usually, but not always follow the Mendelian pattern of inheritance.
- Such abnormalities may affect the genes located on the autosomes (autosomal linked diseases), or affect the genes located on the sex chromosomes (X-linked diseases or sex-linked diseases).
- Most authors prefer the term X-linked diseases rather than the term sex-linked diseases because very little, if any, known disorders are carried on the Y chromosomal genes. Y-linked inheritance is also termed *Holandric inheritance* (Origin [G. holos, entire, + aner, human male]) and implies that an affected male transmits the trait to all his sons but to none of his daughters.
- The Y-chromosome is small and does not carry many genes, few traits are Y-linked, and Y-linked diseases are rare. The main Y gene is called the SRY gene, which is the master gene that specifies maleness and male features. Hairy ear pinna syndrome was postulated to be a Y-linked trait albeit, controversy exists regarding this fact.
- See table (1.5) for the characteristics of single-gene defects. It is postulated that some forms of amelogenesis imperfecta might be carried on the Y chromosome.

Chromosomal abnormalities

- Chromosomal abnormalities can be classified into those, which involve the autosomes, and those, which affect sex chromosomes.
- Each can be subdivided into numerical and structural abnormalities.

- Numerical abnormalities involve the loss or gain of one or two chromosomes. If three, rather than the normal pair, of a particular chromosome, are present, the abnormality is referred to as trisomy.
- If only one of the normal paired chromosomes, is present, this is monosomy.
- Trisomy may affect autosomes or sex chromosomes, while monosomy can affect only the sex chromosomes.
- Monosomy of autosomes is lethal to the cell and no cases of autosomal monosomy have been reported in the literature.
- Structural abnormalities involve translocations or deletions. In translocations, there is an exchange of segments between non-homologous chromosomes. Deletions involve the loss of a segment of a chromosome.
- See also table (1.4).

Multifactorial inheritance

- After Mendel, it was noted that some traits and diseases do not follow exactly the Mendelian mode of inheritance.
- For example some diseases may show an incidence rate of 5% in a certain population, clearly, this is much below the anticipated incidence of at least 25% as proposed by Mendel's law.
- Also, some normal traits such as intelligence, stature and skin color show endless possibilities. For example, the stature of any person in a certain population can be any value between 160.1, 160.2, 160.3, 160.4 or 180.5 cm.
- It has been suggested that such traits are caused by many genes (*polygenic*) plus the effect of environment, so-called multifactorial inheritance.

Chapter 1. Developmental Disturbances: Back to Basics

- In polygenic traits, there is more than one gene controlling the same trait.
- For example, one can assume that for the stature of an individual there are 4 genes (the exact number is not precisely known). The first gene will make the individual 160 cm, the second gene will add 10 cm, the third will add another 10 cm and the fourth will further add 10 cm so that the individual with all the 4 genes will be 190 cm. Such an effect is termed additive genetic effect and the process is termed quantitative genetics (unlike the single gene defects which are termed qualitative genetics). Clearly, if the individual possesses the 4 genes and hence acquires the genetic potentiality to be 190 cm but unfortunately was malnourished in childhood, then he will not be capable of achieving the proposed stature of 190 cm.
- The latter example shows how the environment interacts with the genetic makeup of an individual to determine the final state of any trait.
- Abnormal traits that may be inherited in this way include certain common congenital abnormalities, certain psychiatric disorders, such as schizophrenia and manic depressive psychosis, and certain "diseases of modern society" such as hypertension, diabetes mellitus, ankylosing spondylitis, rheumatoid arthritis, peptic ulcer, and ischemic heart disease. Each of these characteristics is believed to be the result of the action of many genes each of small but additive effects plus the effects of the environment.
- See table (1.6) for the main characteristics of multifactorial inheritance.

Table 1.4: Characteristics of Chromosomal Abnormalities

Chromosomal Abnormalities

- Can affect autosomes or sex chromosomes
- May be numerical or structural abnormalities
- Numerical abnormalities may involve gain or loss of chromosomes
- Gain of one chromosome is termed trisomy, while loss of a single chromosome is termed monosomy
- Autosomal monosomy is lethal to the developing individual and no cases have been reported
- Structural abnormalities may involve deletion, duplication or translocation of a part of a chromosome

Note

Table 1.5: Characteristics of Single Gene Defects

Single Gene Defects

- Usually follow Mendelian pattern of inheritance
- May be sex-linked or autosomal
- May be dominant, recessive or of incomplete dominance
- May show varying degrees of expressivity
- May show varying degrees of penetrance
- May show sex limited features such as male pattern baldness

Note

Chapter 1. Developmental Disturbances: Back to Basics

Table 1.6: Characteristics of Multifactorial Inheritance

> **Multifactorial Inheritance**
>
> - Do not follow the Mendelian pattern of inheritance
> - Result from the action of more than one gene and can be modified by the environmental factors
> - Examples are: Hypertension, diabetes mellitus, ankylosing spondylitis. Rheumatoid arthritis, peptic ulcer and ischemic heart disease

Note

1.2 Environmental Factors and Diseases

1.2.1 Teratogens

- Many environmental agents are known in animals, and few in man, which causes congenital abnormalities.
- An agent believed to cause congenital abnormalities is referred to as a teratogen. A teratogen causes malformation only if exposure occurs at a time when the embryo is sensitive to its effects.
- It is proposed that some of these teratogens act in a similar manner to the mutant genes i.e. interfering with processes that are important at certain critical stages of development.

1.2.2 Proven teratogenic agents in man

- Drugs and chemicals
    * Alcohol: Responsible for growth retardation, microcephaly and mental retardation
    * Anti-thyroid: Responsible for hypothyroidism

- ★ Chloroquine: Deafness
- ★ Folic acid antagonists: CNS malformation
- ★ Hormonal pregnancy tests: Various malformations
- ★ Phenytoin: Cleft lip and or cleft palate
- ★ Hypervitaminosis A: Microphthalmia and congenital heart disease
- ★ Smoking: Growth retardation
- ★ Streptomycin: deafness
- ★ Tetracycline: Teeth pigmentation
- ★ Warfarin: Nasal hypoplasia
- ★ Fluorides: Mottled enamel

- Infections
  - ★ Cytomegalovirus: Microcephaly
  - ★ Herpesvirus: Microcephaly and microphthalmia
  - ★ Rubella: Congenital heart disease, deafness, cataracts
  - ★ Toxoplasma: Microcephaly
  - ★ Varicella: Limb hypoplasia
  - ★ Syphilis: Dental anomalies

- Maternal diseases
  - ★ Diabetes mellitus: Sacral agenesis
  - ★ Phenylketonurea: Mental retardation

- Radiation
  - ★ Almost all types or radiation can cause various forms of developmental malformations.

Chapter 2
Developmental Disturbances of Hard Dental Tissues

Tooth development (***odontogenesis***) comprises the following 6 physiologic processes:

1. Stimulation of certain cells to multiply (*initiation and proliferation*)
2. Establishment of tooth pattern (*morpho differentiation*)
3. Differentiation of cells to perform special functions (*histo-differentiation*)
4. Formation of dentin and enamel matrix (*apposition*)
5. Influx of mineral salts and their subsequent crystallization (*mineralization and maturation*)
6. Emergence of the crown into the oral cavity (*eruption*).

2.1 Normal Tooth Development

- The tooth germ is a group of cells that eventually forms a tooth.
- The tooth germ is organized into three parts: the **enamel organ**, the **dental papilla** and the **dental sac** or follicle.
- The cells of the enamel organ are derived from the ectoderm of the first pharyngeal arch, while the dental papilla and tooth sac are derived from the ectomesenchyme of the neural crest.

Chapter 2. Developmental Disturbances of Hard Dental Tissues

- Disorders of development of teeth may be due to disturbances in any of the above-mentioned phases. However, in some abnormalities more than one phase of development may be involved.

2.2 Classification of Developmental Disturbances of Teeth

1. Abnormalities in Number (defective initiation)
   (a) Increase in number (hyperdontia)
      i. Supernumerary Teeth
      ii. Supplemental Teeth
      iii. Predeciduous Dentition
      iv. Post-permanent Dentition
   (b) Decrease in number (hypodontia, oligodontia)
   (c) False anodontia or hypodontia
   (d) True anodontia or hypodontia
      i. Absence of single tooth
      ii. Absence of group of teeth
      iii. Absence of all teeth
         A. Simple anodontia (not associated with any other abnormalities)
         B. Associated with other abnormalities e.g. Streeter's syndrome
2. Abnormalities in Size and Shape (defective morpho and histodifferentiation)
   (a) Abnormalities in size
      i. Macrodontia

ii. Microdontia

(b) Abnormalities in shape

    i. Gemination

    ii. Fusion

    iii. Concrescence

    iv. Dilaceration

    v. Taurodontism

    vi. Dens in dente (Dens invaginatus)

    vii. Dens Evaginatus (Occlusal Enamel Drop)

    viii. Enamel Pearl

    ix. Talon Cusp

    x. Supernumerary Roots

    xi. Congenital Syphilis

3. Abnormalities in Structure (defective apposition and calcification)

    (a) Acquired defects (usually affect enamel and dentin)

        i. Acquired focal enamel hypoplasia (Turner's tooth)

        ii. Acquired generalized enamel hypoplasia

        iii. Dental fluorosis

        iv. Abnormal discoloration

    (b) Hereditary defects

        i. Hereditary defects of enamel

           Amelogenesis imperfecta

        ii. Hereditary defects of dentin

           A. Dentinogenesis imperfecta

           B. Dentinal dysplasia

        iii. Obscure defects

           Regional odontodysplasia (ghost teeth)

Chapter 2. Developmental Disturbances of Hard Dental Tissues

4. Abnormalities in Eruption (defective eruption)
   (a) Early Eruption
   (b) Delayed Eruption
   (c) Teething Problems

2.3 Abnormalities in Number

Abnormalities in number of teeth are usually due to *defective initiation*. These defects are manifested in either increase or decrease in number of teeth. Abnormalities in number of teeth may occur as a part of some syndromes affecting the craniofacial region. Table (2.1) shows some examples of craniofacial anomalies associated with abnormalities in the number of teeth.

2.3.1 Increase in number (Hyperdontia)

Supernumerary Teeth

- Are excess teeth not similar morphologically to any normal teeth
- They are small and conical in shape
- Supernumerary teeth are classified according to their site of eruption into
    1. Mesiodens (between upper centrals)
    2. Paramolar (on the buccal surface of upper molars, particularly second molars)
    3. Distomolar (distal to third molars)

Supplemental Teeth

- Are excess teeth which are similar morphologically to normal teeth

- May result from dichotomy or due to extra budding of enamel organ from the dental lamina
- Most common sites are:
  - ★ Upper lateral incisors
  - ★ Lower premolar region
  - ★ Distal to the lower third molar
- Other forms of supplemental teeth are either pre-deciduous or post-permanent dentition
- Supernumerary and supplemental teeth are a common finding in the syndrome known as cleidocranial dysplasia.

Pre-deciduous Dentition (natal and neonatal teeth)

- These teeth are not prematurely erupting deciduous series
- Teeth that are present at birth are called natal teeth
- While those that erupt during the first month of life are called neonatal teeth

Post-permanent Dentition

- It is that dentition formed after the permanent dentition
- These are not impacted or embedded permanent teeth that erupt after the insertion of dentures
- Their enamel organs are presumed to arise from the dental lamina after giving the enamel organ of the permanent series

Chapter 2. Developmental Disturbances of Hard Dental Tissues

Cleidocranial Dysplasia

Definition:

Is a developmental bone disease characterized by defective formation of the clavicles with other dental and cranial abnormalities.

The disease was initially thought to involve only membranous bone but now is known also to affect endochondral ossification and to represent a generalized disorder of skeletal structures.

Etiology:

- Autosomal dominant
- 40% of cases appear to represent spontaneous gene mutation
- The defect was mapped to the CBFA1 gene of chromosome 6p21
- This gene normally guides osteoblastic differentiation and bone formation

Clinically:

- Partial or complete absence of the clavicles
- Short stature
- Large head with pronounced frontal and parietal bossing
- Ocular hypertelorism
- Depressed nasal bridge
- Delayed closure of fontanels with presence of many wormian bones

Dental manifestations:

1. Delayed shedding of deciduous teeth

2. Delayed eruption of permanent teeth
3. many unerupted supernumerary or supplemental teeth
4. Many of the unerupted teeth will be seen to have hooked roots.
5. Many teeth may show different degrees of enamel hypoplasia.
6. Some teeth will assume a conical shape.
7. Multiple dentigerous cysts develop in relation to some of the unerupted teeth.
8. Gemination may be observed.
9. The maxilla is narrow and v-shaped with a high arched palate.
10. Absence of cellular cementum is usually found

2.3.2 Decrease in Number (Hypodontia, Oligodontia, Anodontia)

False anodontia or hypodontia:

False anodontia is the failure of eruption rather than failure of formation of a single tooth or group of teeth. The possible causes of eruption failure are discussed later.

True anodontia or hypodontia:

1. **Absence of single tooth**
    (a) Maxillary lateral incisor
    (b) Lower premolars
    (c) Third molars
2. **Absence of group of teeth**
3. **Absence of all teeth (total anodontia)**
    (a) Simple (not associated with any other abnormalities).

(b) Associated with other abnormalities such as ectodermal dysplasia.

Hereditary Ectodermal Dysplasia, (ED, Streeter's Syndrome[1])

- EDs are heritable conditions in which there are abnormalities of at least two or more ectodermal structures such as the hair, teeth, nails, sweat glands and some cranio-facial structures
- Ectodermal Dysplasia (ED) is not a single disorder, but a group of closely related conditions.
- The three most prevalent types of ectodermal dysplasias are:
  1. X-linked anhidrotic (or hypohidrotic) ectodermal dysplasia (EDA), which is the most common form, also known as Christ-Siemens-Touraine Syndrome.
  2. Autosomal recessive anhidrotic (or hypohidrotic) form was also described. Phenotypically the features were indistinguishable from those in males with the X-linked form.
  3. Autosomal dominant hidrotic ectodermal dysplasia (also known as Clouston ectodermal dysplasia) was also described (hidrotic means normal sweating).
- In general the most common manifestations of ectodermal dysplasia are:
  ★ Males usually show the whole manifestations of the syndrome
  ★ While carrier females are free or show the mildest form

---
[1]The term Streeter's syndrome is an obsolete and abandoned name and should not be confused with the term Streeter's dysplasia (Constriction ring syndrome (CRS)) which is a rare disorder of congenital constricting bands associated with autoamputation of distal extremities such as fingers and toes.

- ★ Females may also show patchy areas of skin devoid of hair and sweat glands together with partial loss of some teeth, a finding indicating lyonization
- ★ Some of the most important manifestations are:
  - * Absent or very thin patchy hair (hypotrichosis).
  - * Absence of sweat glands (anhidrosis), the patient can not tolerate hot weather.
  - * Lack of sebaceous glands (dry skin).
  - * Depressed nasal bridge.
  - * Protrusion of the lips.
  - * Deficient height of the alveolar process.
  - * Defective mental development in some cases
- ★ Dental manifestations include partial or total anodontia with malformation of any teeth that may be present (usually small and peg shaped).

2.4 Abnormalities in Size

2.4.1 Macrodontia

(*Megadontia, megalodontia*)

- Means large teeth.
- Macrodontia may be true or relative.
- Relative macrodontia results form disproportion between size of teeth and size of jaws or skull
- True macrodontia may involve all teeth, group of teeth or single tooth.
- The teeth most commonly affected are the maxillary central incisors, canines followed by maxillary lateral and third molars.

- Etiology: Macrodontia affecting a single tooth is caused by disturbance of morphodifferentiation. Generalized macrodontia is usually attributed to some hormonal imbalance (e.g. pituitary gigantism)
- Macrodontia may occur as a part of some rare diseases e.g. ***otodental syndrome***, and ***insulin-resistant diabetes***.
- Otodental syndrome is a rare autosomal dominant hereditary disease characterized by eye coloboma[2], hearing loss and globodontia[3].
- Unilateral macrodontia (involving group of teeth) is observable in hereditary facial hemihypertrophy, see page (62).

2.4.2 Microdontia

- Means small teeth
- Microdontia may be true or relative
- Relative microdontia results form disproportion between size of teeth and size of jaws or skull
- The most commonly affected single teeth are the maxillary lateral incisors and third molars (upper and lower).
- Females are slightly affected more than males
- Unilateral microdonatia (involving group of teeth) is observable in hereditary facial hemihypoplasia see page (63).
- Microdontia can occur as a part of some rare genetic diseases[4] e.g. ectodermal dysplasia, Down syndrome, Marshall syndrome, Rieger syndrome, focal dermal hypoplasia syndrome, Williams syndrome, Salamon syndrome, cleft lip and palate and congenital hypopituitarism.

---

[2] A coloboma is a hole in one of the structures of the eye, such as the iris, retina, choroid, or optic disc.
[3] Significant enlargement with globe shaped canines and molar teeth.
[4] The detailed discussion of these syndromes is out of the scope of this book

- Also can occur due to some environmental factors such as radiation on the jaws and chemotherapy during tooth development.

2.5 Abnormalities in Shape

2.5.1 Gemination (Schizodontia)

- Is the term applied when one tooth appears as two teeth joined together.
- Results from partial division of the enamel organ.
- The degree of splitting depends upon the timing of the splitting.
- The resultant teeth have a a single root canal.
- Occurs in the deciduous or permanent dentition.
- It is usually seen in the anterior teeth.
- The number of teeth is normal.
- If complete schizodontia occurs two teeth are formed twinning and hyperdontia results.
- May occur as a manifestation of *cleidocranial dysplasia* (see page 18)

2.5.2 Fusion

- Is the term applied when two teeth are joined together.
- Results from the union of two adjacent enamel organs.
- The two teeth may be united along their crowns, roots or their entire length.
- It is usually seen in the incisor area.
- The resultant fused teeth may have two roots or a grooved root, but there are usually two root canals.
- Fusion must involve dentin.

Chapter 2. Developmental Disturbances of Hard Dental Tissues

- The number of teeth is reduced by one, unless that one of the fused teeth was a supernumerary tooth.

2.5.3 Concrescence

- Is the term applied when two teeth are joined along their roots by cementum.
- Trauma or crowding of teeth can cause concrescence.
- Extraction of one tooth can be complicated by extraction of the other.

2.5.4 Dilaceration

- Is the presence of sharp bend or angulations along the long axis of a tooth.
- The condition is thought to be due to trauma during tooth development, with the result that the position of the calcified portion of the tooth is changed and the remainder of the tooth is formed at an angle.
- The curve may occur at anywhere along the length of the tooth.
- Some syndromes and developmental diseases such as *Smith Magenis syndrome*, hypermobility type of *Ehlers-Danlos syndrome* (see page 93), *Axenfeld-Rieger syndrome, congenital ichthyosis* and *cleidocranial dysplasia* (see page 18) have been associated with dilaceration.
- The condition may impose difficulty during endodontic treatment or tooth extraction.

2.5.5 Taurodontism

- A hereditary condition, in which there is enlargement of the tooth trunk on the expense of the root.

- It can occur in deciduous or permanent dentitions, but is more common in the later.
- The third molars are the usually affected teeth and the first molars are the least affected ones.
- The condition is thought to result from failure of the epithelial root sheath of Hertwig to invaginate at the proper level to form the furcation area.

2.5.6 Dens in dente (Dens Invaginatus)

- Is the deep invagination in the lingual surface of upper incisors usually the upper lateral incisor.
- It represents a deep accentuation of the lingual pit.
- The condition appears radiographically as a tooth within a tooth and hence the term "*dense in dente*" was used.

2.5.7 Dens Evaginatus (Occlusal Enamel Drop)

- Dens evagination (sometimes known as occlusal enamel drop) is a developmental abnormality that primarily affects premolars.
- It is characterized by the development of an abnormal globe-shaped projection appearing as an extra cusp centrally located on the occlusal surfaces between the buccal and lingual cusps of premolars.
- Frequently, dens evaginatus is seen in association with another variation known as **shovel-shaped** incisors. This alteration also occurs predominantly in Asians, with a prevalence of approximately 15% in whites but close to 100% in Native Americans. Affected incisors demonstrate prominent lateral margins, creating a hollowed lingual surface that resembles the scoop of a shovel. Maxillary lateral and central incisors are the most frequently affected teeth.

2.5.8 Enamel Pearl

- An ectopic globule of enamel usually found on the bifurcation area of upper molars.
- Sometimes, it contains a dentin core and associated pulp horn.
- It may result from downward displacement of ameloblasts below the amelocemental junction or due to differentiation of cells of the epithelial root sheath of Hertwig into ameloblasts.

2.5.9 Talon Cusp

- An extra cusp on the lingual surface of the cingulum area of an anterior tooth.
- Usually affects upper teeth.
- Usually affects permanent teeth.

2.5.10 Supernumerary Roots

- Supernumerary Roots are most commonly seen in mandibular canines, premolars, and molars (especially third molars). Rarely found in upper and lower anterior incisors.
- Radiographic recognition is important for extractions.
- Treatment: None.

2.5.11 Supernumerary Cusps

- Most common is the Carabelli cusp, develops on the mesiolingual surface of permanent maxillary first molars. no clinical problems, normal variation.
- Other examples are dens evaginatus and talon cusp.

2.5.12 Peg shaped laterals

- A peg lateral is a small, tapered, maxillary lateral incisor.
- The tooth is conical in shape and tapers incisally to a blunt point.
- Peg shaped teeth develop from a single lobe instead of four.
- The peg-shaped laterals are predominantly genetically determined and can also be caused due to endocrinal disturbances.
- May be associated with other dental anomalies such as anodontia.
- Studies of identical twins have indicated that missing teeth and peg-shaped lateral incisor might be a different expression of the same genetic trait i.e. the peg-shaped lateral is an incomplete expression of the genetic tendency for agenesis of the tooth.

2.5.13 Dental Abnormalities of Congenital Syphilis

Overview

- Children born to syphilitic mothers show characteristic abnormalities in the size, shape and structure of some of their permanent teeth.
- The deciduous dentition of such children is normal because it develops at such an early stage of intra-uterine life that abortion results if the expectant mother contracts the disease at that stage of her pregnancy.
- Teeth almost consistently affected in congenital syphilis are the upper first permanent incisors and the first molars, both uppers and lowers. Less frequently lateral incisors or canines may be affected.
- It is postulated that syphilitic organisms show higher affinity for developing teeth germs probably for their increased blood supply.
- Infection of the tooth germ results in distortion of the ameloblastic layer.

Chapter 2. Developmental Disturbances of Hard Dental Tissues

Dental Manifestations of congenital syphilis

1. Hutchinson's teeth

    The incisors are barrel-shaped with rounded incisal edges and a notch in the middle of the incisal edge.

2. Moon's molars.

    The permanent molars may be dome shaped.

3. Mulberry molars.

    The occlusal surfaces of permanent molars may be rough, pitted and exhibit multiple irregular tubercles replacing their normal cuspal pattern.

4. Enamel hypoplasia.

    Defective enamel usually associates the mentioned abnormalities of congenital syphilis.

2.6 Abnormalities in Structure

Etiology

1. **Acquired causes**

    Acquired causes usually affect enamel, dentin and possibly cementum. This is because hard tissue forming cells are all sensitive to environmental factors. Because cementum is invisible clinically, its defects are usually unobserved. The acquired defects are either local or systemic.

    (a) **Local factors**
    - Localized infection
    - Localized trauma

    (b) **Systemic factors**
    - Cytotoxic drugs

- Tetracycline
- Fluorides
- Exanthematous fevers
- Severe gastrointestinal tract disturbances
- Dietary deficiencies e.g. calcium, phosphorus and vitamins (A, C, D)
- Hormonal disturbances (hypoparathyroidism)
- Metabolic disturbances (hypophosphatasia)
- Irradiation
- Syphilis

2. **Hereditary causes**

   Hereditary causes usually affect either enamel or dentin. Differences between hereditary and acquired defects are summarized in table (2.2).

3. **Obscure causes**

   Some dental defects such as regional odontodysplasia have no definite known cause.

Classification of Abnormalities in Structure

1. Acquired defects (Usually affect enamel and dentin):
   (a) Acquired focal enamel hypoplasia (Turner's tooth)
   (b) Acquired generalized enamel hypoplasia
   (c) Dental fluorosis
   (d) Abnormal discoloration

2. Hereditary defects
   (a) Hereditary defects of enamel
       Amelogenesis imperfecta
   (b) Hereditary defects of dentin
       i. Dentinogenesis imperfecta

ii. Dentinal dysplasia
3. Obscure defects
   Regional odontodysplasia (ghost teeth)

2.6.1 Acquired Localized Enamel Hypoplasia

- Is the enamel hypoplasia affecting only one or two teeth
- It is also known as Turner's tooth
- It results from localized trauma or localized infection of a deciduous tooth which impinges upon its developing permanent successor
- The enamel shows pits, grooves, wrinkles with brown pigmentation or may be entirely lost

2.6.2 Acquired Generalized Enamel Hypoplasia

- Is the enamel hypoplasia affecting group of teeth
- It usually results from a systemic factor occurring during the period of tooth development
- It appears clinically as a horizontal line of small pits, grooves or wrinkles with brown pigmentation
- The width of these lines correlates with the duration of the insult
- If the duration of the insult was brief, the line is narrow and vice versa
- Most cases involve teeth which are formed during the first year after birth (Maternal immunity vanishes and acquired immunity not yet fully developed)
- These teeth are permanent incisors, canines and first molars

2.6.3 Dental Fluorosis (Mottled Enamel)

Definition

Is the dental defects resulting from increased level of fluorides in drinking water during the period of tooth development.

Etiology and pathogenesis

- Occurs when the fluoride level reaches 1.5 ppm or more
- Fluorides are toxic to all hard tissue forming cells
- Fluoride combines to form calcium fluoroapatite instead of calcium hydroxyapatite
- The disease is endemic in areas where the communal water supply is 1.5 ppm or more
- The severity of the lesions increases with the increase in the fluoride levels
- There is individual variation in the effect of fluorides, not all individuals of the same community show the same degree of mottling, this may be related to some dietary and drinking habits
- At intermediate levels (2–6 ppm) the matrix is normal in quantity and structure and the defect is mainly in calcification
- At higher levels (> 6 ppm) defective matrix formation starts (the enamel is pitted)
- Deciduous teeth are rarely affected because excess fluorides are taken up by the maternal skeleton
- At higher levels (> 8 ppm) deciduous teeth begin to be affected
- With sever mottling (> 8 ppm) sclerosis of the skeleton may develop
- At exceptionally very high levels, rickets and osteoporosis may develop

Clinically

- Mottling ranges from paper-white or chalky patches to opaque, brown, pitted and brittle enamel
- It is difficult to distinguish fluorotic defects from other enamel defects when the degree of exposure to fluorides are unknown
- Mottled teeth are more resistant to dental caries
- Grading of mottling is as follows:
    * Very Mild: Small paper-white or chalky areas less than 25% of surface
    * Mild: Opaque areas up to 50% of surface
    * Moderate: Paper-white (chalky) or brownish areas involving nearly the whole surface
    * Severe: The enamel is opaque, brown, pitted, brittle and easily chipped away from the tooth surface
- Dean's index is used also to determine the grade of dental fluorosis, thus:
    * Grade I (Questionable): Occasional white flecking over the tooth surface mainly on the incisor tips and cusp tips.
    * Grade II (Mild): White opaque areas involving less than 25% of the tooth surface.
    * Grade III (Moderate): White opaque areas involving more than 25% and less than 50% of the tooth surface.
    * Grade IV (Severe): White opaque areas involving more than 50% of the tooth surface.

Histologically

- Accentuated scalloping of the amelodentinal junction

- Defective calcification of the prisms and the interprismatic substance
- Irregular course of the prisms
- Stains, if present, is localized in the interprismatic substance

2.6.4 Abnormal Tooth Discoloration

Discoloration by exogenous pigments or chemicals

- Diet
- Coffee and tea
- Tobacco
- Excessive use of chlorhexidine

Discoloration by endogenous pigments or chemicals

- Fluorosis (yellowish or brownish discoloration)
- Tetracycline (yellow teeth, becoming grey or brown)
- Hemolytic jaundice of newborn (yellowish or greenish bands of discoloration)
- Porphyries (pink tooth, lavender tooth)
- Erythroblastosis fetalis

Tetracycline pigmentation

- Tetracycline is taken up by calcifying tissues
- A band of tetracycline-stained bone or tooth substance fluoresces bright yellow under ultraviolet light
- The teeth become stained only when tetracycline is given during their development and it can cross the placenta

- Permanent teeth become stained when tetracycline is given during infancy and deciduous teeth become stained when it is given during pregnancy
- Tetracycline is deposited along the incremental lines of the dentin and to lesser extent of enamel
- The teeth are at first bright yellow but become a dirty brown or gray
- The stain is permanent
- In very severe cases, intact teeth may fluoresce under ultraviolet light
- Tetracycline should not be prescribed to pregnant women or children less than 12 years of age

Porphyria

- A group of disorders involving heme biosynthesis, characterized by excessive excretion of porphyrins or their precursors
- May be inherited or may be acquired, as from the effects of certain chemical agents (e.g., hexachlorobenzene).
- Porphyrins may have an affinity to calcium phosphate and its incorporation in deciduous and permanent teeth gives them pink or lavender appearance (pink tooth, lavender tooth). Affected teeth fluoresce bright red under ultraviolet light.

Erythroblastosis Fetalis

- A grave hemolytic anemia that, in most instances, results from development in the mother of anti-Rh antibody in response to the Rh factor (ie, Rhesus factor) in the (Rh-positive) fetal blood
- It is characterized by many erythroblasts in the circulation, and often generalized edema (hydrops fetalis) and enlargement of the liver and

spleen; the disease is sometimes caused by antibodies for antigens other than Rh

- Teeth are green or bluish in color

2.6.5 Hereditary Defects of Enamel

Amelogenesis Imperfecta

Definition

- AI is a heterogeneous group of conditions caused by defects in the genes encoding enamel matrix proteins
- Most of these proteins are involved also in the control of enamel mineralization
- Classification of AI is complex and is based on the pattern of inheritance and clinical picture
- Genetic factors act throughout the whole duration of amelogenesis, therefore all teeth are affected and both dentitions are also affected

Enamel, the Hardest Tissue

- Dental enamel is a highly mineralized tissue with 85% of its volume occupied by unusually large, highly organized, hydroxyapatite crystals
- This highly organized and unusual structure is controlled in ameloblasts through the interaction of a number of organic matrix molecules that include enamelin, amelogenin (AMELX), ameloblastin (AMBN), tuftelin (TUFT1), dentin sialophosphoprotein (DSPP), and a variety of enzymes
- These proteins are formed under the action of several genes. Many of these genes are under heavy research

Classification of Amelogenesis Imperfecta

Modified after Witkop [1].

Clinical Classification

Table (2.3) shows the clinical classification of amelogenesis imperfecta

Pattern of inheritance

Confusingly, it seems that the same mutation can sometimes cause hypoplastic, hypomineralized or hypomaturation forms in different patients

1. Autosomal dominant type
   - Defects in the ameloblastin gene mapped to 4q11-4q21
   - Defects in the enamelin gene, mapped to 4p21
   - Defects in tuftelin gene mapped to 1q21
2. Autosomal recessive type
3. X-linked dominant type
   - Defects in the amelogenin gene, mapped to the Xp22.3
4. X-linked recessive type
5. Y-linked type (postulated but not proven yet, under heavy research)

Hypoplastic Amelogenesis Imperfecta

- The main defect is in the formation of the matrix
- Enamel is hard, and translucent
- Enamel is of normal radiopacity
- Enamel is randomly pitted, grooved or very thin
- The defects tend to be stained

- Teeth tends to be small in size with loss of contact points
- Twisted enamel rods course from the dentinoenamel junction to the enamel surface
- Defective amelogenin
- The main patterns of inheritance are AD, AR, and XD
- In X-linked dominant type:
  * The affected males show almost complete failure of enamel formation
  * The affected females show pitted, ridged or grooved enamel indicating a Lyon effect

2.7 Lyon Hypothesis

- In females at the day 16 of intrauterine life, random inactivation of one of X chromosomes occurs
- The inactivated X forms a rounded condensed mass attached to the nuclear membrane and is termed Barr body (could be seen in the interphase nucleus)
- Thus, a group of somatic cells has active X of the mother and other active X of the father
- This is translated in the enamel as the female patient shows alternate zones of healthy and defective enamel
- Male patients, have a single X, hence completely display defective enamel in both dentitions

Hypocalcified Amelogenesis Imperfecta

- Enamel matrix is formed in normal quantity but poorly calcified (qualitative defect)

- When newly erupted, the enamel is normal in thickness and form, but soft, opaque and chalky
- Teeth become stained and rapidly worn away
- Enamel is more radiolucent than dentin
- The main patterns of inheritance are AD, and AR

Hypomaturation Amelogenesis Imperfecta

- Enamel matrix is formed in normal quantity but poorly matured (qualitative defect)
- When newly erupted, the enamel is normal in thickness and form, but soft and opaque, not as severely as the hypocalcified type
- Teeth become stained and show rapid attrition
- Enamel shows the degree of radiopacity as that of dentin
- The main patterns of inheritance are AD, AR, XD, and XR

Complications of AI

The main clinical problems of AI are esthetics, dental sensitivity, and loss of occlusal vertical dimensions

2.7.1 Hereditary Defects of dentin

Classification

1. Dentinogenesis imperfecta type I (associated with osteogenesis imperfecta)
2. Dentinogenesis imperfecta type II (brown opalescent dentin) (Shields type) (not associated with osteogenesis imperfecta)
3. Dentinogenesis imperfecta type III (Shell tooth) (Brandywine type)

4. Dentinal dysplasia (rootless teeth)

Dentinogenesis Imperfecta

Definition

A group of developmental hereditary defect of dentin

Classification

1. Dentinogenesis imperfecta type I (associated with osteogenesis imperfecta)
2. Dentinogenesis imperfecta type II (not associated with osteogenesis imperfecta) (brown opalascent dentin) (Shields type)
3. Dentinogenesis imperfecta type III (shell tooth) (Brandywine type)

Dentinogenesis Imperfecta Type I

Definition

- Developmental hereditary defect of dentin
- The disease occurs associated with osteogenesis imperfecta

Etiology

- Transmitted as an atuosomal dominant trait
- The gene is closely related to that of osteogenesis imperfecta
- Mutation of the genes COL1A1 and COL1A2 are responsible for this condition
- The former had been mapped to chromosome 17q21.31-q22 while the latter is situated at 7q22.1

- These genes are responsible for the polymerization of procollagen alpha helix into normal type I collagen

Clinically

- Type I occurs associated with osteogenesis imperfecta particularly types III and IV. About 80% of cases of osteogenesis imperfecta types III and IV are associated with dentinogenesis imperfecta
- Type II occurs unassociated with osteogenesis imperfecta
  Both types of dentinogenesis imperfecta (types I and II) are clinically similar except for the absence of OI in the later
- Features:
  - Both dentitions are affected
  - Normal enamel which can be easily chipped away due to defective formation of dentinoenamel junction
  - Teeth are brownish and abnormally translucent
  - Crowns are small, bulbous with constricted necks
  - Short roots
  - dentin is abnormally soft
  - Teeth become worn rapidly to the gum margins

X-ray

- Small teeth
- Bulbous crowns with constricted necks
- Short roots
- The pulp shows progressive obliteration with poorly formed dentin

Histologically

- Normal enamel
- Loss of scalloping of the dentinoenamel junctions
- The earliest formed dentin (mantle dentin) is normal
- The deeper dentin layers show the following:
  - Poor calcification
  - Many entrapped cells (osteodentin)
  - Large areas of interglobular spaces
  - Large areas of atubular dentin
  - Irregular dentinal tubules
- Progressive obliteration of the pulp with this malformed dentin

Treatment

- Preventing excessive loss of enamel and dentin and toward improving the teeth esthetically.
- This can be accomplished with appropriate restoration such as metal / porcelain crowns.
- Teeth do not make good abutments for partial dentures because root fractures may occur from the functional stress.
- In severe cases full dentures are usually inevitable.

Dentinogenesis Imperfecta type II

- Etiologically DI-II is distinct from DI-I as the former is caused by mutation in the DSPP gene (125485), encoding dentin sialoprotein and dentin phosphoprotein. The gene was mapped to 4q21.1 – q25
- On the other hand, DI-II is closely related to DI-III as both conditions are considered as allelic variants (different mutations in the same gene)

- Clinically, DI-II is similar to DI-I except for the absence of osteogenesis imperfecta, however DI-II is much more common than DI-1 (frequency may be 1 in 6000 – 8000 children)

Dentinogenesis Imperfecta type III

(Shell tooth, Brandywine type, DI-III)

- A developmental defect of dentin considered as a type of DI-II and probably carried on the same gene
- DI-III was termed the "Brandywine type", named after the region in Maryland, USA, where an affected kindred originated
- Witkop suggested that DI-II and DI-III were the same entity.
- Linkage studies have indicated that the genes for DI-II and III are both on the long arm of chromosome 4 (4q21-q25), and that the two putative conditions are either the same condition or result from different mutations within the same gene
- In any event, isolated DI (DI-II and DI-III) is a different entity from DI in OI (DI-I), with different causative genetic mechanisms
- DI-III is transmitted as an autosomal dominant trait
- The earliest formed dentin layer (mantle dentin) is formed normally but further dentin formation ceases leaving a huge pulp chamber and a thin shell of dentin around
- Pulp lacks the normal odontoblastic layer and consists of coarse connective tissue incorporated into the deep dentin layer
- Early pulp exposure is a common sequel of caries affecting these teeth
- MacDougall et al. (1999) stated that the manifestations of DI-III can differ from those of DI-II by:
    - ★ The presence of multiple pulp exposures
    - ★ Normal non-mineralized pulp chambers and canals

- ★ The general appearance of "shell teeth"
- ★ The amber (pink) discoloration of the teeth
- ★ Attrition, and fractured enamel
- ★ The classic "shell teeth" appearance on radiographs.

Dentinal Dysplasia (Rootless Teeth)

Definition

- A developmental dentin malformation which was originally termed "rootless teeth"
- The disorder has been classified into type I, Radicular dentin dysplasia and type II, coronal dentin dysplasia
- Type I is much more common than type II

Etiology

Transmitted as an autosomal dominant trait

Clinically

Type I (radicular):

- Affects both deciduous and permanent dentitions.
- Normal coronal morphology and color.
- Very short and conical tapered roots.
- Normal eruption pattern.
- Early exfoliation of affected teeth due to short roots.

- The pulp chamber is obliterated by defective dentin with the characteristic crescent-shape radiolucency of the pulp chamber (half moon shaped) particularly in permanent teeth.
- Apical radiolucencies without apparent cause postulated to result from pulpal necrosis.

Type II (coronal):

- Affects deciduous and permanent dentitions.
- Normal morphology and shapes of crowns and roots.
- Primary teeth are amber in color and then tends to be brown opalescent with aging.
- Permanent teeth are of normal color.
- Both primary and permanent dentitions show enlarged pulp chambers with many pulp stones.
- In permanent teeth, the large pulp chambers are typically described as thistle tube appearance in which there is sudden constriction at the base ending with a very narrow root canal and tendency for complete obliteration of the pulp with pulp stones.

Histologically:

- Normal layer of mantle dentin.
- Circumpulpal dentin is atubular with many interglobular dentin.

Table (2.4) illustrates the most important differences between coronal and radicular types of dentinal dysplasia.

2.7.2 Obscure Defects of dentin

Regional Odontodysplasia (Ghost Teeth)

Definition

This is a localized non-hereditary disorder affecting a group of teeth in which there are severe abnormalities of enamel, dentin and pulp

Etiology

- Unknown; not hereditary
- Suggested factors are local circulatory disturbance, trauma, nutrition, infection and metabolic abnormalities. The theory of circulatory disturbance is suggested as there have been many cases reported with vascular nevi or hemangiomas on the affected side.
- Facial vascular nevi, on the ipsilateral (same side) is sometimes noted
- Females are slightly more affected than males (1.4:1)
- No racial predilection

Clinically

- The most common site is the upper lateral incisor, canines and premolars
- One or two quadrants may be affected
- One or both dentitions may be affected
- Teeth show severe deformed crown and root morphology
- Enamel is very thin, pitted, pigmented and rough
- The abnormal teeth may fail to erupt
- Teeth are susceptible to caries and fracture

- The condition can affect both primary and permanent dentition. If primary teeth are affected, the permanent teeth are affected as well.

X-ray

- Due to lack of adequate calcification, the teeth appear as radiolucent "shells" on x-ray, with thin enamel and dentin
- Large pulp chambers justifying the term "Ghost teeth"

Histologically

- Thin, irregular enamel with loss of prismatic structure
- dentin show disorganized tubular structures, many clefts and many interglobular dentin

2.8 Disturbances in Eruption

2.8.1 Early Eruption

- Show genetic and racial predilection
- Usually affects deciduous dentition
- It is questionable whether early loss of deciduous teeth can slightly accelerate the eruption of their permanent successors
- Occurs in facial hemihypertrophy and affects the enlarged half of the face
- The condition is of no clinical significance

2.8.2 Delayed Eruption

Local Causes

1. Loss of space and overcrowding of teeth
2. Abnormal position of the tooth germ (usually lower third molars and upper canines)
3. Presence of supplemental and supernumerary teeth
4. Retention of deciduous teeth
5. Eruption cyst
6. Dentigerous cyst

Systemic Causes

1. Rickets
2. Cretinism
3. Cherubism (familial fibrous dysplasia)
4. Cleidocranial dysostosis
5. Hereditary gingival fibromatosis (elephantiasis gingivae)
6. Irradiation

Complications affecting unerupted or partially erupted teeth

1. Often no clinical effects
2. Pericoronitis
3. Cyst formation
4. Resorption of adjacent teeth
5. Root resorption of the affected tooth
6. Hypercementosis of the affected tooth

2.8.3 Teething Problems

- The idea that teething, the normal eruption of infant's teeth, can cause systemic symptoms or serious illness is a myth
- The time of teething coincides with a period of naturally low resistance to infection and declining maternal immunity
- So that infection during the period of teething is merely coincidental

2.9 Multisystem Disorders Affecting Teeth

Many multisystem disorders show some dental abnormalities. Most of these disorders are discussed in their relevant system chapters. Although, most of these disorders are rare, the following disorders are the most important.

- Ehlers-Danlos Syndrome (Floppy Joint)

  See chapter "Developmental Disturbances of Oral & Para-Oral Tissues, page (93)"

- Gardner's Syndrome (Familial Adenomatous Polyposis)

  See chapter "Developmental Disturbances of Oral & Para-Oral Tissues, page (93)"

- Epidermolysis Bullosa

  See chapter "Developmental Disturbances of Oral & Para-Oral Tissues, page (77)"

- Hypophosphatasia

  See chapter "Developmental Disturbances of Oral & Para-Oral Tissues, page (93)"

- Early Onset Idiopathic Hypoparathyroidism

  See chapter "Developmental Disturbances of Oral & Para-Oral Tissues, page (96)"

Table 2.1: Examples of craniofacial anomalies and developmental syndromes associated with abnormalities in the number of teeth. Most of these syndromes are discussed in the following chapters.

> **Always Remember**
>
> - **Hypodontia**
>   - Cleft lip/palate
>   - Crouzon syndrome
>   - Down syndrome (trisomy 21)
>   - Hereditary ectodermal dysplasia
>   - Ellis-van Creveld syndrome (chondroectodermal dysplasia)
>   - Oral-facial-digital syndrome
>   - Van der Woude syndrome
> - **Hyperdontia**
>   - Cleft lip/palate
>   - Cleidocranial dysplasia
>   - Gardener syndrome (polyposis coli, Familial Adenomatous Polyposis (FAP))
>   - Oral-facial-digital syndrome
>   - Ehlers-Danlos syndrome Type III
>   - Incontinentia pigmenti
>   - Marfan syndrome

Chapter 2. Developmental Disturbances of Hard Dental Tissues

Table 2.2: Differences Between Hereditary and Acquired Defects of Enamel

Hereditary Versus Acquired Defects

Hereditary Defects	Acquired Defects
Affect enamel or dentin	Affect enamel and dentin
Affect both dentitions	Affects one dentition usually the permanent
Usually affect all teeth	Usually affect single or group of teeth
vertically or randomly oriented pits or defects	horizontally oriented pits or defects

Note

Table 2.3: Classification of Amelogenesis Imperfecta

Always Remember

1. Hypoplastic type (AD, AR, XD)
2. Hypomineralized type (AD, AR)
3. Hypomaturation type (AD, AR, XD, XR)
4. Hypoplastic/hypomaturation type (AD)

AD: Autosomal dominant, AR: Autosomal recessive, XD: X-linked dominant, XR: X-linked recessive

Note

Table 2.4: Differences Between Coronal and Radicular Dentinal Dysplasia

Always Remember

Defect	Type I	Type II
Nature	Radicular	Coronal
Etiology	Autosomal dominant	Autosomal dominant
Dentition affected	Deciduous + permanent	Usually deciduous
Crown	Nearly normal	Opalescent
Roots	Short + conical	Nearly normal
Pulp	Complete obliteration + stones	Incomplete obliteration + stones
Apical radiolucencies	Present	Absent
Differentiation from DI	Easy	Difficult

Chapter 3
Developmental Disturbances of Oral & Para-oral Tissues

In this chapter the developmental disturbances of soft and hard non-dental tissues that are related to the oral and para-oral structures are to be discussed.

3.1 Developmental Disturbances of Face

3.1.1 Treacher Collins Syndrome

(Mandibulo-facial dysostosis)

Definition

- A developmental malformation affecting face. The severe form of the disease is known as *Franceschetti's* syndrome.
- Treacher Collins syndrome constitutes one member of what was known as the first arch syndrome.

Etiology

The disease is hereditary, transmitted through a dominant autosomal gene with high penetrance. The mutant gene was identified on the long arm of the chromosome 5 (5q32-33.1) and was termed treacle gene.

Clinically

1. Colobomata of the lower eye lids with atrophy of the outer third of the eyelid.
2. Antimongoloid slant of the palpebral fissure .
3. Hypoplasia of the zygomatic bone resulting in flattening appearance of the face.
4. Hypoplasia of the mandible.
5. Deformity of the ear pinna.
6. Deformity or absence of the external auditory meatus leading to deaf-mutism.
7. Abnormal growth of hair in front of the ears.
8. Flattened frontonasal angle.
9. Cleft lip and/or palate.
10. Incomplete forms of the disease may occur.

3.1.2 Pierre Robin Syndrome

(Pierre Robin sequence, mandibular dysostosis with glossoptosis syndrome)

Definition

- A developmental malformation characterized by mandibular hypoplasia, cleft palate and glossoptosis.

- Until 1974, the triad was known as Pierre Robin syndrome; however, the term syndrome is now reserved for those cases with the simultaneous presence of multiple anomalies. The term sequence has been introduced to describe any condition that includes a series of anomalies caused by a cascade of events initiated by a single malformation.

Etiology

Two postulates exist:

1. The first one is that the disease is hereditary mediated through mutation near the SOX9 gene.
2. The other theory (mechanical theory, oligohydramnios theory) assumed that the disease results from oligohydramnios by which the weight of the body is forced on the vertex of the head thus allowing the mandible to come in forceful contact with the shoulder and the sternum. This condition will in turn results in failure of the tongue to descend into its normal lower position with consequent clefting of the palate. The presence of a shoulder impression on the body of the mandible and the characteristic U-shaped cleft palate lend support to this theory.

Clinically

- Hypoplasia of mandible. Sometimes the mandible is not hypoplastic but there is right angle gonial angle (mandibular angle) instead of being obtuse. There is also a shoulder impression on the body of the mandible.
- Glossoptosis (ptosis in Greek means downward displacement) in which the tongue may fall back to touch the posterior wall of the pharynx producing asphyxia.
- Cleft palate.

3.1.3 Crouzon Syndrome

(cranio-facial dysostosis)

Definition

A developmental disorder characterized by craniosynostosis and cranio-facial malformation.

Etiology

- Inherited in an autosomal dominant pattern
- It is suggested that mutation of fibroblast growth factor receptor FGFR-2 gene could be responsible for Crouzon syndrome
- Moreover, the mutation in the transmembrane region of FGFR-3 was detected in this syndrome

Clinically

- Coronal and sagittal sutures show early ossification
- Anteroposterior diameter of the skull is smaller than transverse diameter (broad face and skull).
- Hypoplastic maxilla
- Progressing optic nerve atrophy leads to vision impairment because of the intracranial hypertension.
- Impairment of hearing
- Malocclusion
- Short upper lip with possible cleft lip
- Widely spaced eyes (hypertelorism), shallow orbits and protruding eyeballs

- Possible unilateral or bilateral posterior crossbite

3.1.4 Cleft Lip and Palate

Definition

These are congenital clefts of varying degrees, which may affect lip, alveolus or palate.

Classification of Clefts

Many classifications were advocated based upon etiological, anatomical, surgical and clinical points of view. However, the following ones are adopted:

Etiologic Classification

1. Syndromic (30% of cases) occurring associated with genetic syndromes.
    (a) Treacher collins syndrome
    (b) Pierre robin syndrome
    (c) Apert's syndrome
    (d) Van der Woude syndrome (see later in this chapter)
2. Non-syndromic (70% of cases)

Anatomical Classification

1. Pre-alveolar clefts (cleft lip) 22%
    (a) Unilateral
        i. Complete
        ii. Incomplete
    (b) Bilateral

i. Complete

ii. Incomplete

iii. Mixed

(c) Median (hare lip)

2. Alveolar clefts:

    (a) Unilateral

    (b) Bilateral

3. Post-alveolar clefts: (cleft palate) 20%

    (a) Cleft uvula (bifid uvula)

    (b) Cleft uvula and soft palate

    (c) Cleft uvula, soft palate and hard palate till the incisive foramen.

    (d) Cleft uvula, soft palate, hard palate till the incisive foramen then the cleft includes the alveolus unilaterally.

    (e) As above but the cleft includes the alveolus bilaterally (the condition often termed complete median cleft palate, alveolus and lip).

    (f) Submucous cleft palate

4. Median clefts of lower lip are rare

Etiology

Syndromic clefts:

- Are usually due to single gene defect and follow Mendelian rules of inheritance.
- The following genes are candidates for developing oro-facial clefts:
- IRF6 (interferon regulatory factor-6) associated with Van der Woude syndrome[1], the exact function is unknown.

---

[1] An autosomal dominant disorders characterized by congenital lip pits, cleft lip with or without cleft palate, hypodontia, congenital heart disease cerebral abnormalities.

- PVRL1 (poliovirus receptor related-1) responsible for autsomal recessive CLP-ectodermal dysplasia syndrome.
- P63 (homologue for P53 tumor suppressor gene). Its mutations were found to cause CLP in mice.

Non-Syndromic clefts:

- Are due to multifactorial inheritance.
- Multifactorial inheritance are diseases in which genetic and environmental factors play an influential role.
- Do not follow the Mendelian pattern of inheritance.
- Result from the action of more than one gene and can be modified by the environmental factors.
- The environmental factors responsible for cleft lip and palate are not known precisely, however the following factors were suggested:
    * Alcohol consumption
    * Smoking
    * Altitude hypoxia
    * diabetes
    * Age > 40 years
    * Vitamin A excess or deficiency
    * Folic acid deficiency
    * Zinc deficiency
    * Corticosteroids (proven in experimental animals)
    * An interesting finding was that folic acid could reduce the incidence of clefts in genetically prone individuals

Clinically

Cleft lip:

- Incidence: 1: 500–2500 of live births depending on race, geographic location, maternal age and prenatal exposures to teratogenic agents.
- Population differences have been reported, with the highest rates in Asians and Native Americans (1 in 500 births) and the lowest rate in Africans (1 in 2,500 births)
- Sex: Males are affected more than females 2:1.
- The relative frequency of cleft lip is about 22% of all cases of clefts.
- Usually occurs in the left side three times more than the right side.
- The incomplete form takes the form of a notch in the lower border of the lip while the complete form the lip is completely bisected into two parts.
- In cases of complete bilateral cleft of the upper lip the median piece of tissue (prolabium) is isolated, devoid of muscle and shows no filtrum.

Cleft alveolus

- In cases of complete bilateral clefts of the alveolus, clefting of the lip is usually found and the premaxilla with the prolabium are isolated and remains suspended from the nasal septum
- During surgical correction, fracture of the premaxilla is a probability which should be avoided

Cleft Palate

- Incidence: 1: 2000 of live births
- Sex: Females are affected more than males (2-1)
- The relative frequency of cleft palate is about 20% of all cases of clefts, while combined cleft lip and palate is about 58%

- Fusion of the palate starts form the incisive foramen area and runs posterior toward the uvula

Submucous cleft palate

- Submucous clefts are an abnormality of the attachment of the muscles of the soft palate beneath an intact mucosa.
- They are present in approximately 1 in 1200 births but frequently missed. The chief effects are slowness in feeding and nasal regurgitation. Middle ear infections and speech defects can result from defective muscle attachments. Symptoms are absent in around 10% of cases.
- Clinically, a Submucous cleft is visible as a translucent area along the midline of the soft palate and frequently a bifid uvula. On palpation, a notched posterior nasal spine may be felt. The diagnosis can be confirmed by imaging techniques.

3.1.5 Oblique Facial Cleft

- This is a developmental congenital cleft, which runs from the inner canthus of the eye to the ala of the nose along the path of the nasolacrimal duct, and often extends into the lip and primary palate.
- The cleft is due to failure of fusion of the lateral nasal and the maxillary processes.

3.1.6 Transverse Facial Cleft

- This is a cleft running from the angle of the mouth to the ear
- Due to failure of fusion between the maxillary and mandibular processes.

3.1.7 Macrostomia

- Macrostomia means large mouth
- Due to early arrest of fusion between maxillary and mandibular processes.

3.1.8 Microstomia

- Microstomia means small mouth
- Due to excessive closure of the maxillary and mandibular processes.

3.1.9 Facial Hemihypertrophy (Hemifacial Hypertrophy)

Definition

This is a congenital malformation in which one half of the face and jaw are enlarged.

Etiology

The exact etiology is not precisely known. Vascular and neurogenic factors are supposed to cause this anomaly.

Clinically

- Teeth on the affected side are larger than normal, while the roots may be normal.
- Early shedding of deciduous teeth and early eruption of permanent teeth on the affected side is reported in some cases.

3.1.10 Facial Hemihypoplasia (Hemifacial Atrophy)

Definition

A characteristic loss in the soft tissues below the skin, usually on one side of the face, in some severe cases, the underlying bone is also affected.

Clinically

- Starts in 1st or 2nd decade of life
- Left side more commonly affected
- Affected side may be hyperpigmented
- Hollowing of cheek and the orbit
- Jaw bones and roots of teeth on affected side my exhibit delayed development and retarded tooth eruption

Radiographically

Deficient root development or root resorption

Etiology

Peripheral nerve dysfunction, trauma or infection of the growth centers, and genetic causes have been proposed

Prognosis

The condition progresses slowly for a few years and remains stable thereafter

3.2 Developmental Disturbances of Jaws

3.2.1 Agnathia (Aplasia of Mandible)

- This is a very rare developmental malformation in which there is partial or complete absence of either jaw particularly mandible.
- Absence of the ramus with its condyloid process is more common than complete absence of the jaw and is usually associated with deformity of the ear pinna.

3.2.2 Micrognathia (Mandibular Dysostosis)

Definition

Means a small jaw

Types

1. False, pseudo, apparent or relative micrognathia

    Which is due to disproportion between size of the jaw and size of the skull or teeth, and the jaw is still within the normal range of size.

2. True micrognathia, which may be

    (a) Congenital: This is usually hereditary and is usually associated with some craniofacial malformations such as Treacher Collins syndrome and Pierre robin syndrome.

    (b) Acquired: which is usually due to trauma, irradiation or infection in the region of the mandibular growth centers particularly the condylar centers.

3.2.3 Macrognathia

Definition

Means large jaw and can results in prognathism

Types

1. False, pseudo, apparent or relative:

    Which is due to disproportion between size of the jaw and size of the skull or teeth as in Crouzon syndrome.
2. True macrognathia, which may be:

    (a) Congenital: which is usually hereditary.

    (b) Acquired, due to acromegaly, tumors, infections or diseases affecting the jaw e.g. Paget's disease of bone.

3.3 Developmental Disturbances of Palate

3.3.1 Cleft Palate

Has been discussed before

3.3.2 Torus Palatinus

- This is a hereditary condition in which there are multiple bony exostoses or projections in the midline of the palate covered by thin mucosa.
- Histologically they consist of compact bone or a core of cancellous bone covered by compact bone. The overlying mucosa may be stretched.

Tori, if large can interfere with the stability of upper dentures and may need surgical removal or denture relief.

Torus mandibularis is a unilateral or bilateral bony projection presents on the lingual aspect of the mandible and can interfere with the stability of lower dentures.

3.4 Developmental Disturbances of Lips

3.4.1 Cleft Lip

Has already been discussed before.

3.4.2 Double Lip

- Is the condition characterized by presence of a fold of tissue on the mucosal side of the lip
- The condition usually affects the upper lip more often than the lower lip
- The condition may be congenital or acquired later on life as in case of Ascher syndrome
- Congenital cases may result from malformation of the labial sulcus
- Treatment by surgical excision if necessary.
- **Ascher syndrome:** is a condition of unknown etiology characterized by:
    1. Double lip
    2. Edema of the upper eyelids (blepharochalasis)
    3. Non-toxic thyroid enlargement

3.4.3 Congenital Lip Pits and Fistulae

Definition

Congenital lip pits are epithelial lined pits or depressions found on the vermilion border of the lip. Lip fistulae are epithelialized tracts connecting the vermilion border with the inside surface of the lip.

Etiology

- The disease is hereditary and transmitted as a dominant autosomal trait.
- Can occur as a part of *Van der Woude* syndrome (see page 58).

Clinically

- Usually affecting the lower lip.
- May be single or multiple.
- May be present near the midline or near the oral commissures.
- Pressure may elicit a mucous secretion from the base of the pits due to the occasional opening of a minor salivary gland in the base of the pit.

3.4.4 Cheillits Glandularis

Definition

This is the condition in which there is persistent inflammation of the labial salivary glands.

Etiology

- The cause of this condition is poorly understood, most probably not developmental.
- Chronic exposure to sun, dust and wind is supposed to a play a role in the etiology.

Clinically

- The lower lip is usually affected.
- Males are affected more than females.
- The lip gets enlarged, firm and everted thus exposing the orifices of the labial salivary glands, which becomes dilated and inflamed producing red dots.
- The condition is considered by some authors to be a precancerous condition.

3.4.5 Cheillitis Granulomatosa

Definition

A condition in which there are multiple granulomata affecting the lip.

Etiology

The exact cause of the disease is unknown, the disease is considered by some authors to be a type of sarcoidosis.

Clinically

- The lower lip is usually affected.

- Rare cases show involvement of the upper lip, chin, tip of nose and forehead.
- The lip is enlarged, firm and everted.
- Enlargement of the submental, submandibular and cervical lymph nodes may occur.

Histologically

The lesion consists of:

- Granulation tissue which consists of delicate collagen fibrils, proliferating fibroblasts and proliferating capillaries.
- Chronic inflammatory cell infiltration.
- Epithelioid cells.
- Langhans giant cells.
- No caseation.

Treatment

The lesion may respond to intralesional injections of corticosteroids

3.4.6 Melkersson - Rosenthal Syndrome

This is a developmental disorder characterized by:

1. Cheillits granulomatosa
2. Fissured tongue
3. Facial paresis

3.4.7 Xeroderma Pigmentosa

Definition

This is a condition in which there is increased sensitivity of the skin to the ultraviolet rays of sun.

Etiology

Hereditary, transmitted as a recessive autosomal trait. The inherited defect seems to be in the DNA repair mechanism.

Clinically

- Exposure to sun results in erythema of the skin associated with hyper-pigmentation resembling freckles.
- This is followed by atrophy of the skin and appearance some of multiple papules, which may turn, into multiple squamous cell carcinomas or malignant melanomas.

Histologically

- Hyperkeratosis.
- Atrophy of the prickle cell layer.
- Atrophy of some rete pegs and elongation of others.
- Melanin pigmentation of the basal cell layer.

3.4.8 Peutz - Jeghers Syndrome

(PJS, Multiple intestinal polyposis syndrome with melanin pigmentation)

Definition

This is a hereditary disease characterized by presence of multiple polyps in the small intestine associated with circum-oral, circum-nasal, circum-ocular melanin pigmentation. Melanin pigmentation may also be present in the oral mucosa and on the dorsum of hands and feet.

Etiology

- Hereditary, transmitted as a simple Mendelian dominant autosomal trait.
- The putative gene STK11 (LKB1) is located on the chromosome 19 and is considered as a tumor suppressor gene inherited in an autosomal dominant pattern.
- This means that anyone who has PJS has a 50% chance of passing the disease on to their offspring.

Clinically

- Many patients with this syndrome have frequent episodes of abdominal pain and signs of minor obstruction.
- Recent trends suppose that this condition is precancerous. Patients with the syndrome have an increased risk of developing carcinomas of the liver, lungs, breast, ovaries, uterus, testes and other organs.

3.5 Developmental Disturbances of Oral Mucosa

3.5.1 Fordyce's Granules (Spots)

- A developmental condition in which there are ectopic sebaceous glands in the oral mucosa, which should normally be devoid of them.
- These sebaceous glands appear as yellowish spots, which may be raised above the surface, scattered along the line connecting the oral commissures with the retromolar area (linea alba buccalis). They may grow in size with age.
- Fordyce's granules are present in around 80% of populations and hence are considered by some to be normal variants of oral mucosa.
- They may result from inclusion of ectoderm possessing the potentiality to form skin appendages at the line of fusion of maxillary and mandibular processes.
- Histologically the lesion consists of normal sebaceous gland follicles, with or without well formed ducts, lying free in the dermis.
- The term ectopia or heterotopia by definition is the presence of normal tissue in an abnormal anatomical site.

3.5.2 Leukoedema

- Is a bilateral, diffuse, translucent white thickening of the oral mucosa
- The thickening is soft, pliable and can not be wiped off
- The thickening disappears upon stretching and reestablishing itself when released
- The buccal mucosa is the most common site
- It is a variation of normal, present in 90% of blacks and variable numbers of whites.

- The cause of this normal variation is not precisely known
- Histologically, there is acanthosis with intercellular edema of the spinous cell layer.
- Treatment is unnecessary but reassurance may be required.

3.5.3 White Spongy Nevus

(Familial White Folded Gingivostomatitis, Cannon's Disease)

- An autosomal dominant condition of the oral cavity characterized by soft, white or opalescent, thickened and corrugated folds of mucous membrane.
- The condition resembles leukoplakia, but the lesion tends to be soft and spongy upon palpation.
- The disorder may appear at birth, in infancy, or in childhood, and reaches full severity at puberty when it should remain stationary.
- The lesion usually affects the buccal mucosa; however in rare cases the entire oral mucosa may be affected.
- A *nevus* by definition is a developmental malformation of skin or mucous membrane arising form cells native to skin or mucous membrane and simulating a neoplasm.
- Nevi in general are of three types, keratotic (white spongy nevus), melanotic and vascular (e.g. hemangioma and lymphangioma).
- Nevi, in general, are considered to be one of the types of hamartomas.
- The term hamartoma by definition is a developmental malformation appearing in a tumor like condition due to presence of normal cells in normal sites but in an exaggerated amount.
- Treatment is unnecessary but reassurance may be required.

Histologically

- Acanthosis (increased thickness of prickle cell layer).
- Inter and intra-cellular edema of the prickle cell layer giving the characteristic picture of *basket weave appearance*.
- Some degree of hyperkeratosis.
- Chronic inflammatory cell infiltration of the connective tissue (secondary phenomenon due to chronic trauma of the lesion and defective protective function of the epithelium; the lesion is primarily a developmental condition and not an inflammatory one).

3.5.4 Hereditary Benign Intraepithelial Dyskeratosis

(Witkop's disease, red eye)

Definitions

- Dyskeratosis by definition is an abnormal keratinization of epithelial cells.
- Two types have been recognized, malignant and benign. Malignant dyskeratosis is that type of keratosis usually found in malignant and premalignant conditions, while benign dyskeratosis is the type usually found in some benign conditions such as hereditary benign intraepithelial dyskeratosis and Darier's disease.
- Hereditary benign intraepithelial dyskeratosis is an autosomal dominant condition consisting of white spongy lesions of the buccal mucosa, floor of the mouth, ventral and lateral surfaces of the tongue, gingiva and palate.

- Transient gelatinous plaques form over the cornea, which may produce conjunctivitis and temporary blindness, and hence the term red eye was sometimes proposed for such disease.
- Treatment is unnecessary but reassurance may be required.

Histologically

- The lesion is similar to white spongy nevus except for the presence of eosinophilic dyskeratotic cells in the prickle cell layer. Most of these cells show perinuclear condensation of keratin.
- Some degree of hyperkeratosis.
- The descriptive term "cell within cell dyskeratosis" was given for these eosinophilic dyskeratotic cells.

3.5.5 Darier's Disease

(Keratosis follicularis, Follicular keratosis, Keratosis vegetans, DD)

- Keratosis follicularis is a hereditary skin disease characterized by hyperkeratotic papules usually in seborrheic regions with various nail abnormalities.
- The disease is autosomal dominant and caused by mutations in the ATP2A2 gene.
- Abnormal cell-cell adhesion and abnormal epithelial keratinization are the primary features of DD
- Electron microscopy reveals loss of many desmosomes and breakdown of desmosome keratin intermediate filament attachment.
- Mutations in the ATP2A2 gene cause functional disruptions of the adhesion between keratinocytes and affect cellular differentiation in the epidermis

- DD most commonly begins in the first and second decades of life.
- The lesions may first appear as skin-colored papules, which soon become yellowish brown, greasy, warty papules. These lesions are especially common in the seborrheic areas, such as the forehead, the scalp, the nasolabial folds, the ears, the chest, and the back.
- Involvement of the hands is very common (about 95%).
- Mucosal lesions are detected in about 15% of patients, and they appear as white papules with a central depression. These lesions are most commonly found in the mouth, and they give the mucosa a sandpaper texture or cobble stone appearance. At times, these lesions may affect the salivary glands and cause obstruction
- **Histologically**: The disease is characterized by:
  * Hyperkeratosis.
  * Acanthosis.
  * Benign dyskeratosis. Two types of dyskeratotic cells are present: corps ronds and grains. Corps ronds are predominantly located in the prickle and granular cell layer. Corps ronds are characterized by an irregular eccentric and sometimes pyknotic nucleus, a clear perinuclear halo, and a brightly eosinophilic cytoplasm. Grains are mostly located in the stratum corneum, and they consist of oval cells with elongated cigar-shaped nuclei and abundant keratohyalin granules.
  * Acantholysis (loss of attachment between epithelial cells). Acantholysis results in the formation of suprabasilar clefts which may contain many acantholytic cells.
- **Treatment:**
  * No effective treatment.
  * Systemic and sometimes topical retinoids such as isotretinoin, is the most effective medical treatment.

- ★ Long-term treatment with oral retinoids may be required. Unfortunately, prolonged use of oral retinoids can cause significant adverse effects, and many patients have to stop taking them because of the toxicity.
- ★ Doxycycline was also effective in controlling the disease. Doxycycline belongs to the tetracycline family. In addition to their antibiotic potential, tetracyclines and their analogues exhibit anti-inflammatory properties by inhibiting granulocyte chemotaxis.

3.5.6 Epidermolysis Bullosa

- A group of inherited chronic skin diseases in which large bullae and erosions result from slight mechanical trauma affecting skin and oral mucosa. Theses bullae and erosions will be followed by scarring. Tooth brushing increases bullae formation. Dystrophy of nails was described in some cases
- There are more than one mode of inheritance for EB with many gene mutations, thus EB has a highly variable molecular etiology and represents a collection of different diseases. The majority of cases are autosomal dominant, but recessive inheritance was also described for some cases.
- The disease may be related to genetic defect in the basal cells, desomosomes, or anchoring connective tissue filaments. Circulating antibodies are not evident.
- Onset of EB is at birth or shortly after. The exception occurs in mild cases of EB, which may remain undetected until adulthood or occasionally remain undiagnosed.
- Dental manifestations include pitted or thin enamel which may lack prismatic structure, smooth amelodentinal junction and delayed or failure of eruption of teeth

- **Histologically**, there are many sub-epithelial bullae which heal with fibrosis leading to extensive scarring.
- EB is a genetic disease and no drugs are known to correct the underlying molecular defects. Prolonged use of steroids is contraindicated in the treatment. Steroid-induced complications prohibit their use. No other drugs, including phenytoin and tetracycline, have improved the blistering or epithelial disadhesion in EB significantly or consistently
- **Oral care**: Good dental hygiene is essential for patients with EB, and regular visits to the dentist are recommended. If possible, a dentist familiar with EB should be consulted. Despite their best efforts, many patients with EB develop dental caries because of enamel defects. In addition, significant oral mucosal involvement can accompany severe forms of EB. Avoid harsh tooth brushing and intensive mouthwashes containing alcohol. Normal saline rinses can help gently clean the mucosal surfaces

3.5.7 Hereditary Hemorrhagic Telangiectasia

(Rendu-Osler-Weber Disease)

- Autosomal dominant disease of blood vessels.
- Onset may be delayed until adult life
- Pinhead or spider-like telangiectases of the mouth, skin and sometimes of viscera
- Severe epistaxis often early
- Sometimes oral bleeding from lips or tongue
- Hemostatic function is normal
- Little risks with extractions
- Laser therapy is adopted for treatment

3.5.8 Dyskeratosis Congenita

X-linked recessive disease which occurs only in males and characterized by the triad:

1. Premalignant leukoplakia of the oral mucosa.
2. Dystropy of nails.
3. Pigmentation, atrophy and telangiectasia of the skin.

3.5.9 Fanconi's Syndrome

- An autosomal recessive hereditary condition characterized by:
    1. Dyskeratosis Congenita
    2. Hypersplenism
    3. Oral and anal lesions may progress into carcinomas.
- Shows higher incidence in Ashkenazi Jews.

3.5.10 Pachyonychia Congenita

- A hereditary condition characterized by:
    * Abnormal thickening of fingernails
    * Oral white patches which are not premalignant
    * Hyperkeratosis on the palms and soles and natal teeth
- The mode of inheritance is autosomal dominant. However, autosomal recessive inheritance was also mentioned in the literature
- Oral lesions of pachyonychia congenita should be differentially diagnosed form natal candidiasis, while those of pachyonychia tarda should be differentially diagnosed from oral leukoplakia.

3.5.11 Plumer-Vinson Syndrome

(Paterson-Kelly Syndrome)

Characterized by:

- Iron deficiency anemia
- Atrophy of the mucosa of the oral cavity, pharynx and esophagus
- Atrophy of tongue papillae with glossitis
- Dysphagia due to atrophy causing burning sensation of the esophagus associated with degeneration of the esophageal muscles
- Atrophy of the epithelium is thought to be due to iron depletion
- The disease is a risk factor for oral and pharyngeal cancer

3.6 Developmental Disturbances of Tongue

It is to be noted that some of the lesions to be mentioned here are in fact not strictly of developmental nature. They are discussed for their relevancy to the subject.

3.6.1 Aglossia

Aglossia is the congenital absence of tongue, a condition that is extremely rare. It is due to failure of development of the two lateral lingual swellings. In such cases a small nodular elevation may be found and took the place of the normal tongue; this probably represented the tuberculum impar. Speech, mastication and deglutition will be impaired. Aglossia is usually associated with agnathia.

3.6.2 Microglossia

This is a condition in which the tongue is markedly small. No impairment of functions was detected and the condition is of little clinical significance.

3.6.3 Macroglossia

- This means an enlargement of the tongue. In extreme cases, the tongue may fill the entire mouth or may even protrude from it. The edges of the tongue are crenated where they fit against the interdental spaces. Macroglossia may be congenital or acquired.
- Congenital macroglossia may be due to several conditions e.g. mongolism, cretinism, or hemangioma and lymphangioma of the tongue.
- Acquired macroglossia is commonly observed in amyloidosis, myxodema and acromegaly or may be due to edema, inflammation or tumors of the tongue.
- Clinically: Macroglossia is of little clinical significance except for the fact that it can cause spacing and outward drifting of teeth

3.6.4 Ankyloglossia (Tongue Tie)

- Ankyloglossia is the condition in which the tongue is restricted in its movement. The condition may be superior (the tongue is tied to the palate) or inferior (the tongue is tied to the mouth floor).
- In superior ankyloglossia the dorsum of the tongue is attached to the palate by a membrane. Superior ankyloglossia is always associated with cleft palate (the reverse is not true).
- Inferior ankyloglossia may be complete or incomplete (partial). Complete inferior ankyloglossia is a rare condition and results from failure of separation of the tongue form the mouth floor.

- Partial inferior ankyloglossia is a much more common condition in which the tongue is restricted in its movement due to short lingual frenum or a frenum, which is attached very near to the tip.
- Acquired ankyloglossia may be due to trauma, infection or tumors of the tongue.
- A more serious condition, although very rare, is the tongue hypermobility due to long lingual frenum, which may allow the tongue to slip back and obstruct the airway. Few deaths from suffocation have been reported in such cases. The condition may occur as a part of the syndrome known as Pierre Robin syndrome that was discussed earlier.

3.6.5 Lingual Varicosities (Lingual Varices)

- Tortuous dilated veins being observed on the undersurface of the tongue and tend to be more prominent with age.
- This is an asymptomatic condition and requires no treatment.

3.6.6 Prominent Circumvallate Papillae

- A condition affecting the dorsum of the posterior tongue in which large, mushroom-shaped circumvallate papillae are observed; once properly diagnosed, no treatment is necessary.
- The circumvallate papillae form a "v-shaped" row crossing the dorsum of the tongue near its base.
- Sometimes these papillae are enlarged to the point that they resemble a row of mushrooms.
- Sometimes, inflammation of the lateral circumvallate papillae or foliate papillae may occur due to rubbing of the tongue against a sharp broken down molars or restorations. The area then may become painful.

- Removal of the cause will result in regression of the condition. If the lesion does not resolve after removal of the cause, it should be biopsied immediately as this area is a common site for tongue cancer.

3.6.7 Lingual Tonsils

(Prominent Foliate Papillae, Foliate Papillitis)

- The foliate papillae are bilateral, pink nodules on the lateral borders of the tongue at the junction of the anterior two thirds and the posterior one third. They enclose lymphoid follicles which sometimes become hyperplastic or inflamed. Their appearance may alarm patients who need to be reassured that they are normal structures.
- The condition may occur as a result of trauma from teeth or dentures or as a result of reactive hyperplasia of the lymphoid tissue
- The condition may resemble oral SCC, their location and bilateral occurrence usually establish the correct diagnosis without biopsy.
- Tonsillar tissue consists of a collection of lymphocytes guarding the entrance of the oral pharynx. Several of these are large and discrete enough to qualify as "tonsils".
- Because the tongue must be extended out and to one side for the lingual tonsils to be seen, they are seldom observed except during clinical cancer detection examinations. Considering the high risk location of such a "lesion" biopsy and subsequent microscopic examination may be necessary to be certain that the "abnormal" tissue is really a lingual tonsil. Once the diagnosis is confirmed, no further treatment is necessary.

3.6.8 Cleft Tongue (Bifid Tongue)

- A congenital defect in which there is a complete or partial fissure or cleft of the tongue running from the tip backwards.
- In the complete cleft, the tongue is completely bisected into two halves, while in the partial cleft; there is a deep groove or fissure on the dorsum of the tongue on the site normally occupied by the median lingual raphe.
- *Bifid tongue* is the condition in which, only, the tip of the tongue is split into two parts.
- In case of partial cleft tongue, the depth of the fissure in devoid off papillae and hence with food accumulation, inflammation of the fissure may ensue. Cleft tongue results from failure of fusion of the two lateral lingual swellings.

3.6.9 Fissured Tongue

(Lingual Pelicata, Scrotal Tongue)

- A condition in which there are multiple fissures or grooves on the dorsum of the tongue. The condition is congenital; its severity was observed in some studies to increase with age suggesting that some factors e.g. smoking, vitamin deficiency or psychological stresses may play a role.
- The arrangement of the fissures varies; it may be transverse, crebriform, folacious or irregular.
- The depths of the fissures are seen to be devoid of papillae.
- On microscopic examination the epithelium shows inflammatory hyperplasia with chronic inflammatory cell infiltration of the underlying connective tissue. The inflammatory changes are thought to be due to

food accumulation in the depths of fissures concomitant with lack of the protective effect normally offered by the papillae.

3.6.10   Median Rhomboidal Glossitis

- This is a congenital malformation due to persistence of the tuberculum impar on the dorsum of the tongue resulting from failure of the two lateral lingual swellings to submerge it before they fuse together.
- Chronic candidal infection was proposed as the etiologic factor but without substantial evidence. The condition appears as a reddish depapillated smooth or mamelonated painless swelling on the dorsum of the tongue just in front of the foramen caecum. It has no clinical significance apart from the fact it may sometimes be confused with carcinoma of the tongue.
- **Histopathology**: There may be an inflammatory hyperplasia of the epithelium with chronic inflammatory cell infiltration of the underlying connective tissue. The inflammatory reaction is a secondary phenomenon resulting from lack of the protective action of papillae.

3.6.11   Glossitis Areata Exofoliativa

(Geographic Tongue, Erythema Migrans, Benign Migratory Glossitis, Wandering Rash of the Tongue)

- This is a condition of unknown etiology.
- Familial history was described in some cases.
- Concomitant psoriasis was also described in some patients.
- Many authors deny the developmental nature of the condition.
- Clinically there are small rounded or ovoid patches on the anterior 2/3 of the tongue. The patches are smooth and red dotted due to disappear-

ance of filliform papillae and persistence of the fungiform papillae. The patches show slightly elevated and irregular yellowish borders. When a patch reaches the border of the tongue, it may creep round to the undersurface; and when one patch meets another, one of them may recede and the other continues to spread, or they may coalesce together. Each patch has a life history of about one week, after which it disappears only to appear at another site and the whole condition may regress spontaneously, but only to recur later. Most patients have no symptoms but some adults complain of soreness.

- **Histopathology:** There is thinning of the epithelium in the center of the lesion and there may be hyperplasia and hyperkeratosis at the periphery. There is chronic inflammatory cell infiltration of the connective tissue.

3.6.12 Hairy Tongue (Black Hairy Tongue)

- This is a condition in which there is elongation of the filiform papillae.
- The condition may be attributed to either excessive proliferation of the filiform papillae or impaired desquamation or both.
- The elongated papillae may cover the whole dorsum of the tongue or only a part of it. They vary in color from yellowish to various shades of brown to black.
- The color is due to extrinsic causes e.g. food, drugs, or the action of some chromogenic bacteria e.g. aspergillus niger.
- The exact etiology of the condition is not precisely known, however many factors are blamed, but without a substantial evidence. Smoking, excessive use of antiseptic mouthwashes and defective diet were among the factors blamed for this condition.

3.6.13 Black Tongue

- A condition in which the tongue acquire a black stain without overgrowth of papillae
- Pathogenesis:
  - ⋆ Drugs as iron compounds used in the treatment of anemia
  - ⋆ Sucking of antibiotic lozenge which may be attributed to the action of aspergillus niger
- The condition is transient and regresses to normal after removal of the etiologic factor. Black tongue is not a developmental condition and is mentioned here for its relevancy to black hairy tongue

3.6.14 Furred Tongue

- A condition in which the tongue becomes coated with desquamated cells and debris
- Pathogenesis:
  - ⋆ Heavy Smoking
  - ⋆ In many systemic upsets, especially of the gastrointestinal tract
  - ⋆ Conditions in which the mouth becomes dry with little food intake
  - ⋆ During childhood fevers
- Furred tongue is not a developmental condition and is mentioned here for its relevancy to hairy tongue and the possibility of being confused with it.

3.6.15 Thyroglossal Tract Cyst

- This is a developmental condition arising as a result of cystic degeneration of the remnants of the thyroglossal tract and its failure of complete regression.
- The condition may occur anywhere along the course of the tract from the foramen caecum of the tongue to the thyroid gland and, hence it is classified into suprahyoid and infrahyoid. The condition appears clinically as a fluctuant painless swelling situated in the midline of the tongue or in the neck. The characteristic finding is that the lesion moves with the tongue movement. Sometimes the cyst will rupture establishing communication with the overlying skin and resulting in a thyroglossal tract fistula.
- **Histopathology**: The cyst may be lined by stratified columnar epithelium. Patches of thyroid and lymphoid follicles may be present in the underlying connective tissue wall. The cystic cavity contains mucoid fluid, which frequently contains cholesterol crystals.

3.6.16 Lingual Thyroid Nodule

- Is the ectopic presence of thyroid tissue in the tongue substance.
- It is known that thyroid gland develops as a result of differentiation of the caudal (lower) end of the thyroglossal tract, which originally arises from the foramen caecum of the tongue.
- Differentiation of the cranial (upper end) of the tract, or differentiation of both, the cranial and the caudal end of the tract will result in the formation of the lingual thyroid nodule. In the first case (differentiation of only the cranial end of the tract), the lingual thyroid nodule will represent the only thyroid tissue of the body, and should not be removed (un-

less it gives rise to serious complications when it can be transplanted to the neck).

- In most cases the condition is of little clinical significance unless in cases of thyroid insufficiency where it may gets enlarged and causes fullness of the throat.

3.7 Developmental Disturbances of Salivary Glands

3.7.1 Aplasia

This is the complete absence of one or more of the major salivary glands. The condition results from failure of the terminal portion of the gland bud to differentiate into salivary tissue. No hereditary basis has been established. The condition is of no clinical significance unless the remaining salivary glands fail to compensate for the decrease in saliva production, in which case, xerostomia will result.

3.7.2 Atresia

This is the condition in which there is congenital absence or occlusion of one or more of the ducts of one of the major salivary glands. The condition results from degeneration or failure of canalization of the proximal part of the salivary gland analage after the distal part has differentiated into salivary gland tissue. Its clinical significance is similar to that of aplasia.

3.7.3 Aberrancy

This is the condition in which normal salivary gland tissue develops in an anatomically abnormal position. The most common site for this condition to occur is the lingual surface of the body of the mandible and in such case, the condition will be known as Latent bone cyst.

3.7.4 Latent Bone Cyst

(Static bone cyst, Stafne bone cyst, Developmental lingual mandibular salivary gland inclusion cyst or depression).

- This is a developmental ectopic condition, in which a part of the submandibular or rarely the sublingual salivary gland develops in a bony cavity or depression in the lingual surface of the body of the mandible. This ectopic portion maintains its connection with the parent gland through a stalk or duct passing through a small opening on the lingual surface of mandibular cavity.
- The condition was first described by Stafne as a radiolucent area surrounded by a radio-opaque margin situated in the body of the mandible just above the lower border and below the inferior alveolar canal. The condition is static and never increases in size. Injecting a radio-opaque material through the duct of the parent gland could elucidate the nature of the lesion.

3.8 Developmental Disturbances of Gingiva

3.8.1 Fibromatosis Gingivae

(Elephantiasis Gingivae, Hereditary Gingival Fibromatosis)

- This is the condition in which there is diffuse fibrous enlargement of the gingiva. The condition is frequently associated with the syndrome known as **hypertrichosis**. The condition is inherited as an autosomal dominant trait.

- **Clinically:** The gingiva starts to enlarge in infancy or even as late as the ninth year. The enlargement usually affects both jaws; however, it is greater in the maxillary than in the mandibular gingiva. The enlargement is diffuse, firm, smooth or modulated with no apparent signs of inflammation. The condition may interfere with the eruption of teeth and can be regarded as a potential cause of partial or total anodontia.

3.8.2 Gingival Cyst of Adult

- This is a developmental soft tissue cyst that occurs in the free or attached gingiva of adults and should be differentiated from gingival cyst of newborn (Bohn's nodules) which occurs only on the alveolar crest of the newborn. Gingival cyst of adult should be also differentiated from the developmental lateral periodontal cyst, which is an intra-bony cyst with a positive X-ray picture. The gingival cyst of adult arises as a result of cystic degeneration of the remnants of the dental lamina or the remnants of epithelial rests of Malassez.
- **Clinically**: The cyst appears as a small, painless and fluctuant swelling in the free gingiva, attached gingiva or sometimes in the interdental papilla. Its size rarely exceeds 1 cm in diameter and may resemble a superficial mucocele.
- **X-ray picture**: The cyst is a soft tissue cyst and does not manifest itself in X-ray films.
- **Histologically**: The cyst is lined by stratified squamous epithelium, which may show some degree of keratinization.

3.8.3 Gingival Cysts of Newborn (Bohn's Nodules)

- These are small whitish swellings occurring on the alveolar crest of newly born infants. They are small cysts thought to arise from cystic degener-

Chapter 3. Developmental Disturbances of Oral & Para-Oral Tissues

ation of remnants of the dental lamina. If a gingival cyst of newborn persists till the time of eruption of teeth and interferes with the process of eruption, then it may be termed eruption cyst or eruption hematoma. Eruption cyst is considered by some authors to be a type of dentigerous cysts (for further details, see page (182).

- **Histopathology**, the cyst is usually lined by stratified squamous epithelium, which may show some degree of keratinization.

3.8.4 Epstein's Pearls

- Epstein's pearls are small whitish swellings found on the soft tissues of the midpalatine raphe.
- It is postulated that Epstein's pearls arise due to cystic degeneration of the non-odontogenic epithelium entrapped at the line of fusion of the two palatine processes. Although, Epstein's pearls are not gingival disease, they are mentioned here because they are frequently confused with *Bohn's nodules*.

3.9 Multisystem Disorders Affecting Oral and Para-Oral Tissues

3.9.1 Cleidocranial Dysplasia

Refer to the chapter: "Developmental Disturbances of Hard Dental Tissues, on page 18".

3.9.2 Gardener's Syndrome (Polyposis Coli)

- Gardener's syndrome is a developmental hereditary disease characterized by presence of multiple polyps in the large intestine particularly the colon area.
- Autosomal dominant inheritance was established in many cases.
- The disease is caused by mutations of the tumor suppressor APC gene
- The condition begins usually in late childhood; polyps increase in numbers, causing symptoms of chronic colitis, and carcinoma of the colon almost invariably develops in untreated cases.
- The disease is also characterized by presence of multiple osteomata and fibromata affecting the skull, jaw bones and sometimes the oral mucosa.
- There are also multiple supernumerary and supplemental teeth, many of them remain impacted.

3.9.3 Ehlers-Danlos Syndrome (Floppy Joint)

- This group of collagen disorders is characterized by hypermobile joints, loose hyperextensible skin, fragile oral mucosa, early onset periodontitis and recurrent dislocation of the temporomandibular joints.
- Dental manifestations are dilaceration, small teeth with short roots and multiple pulp stones.
- The most common form is inherited as an autosomal dominant trait; some autosomal recessive and X-linked cases have been also described.

3.9.4 Hypophosphatasia

- Is a hereditary disease characterized by deficiency of alkaline phosphatase

- Etiology: Autosomal recessive
- Alkaline phosphatase plays a role in bone formation and mineralization but the exact mechanism is unclear
- Early loss of primary teeth primarily due to lack of cementum on the root surfaces
- Bone abnormalities that resemble rickets
- Clinically: Similar to rickets
  * Short stature
  * Bowed legs
  * Waddling gait
  * Open fontanelles
- Oral manifestations:
  * Premature loss of primary teeth without evidence of significant inflammatory response
  * Alveolar bone loss
  * Absence of cementum
  * Enlarged pulp chambers
- Treatment:
  * Symptomatic because the lack of alkaline phosphatase can not be corrected
  * Prosthetic appliances are indicated to replaced missing teeth

3.9.5 Hereditary Hypophosphatemia

(Vitamin D-Resistant Rickets)

- Is a hereditary disease characterized by defective vitamin D metabolism
- **Etiology:** X-Linked dominant, therefore males are affected more severely than females

- Caused by mutations in a gene known as PHEX located on the human X chromosome at location Xp22.2-p22.1 (phosphate regulating gene with endopeptidase activity on the X chromosome)
- The PHEX protein regulates another protein called fibroblast growth factor 23 (produced from the FGF23 gene). Fibroblast growth factor 23 normally inhibits the kidney's ability to reabsorb phosphate into the bloodstream.
- The resulting overactivity of FGF-23 reduces vitamin D 1α-hydroxylation and phosphate reabsorption by the kidneys, leading to hypophosphatemia.
- Clinically:
    - In addition to the rachitic features,
    - Short stature
- Laboratory Findings:
    - Hypophosphatemia
    - Diminished renal re-absorption of phosphates
    - Decreased intestinal absorption of calcium
- Oral manifestations:
    - Large pulp chambers with extension of pulp horns to the amelo-dentinal junction
    - Multiple microclefts in the enamel allowing the oral bacteria to gain access to the dentinal tubules with subsequent pulp infection and periapical abscesses
- Treatment and Management:
    - Multiple daily doses of phosphates
    - Daily doses of calcitriol
    - Endodontic treatment for pulpally involved teeth

3.9.6 Early Onset Idiopathic Hypoparathyroidism

- A rare condition associated with ectodermal defects
- Hypoplastic and ridged enamel, short blunt roots and persistently open apices
- Defective nails
- Absent hair
- Chronic candidosis
- May develop other endocrinal deficiencies

3.9.7 Oral Facial Digital Syndrome *(OFDS)*

(Papillon-League and Psaume syndrome)

Definition

- OFDS is an X-linked hereditary disorder characterized by malformations of the face, oral cavity, and digits with polycystic kidney and involvement of the central nervous system.
- The disease is lethal in males very early in development.
- OFDS is a generic term for at least 10 distinctive genetic disorders, the presentation of signs and symptoms is extremely varied, making diagnosis difficult. OFDS type I is the most common of all of these disorders.

Clinical Features

Inheritance: X-linked dominant

Growth: Short stature

Face: Frontal bossing, facial asymmetry, micrognathia, retrusion of mandible

Ears: Low-set ears, hearing loss

Eyes: Epicanthus, hypertelorism, telecanthus, Down-slanting palpebral fissures

Nose: Broad nasal bridge, hypoplastic alar cartilage,

Mouth: Hyperplastic oral frenuli,

Buccal frenuli, median cleft lip, pseudocleft of the upper lip, lobulated tongue, bifid tongue, tongue nodule, cleft palate, high-arched palate

Teeth: Dental caries, anomalous anterior teeth, enamel hypoplasia, supernumerary teeth, missing teeth

Hands: Abnormalities of the fingers, syndactyly, brachydactyly, polydactyly, X-ray shows irregular pattern of radiolucency and/or spicule-like formation in metacarpals and phalanges

Feet: Abnormalities of the toes, polydactyly, preaxial or postaxial (rare)

Molecular Basis: Caused by mutation in the OFD1 protein gene

3.9.8 Mongolism (Down's syndrome, Trisomy 21)

Overview

Mongolism is a chromosomal abnormality resulting from the presence of 3 homologous chromosomes of the chromosome 21 in each cell of the human body.

Clinically

Down's syndrome is characterized by mental retardation, congenital abnormalities of heart and joints, sexual underdevelopment, and the mongoloid slant of the eyes. Increased incidence of *Alzheimer* disease in cases more than 30 years of age.

Oral manifestations are:

1. Macroglossia
2. Macrognathia
3. Fissured tongue
4. High arched palate
5. Microdontia
6. Enamel hypoplasia
7. Excessive salivation
8. Decreased incidence of caries (probably due to increased salivation)
9. Increase incidence of periodontal disease (probably due to impaired immune response)

Chapter 4
Dental Caries

Dental caries or tooth decay is the major health problem in most countries and represents the most common cause of tooth loss.

4.1 Definition

Dental caries is a progressive, mostly irreversible bacterial damage affecting hard tooth structure exposed to oral environment.

4.2 Classification of dental caries

1. Pit and fissure caries
    - Is the most common type of dental caries.
    - It appears on the occlusal and buccal surfaces of molars in primary and permanent dentition.
    - This form of caries is the most destructive because it quickly goes deeply into the dentin.
2. Smooth surface caries
    - Is less common and essentially occurs on the interproximal areas of the teeth that are not self-cleansing.

- On occasion the cervical regions of the buccal and lingual surfaces of the teeth will become involved.

3. Cemental (root) caries
    - Is nearly always exclusively found in the older population, particularly in those with gingival recession, hence sometimes termed "senile caries".
    - This type of carious lesion represents considerable difficulties to the clinician because it is located in a region of the tooth where there is little tooth structures overlying the pulp.

4. Recurrent caries (secondary caries)
    - Is the term applied to caries that arises around an existing restoration.
    - Lesions usually arise as a result of an alteration in the integrity of a restoration that results in marginal leakage.

5. Residual caries: Is the demineralized tissue that has been left behind before a filling is placed.

6. Arrested caries or inactive caries: Is the caries that stopped progression due to change in the environmental factors responsible for caries progression.

7. White spot caries (lesion): Described an early, initial or incipient lesion.

8. Hidden caries (Occult caries): A term used to describe lesions in dentin that are missed on a visual examination but are large enough and demineralized enough to be detected radiographically.

9. Acute (rampant) and chronic caries
    - Acute (rampant) and chronic caries are terms used to denote the rate that dental caries progresses in patients. Young patients are most susceptible to acute or rampant caries because they have teeth with large pulpal chambers wide and short dentinal tubules

containing little or no sclerosis. In these patients the condition is often combined with a diet rich in refined carbohydrates.

- Chronic caries is most common in older patients whose teeth have smaller pulpal chambers, usually with additional deposits of a denser and lesser tubular dentin on the pulpal walls, referred to as secondary dentin.

4.3 Sequelae of caries

1. Sequelae In hard tooth structure
   (a) Destruction of enamel
   (b) Destruction of dentin
   (c) Translucent dentin formation (sclerotic dentin)
   (d) Formation of dead tracts
   (e) Reparative (reactionary) dentin formation
2. Sequelae in the pulp and para-dental tissues
   (a) Pulp hyperemia
   (b) Acute pulpitis
   (c) Chronic pulpitis
   (d) Chronic hyperplastic pulpitis
   (e) Apical periodontists
   (f) Acute periapical abscess
   (g) Chronic periapical abscess
   (h) Periapical granuloma
   (i) Periapical cyst
   (j) Osteomyelitis
   (k) Facial cellulitis with its complications

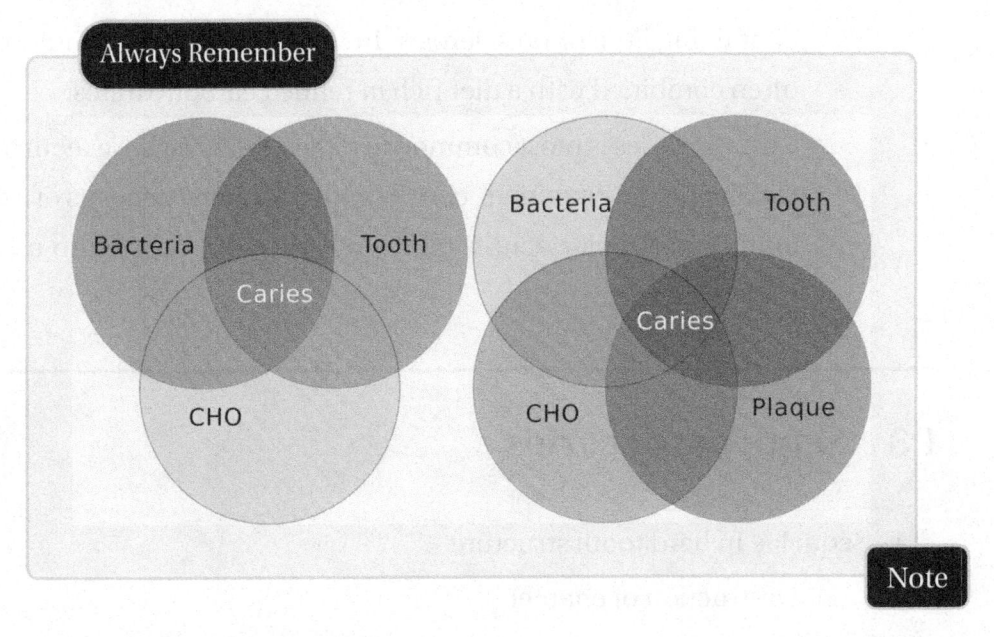

Figure 4.1: Contributing factors for dental caries. Left panel: are the factors essential for pit and fissure caries, while the right panel are the factors necessary for the development of smooth surface caries.

4.4 Etiology of Dental Caries

4.4.1 Contributing factors

For pit and fissure caries 3 factors should be fulfilled. These are a host, carbohydrates and bacteria. While for smooth surface caries to occurs, a fourth factor should added, which is the dental plaque. See figure (4.1) which illustrates the contributing factors for caries.

Host factors

Tooth susceptibility

The following factors may affect the susceptibility of teeth to caries:

1. Position of tooth
   - Malposed teeth are more prone to caries because of creation of stagnation areas.
2. Morphology or form of tooth
   - Pits and fissures increase susceptibility to caries because of creation of stagnation areas.
   - The position and shape of contact areas also influence caries involving proximal surfaces.
3. Structure of teeth
   - No evidence indicating that enamel hypoplasia and\or hypocalcification may increase susceptibility to caries.
   - Caries is prevalent in rich European countries, where enamel hypoplasia and hypocalcification caused by nutritional deficiencies have been virtually disappeared. By contrast caries is very low in some countries where hypoplasia and hypocalcification caused by nutritional deficiencies are widespread.
   - However, it is postulated that caries may progress faster in hypoplastic and\or hypocalcified teeth if compared to normal tooth.
4. Fluorides
   - Teeth with excess fluorides show decreased incidence of caries if compared to normal teeth.
5. Other trace elements
   - Molybdenum increase resistance to caries
   - Selenium decrease resistance to caries.
6. Genetic factors
   - Hereditary has a minor influence on resistance to caries.
   - Breading studies showed that genetically susceptible and resistant strains of rats can be developed.

- In man studies showed that there is a low incidence of caries in certain families which may be due to inheritance of a more favorable tooth shape or anatomy. However, it is difficult to exclude the role of common dietary habits in related persons.

Role of Saliva in Dental Caries

Saliva exerts a protective effect against caries. This effect may be due to:

1. Formation of acquired enamel pellicle
   - The acquired enamel pellicle is derived form salivary mucin.
   - This pellicle protects enamel surfaces from being colonized by oral bacteria as it masks the residual chemical charges found on hydroxyapatite crystals (see the mechanism of dental plaque formation).
2. Washing effect of saliva

   A free flow of saliva has a cleansing effect in the mouth and teeth. In cases of xerostomia, increased incidence of caries occurs.
3. Buffering effect of saliva

   The buffering effect of saliva depends mainly on its bicarbonate and phosphate contents and this is increased at higher rates of flow. In mongolism, decreased caries incidence may be due to increased rate of salivary flow with its associated increase of buffering effect.
4. Salivary antibodies
   - Saliva also contains immunoglobulin A (IgA) which is produced by plasma cells found in salivary glands and modified by the acinar cells. The acinar cells produce a secretory portion which becomes attached to the IgA produced by plasma cells.
   - The whole molecule is now termed secretory IgA. The role of salivary IgA may be:

- Killing or inhibition of bacterial growth.
- Opsonization of bacteria.
- Prevention of adherence of bacteria to tooth surfaces.

5. Antibacterial substances

   Lysozymes, peroxidases and lactoferrin are the main antibacterial substances found in saliva.

Carbohydrates

Importance of carbohydrates

- Carbohydrates are the main component of diet upon which oral bacteria can act and produce acids
- There are many research work confirming that carbohydrates are essential for caries to ensue

Factors affection cariogenicity of carbohydrates

1. Type of carbohydrate

   Carbohydrates are of 3 main types: monosaccharides, disaccharides and polysaccharides.

   (a) Monosaccharides: e.g. glucose and fructose.
   (b) Disaccharides: e.g. sucrose, maltose and lactose. Sucrose has been described as the "arch criminal of caries". This may be due to (see figure ((4.2))):
   - Sucrose is the most frequently consumed carbohydrates.
   - Sucrose is of low molecular weight (unlike starch) and can diffuse rapidly and efficiently into dental plaque.
   - Sucrose consists of glucose, which will be utilized in the formation of dextran and fructose which will be utilized in the

formation of levan. Both dextran and levan are needed for an efficient caries to occur.

(c) Polysaccharides: e.g. starch and glycogen. Polysaccharides are of little or no importance in the etiology of dental caries. This is evidenced by the fact that individuals eating large amounts of polysaccharides (rice in China and coarsely ground cereals in Africa) showed a low prevalence of caries. The low cariogenic effect of polysaccharides may be due to:

   i. They are of larger molecular weight and hence can not diffuse readily and rapidly into dental plaque.

   ii. They need the action of salivary amylase before oral bacteria can act upon them.

2. Total amount of carbohydrate intake

   The total amount of carbohydrate intake particularly sugars showed some little effect on caries. The effect of reducing sugar consumption on caries during war time (World War II) was a slight decline in caries incidence.

3. Frequency of carbohydrate intake

   Frequent intake of carbohydrates between meals will cause an increased caries incidence.

4. Consistency and texture of carbohydrates

   Sticky carbohydrates are more cariogenic because they remain attached to tooth surfaces for longer time.

5. Refinement of carbohydrates

   Refinement by definition is the treatment of carbohydrates in order to make them whiter, remove fibrous material and improve flavor. Most carbohydrates eaten today are refined to some extent. In general the effect of refinement is to increase caries because:

   (a) Removal of fibrous material which possesses cleansing effect.

(b) Concentrate the fermentable fraction of carbohydrates.

(c) Increase adhesiveness of carbohydrates.

However, there are some unrefined, natural carbohydrates which are highly cariogenic e.g. honey.

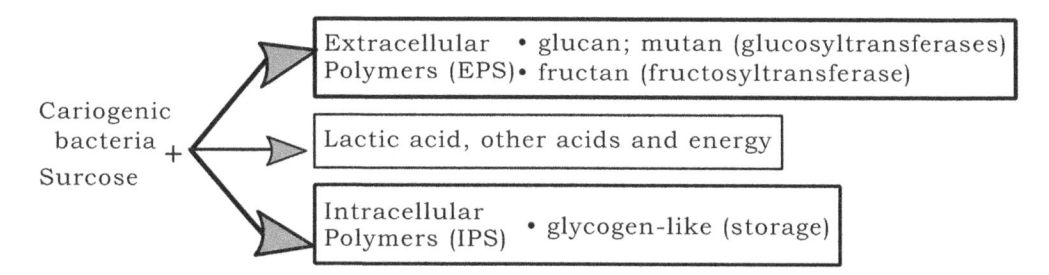

Cariogenic bacteria + Surcose
- Extracellular Polymers (EPS) • glucan; mutan (glucosyltransferases) • fructan (fructosyltransferase)
- Lactic acid, other acids and energy
- Intracellular Polymers (IPS) • glycogen-like (storage)

Figure 4.2: The metabolism of sucrose by cariogenic bacteria.

Micro-organisms

Miller experiment

- Miller was the first to suggest that caries might be caused by the action of bacteria on fermentable carbohydrates.
- He conducted an experiment in which he suspended two sound teeth in two test tubes containing saliva and carbohydrates saliva of course contains oral micro-organisms). After subjecting the contents of one test tube to boiling, he incubated both test tubes at 37 °C. The tooth suspended in the test tube not subjected to boiling suffered extensive caries like lesions, while the other tooth remained caries free.

Orland experiment

- It was Orland, who proved conclusively and beyond any shadow of doubt, in 1954 that for caries to occurs, micro-organisms should be present. He used germ-free rats obtained by caesarean operation under strict aseptic conditions and reared for several generations in completely aseptic incubators; he feed them a sterile but highly cariogenic diet. These rats remained caries free at the time when the same diet produced caries in the control group of rats.

- The next step which was undertaken by Orland in 1955 was the creation of gnotobiote rats. Gnotobiote animals are animals in which a certain known strain of micro-organism was introduced. These gnotobiotic animal studies made it possible to sort out which species of bacteria are cariogenic for these animals and which might, therefore, be cariogenic for man.

Types of bacteria involved in caries

1. Acidogenic bacteria:
    (a) Lactobacilli:
        i. L. acidophilus
        ii. L. caesi
    (b) Streptococci: Viridance group which are also aciduric i.e. can survive an acidic pH which inhibit the growth of other bacteria. These are:
        i. St. mutans
        ii. St. sanguis
        iii. St. salivarius
        iv. St. mitis
        v. St. mileri
2. Proteolytic bacteria:
    (a) Actinomyces:
        i. Act. viscosus
        ii. Act. odontolytics

   iii. Act. Naeslandi

   iv. Act. bovis

   v. Act. Israeli

 (b) Clostridia

 (c) Pseudomonas

3. Chromogenic fungi: e.g. Aspergillus niger (play a role in staining of carious lesions)

Discussion of the role of some bacteria

Lactobacilli

- Lactobacilli are powerful acidogenic bacteria
- They are also powerful aciduric
- They are mild proteolytic
- They are found in all stages of caries
- Their number increase in saliva when caries activity is increased. This was the base for the lactobacillus count test.
- Lactobacilli produced pit and fissure caries in gnotobiote animals but failed to produce smooth surface caries in these animals due to their inability to produce the adhesive extracellular polysaccharides.

Streptococci

- Some strains of streptococci particularly st. mutans were found to be able to produce smooth surface caries in gnotobiote animals.
- This ability was attributed to the fact that streptococci can produce extracellular polysaccharides.
- The extracellular polysaccharides are of two types:
  - ★ **Dextran:**

This is formed from glucose by the action of glucosyletransferase enzyme. Dextran is an insoluble adhesive material.

* **Levan:**

    This is formed from fructose by the action of fructosyletransferase enzyme. Levan is less adhesive than dextran and acts mainly as a store of carbohydrates.

- Function of bacterial polysaccharides:
    1. Increase adhesiveness of dental plaque and allow bacteria to adhere together and to enamel surface.
    2. Act as a store of carbohydrates after the dietary carbohydrates are washed away from the mouth.
    3. Increase thickness of dental plaque.
- Streptococci also can form intracellular polysaccharides which are glycogen (amylopectin) which act as a store of carbohydrates.
- Streptococci are also powerful acidogenic bacteria.

Conclusions

- Evidence from the current review strongly supports a central role of the mutans group of streptococci in the initiation of caries on the smooth surfaces and fissures of the crowns of the teeth of adults and children, and suggests a potent etiologic role of them in the induction of root surface caries also.
- Lactobacilli are also implicated as important contributory bacteria in tooth decay, but their role in induction of lesions is not well supported.
- Evidence that other streptococci, enterococci, or actinomycetes are contributing etiological agents of dental caries in humans is equivocal at best.

- The mutans streptococci are spread vertically in the population, mostly but not exclusively, from mothers to their children. These findings suggest strategies for improvement of the dental health of both children and adults.

Dental plaque

Definition

An adhesive non-visible biofilm[1] firmly adherent to tooth surfaces and consists of microbial population embedded in a matrix of polymers of bacterial and salivary origin.

Types

1. Subgingival
2. Supragingival

Importance

Involved in 2 main diseases in the oral cavity, depending on the bacterial population of the plaque and its site:

1. Dental caries
2. Periodontal disease

Composition

1. Microorganisms

---
[1] A biofilm is a community of microorganisms growing on a surface

2. Matrix which is formed of Protein: derived from saliva and gingival crevicular fluid
3. Carbohydrates: derived from saliva and bacterial polysaccharides
4. Inorganic component mainly Ca, P, and K
5. Water

Mechanism of Formation

1. Acquired enamel pellicle
   It is formed by selective adsorption of certain salivary mucins (acidic proline rich glycoproteins) to the hydroxyapatite crystals of enamel. This process does not depend on the presence of microorganisms and thus the pellicle is often termed germ free pellicle. The pellicle is approximately 10 mm in thickness. It should be noted that microorganisms can not colonize directly on the mineralized tooth surface.

2. Colonization phase
   Within 24 hours st. sanguis, st. mutans and some strains of actinomyces viscous begin to invade the pellicle

3. Maturation phase
   After 48 hours filamentous organisms start to appear and to proliferate to form the second largest population after the streptococci.

Mechanism of Action of Plaque

- Allow adhesion of bacteria and their products (acids) on the surfaces of teeth. Thus allowing a concentrated attack to be made on enamel surface by the action of acids.
- Prevent escape of acids and entry of salivary buffers.

Factors Affecting Cariogenicity of the Plaque

1. Thickness

    Thickness of the plaque is the most important factor affecting its cariogenicity. Plaque can not produce caries unless it acquires a critical thickness. The factors affecting thickness are:
    - (a) Size and distribution of sheltered areas
    - (b) Use of oral hygiene methods
    - (c) Functional mouth movements
    - (d) Types of carbohydrates consumed by the patient

2. Bacterial population of the plaque

    Type of bacteria populating the plaque will determine to a large extent its cariogenic effect and whether the formed plaque will be involved in periodontal disease or in caries process.

Acid Production in the Plaque - Stephan Curve

After brief exposure to carbohydrates (as rinsing with 10% sucrose solution for 10 seconds) a rapid fall of pH to the critical level occurs within 2–5 minutes. The critical pH is the pH at which enamel demineralization occurs. It lays around 5.5 then the pH will continue to fall more below this critical pH for another 15–20 minutes. Then it will return to normal resting level after 1 hour. This is illustrated in figure (4.3).

Biochemical Reactions in the Plaque

1. Acid production
2. Formation of extracellular polysaccharides which are dextran and levan. Dextran is a polymer of glucose formed by the action of glucosyltransferase enzyme while levan is a polymer of fructose formed by the action

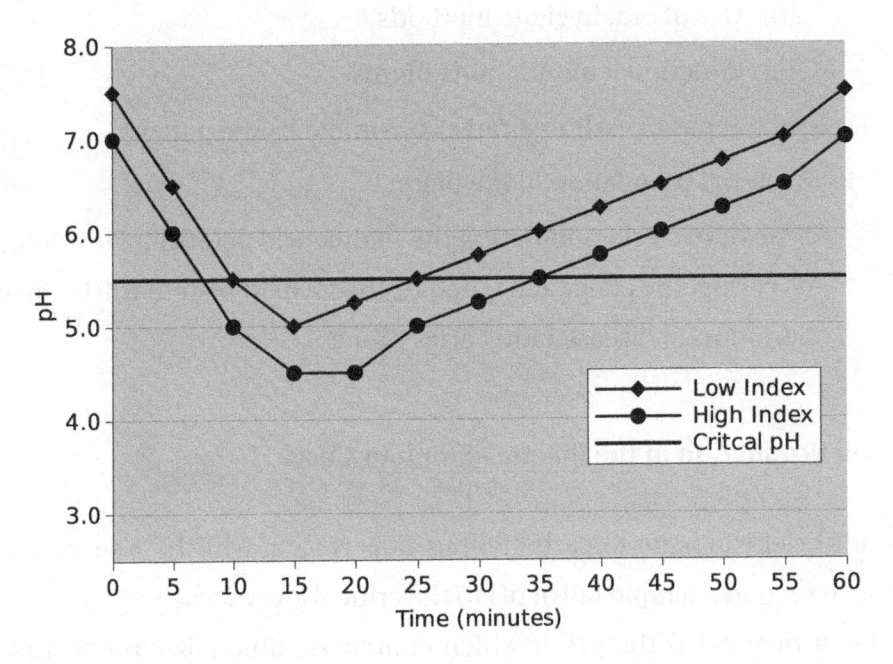

Figure 4.3: Acid production in the plaque of two populations of high and low caries index as supposed by Stephan (modified from Stephan curve).

of fructosyltransferase enzyme. Their functions in the dental plaque are:

    (a) Increase adhesiveness of the plaque

    (b) Act as a store of carbohydrates

    (c) Increase thickness of the plaque

3. Formation of intracellular polysaccharide which is glycogen

4.4.2 Theories of Dental Caries

Acidogenic theory

(Miller's theory) (Chemicoparasitic theory)

1. Acidogenic bacteria + carbohydrates → acids, these acids are mainly lactic acids which diffuse into enamel through the organic matrix of enamel.
2. Acids + inorganic part of enamel → demineralization.
3. Acids + inorganic part of dentin → demineralization.
4. Proteolytic bacteria + organic matrix of dentin → digestion and dissolution.

Proteolytic theory

Proteolytic bacteria act on the organic matrix of enamel liberating sulfuric acid from the sulfated mucopolysaccharides of organic matrix. These acids then demineralize enamel. Points against this theory are:

1. No explanation of the role of carbohydrates
2. Pure proteolytic bacteria failed to produce caries in gnotobiote animals.
3. The amounts of acids formed are to little to affect enamel

Proteolosis-chelation theory

Chelation is the ability of certain organic compounds to associate with other ions or atoms by covalent bonds. This theory postulates that proteolytic bacteria act on the organic matrix of enamel liberating chelating agents. These chelating agents then demineralize enamel by binding to calcium and phosphates. An example of chelating agents is EDTA (ethylene diamine tetra-acetic acid) used to prevent blood clotting by binding to serum calcium.

Points against this theory are:

1. No explanation of the role of carbohydrates.
2. Pure proteolytic bacteria failed to produce caries in gnotobiote animals.
3. This theory assumes that caries could occur at an alkaline pH, a condition which is difficult to prove.

4.5 Pathology of enamel caries

4.5.1 Macroscopic Picture

Clinical picture of caries enamel

- At first the lesion appears as a white chalky area.
- Then it becomes rough to the probe.
- And staining will occurs due to the action of some chromogenic bacteria.
- Later on cavitations will occurs.
- The carious lesions are cone shaped in which the base is toward the dentinoenamel junction and the apex toward the surface in pit and fissure caries. In smooth surface caries the base of the cone is toward the surface and the apex toward the dentinoenamel junction.

4.5.2 Microscopic Picture

Using polarized light technology, electron microscopy, micro-hardness tests and microradiography, it was evident that caries of enamel occurs in 4 phases:

1. Initiation phase
2. Bacterial invasion
3. Destruction phase
4. Phase of secondary enamel caries

Initiation phase

This phase is due to the action of acids only.

In this phase 4 zones was described:

1. Translucent zone
    - Lies at the advancing front of the carious lesion.
    - It is due to initial demineralization.
    - It contains pores accounting for 1 -2 % of enamel volume.
    - This zone appears translucent only when seen with quinoline or Canada balsam media which have the same refractive index as that of enamel. The molecules of the media will fill these pores and thus the zone appears translucent.
2. Dark zone
    - It lies superficial to the translucent zone.
    - It results from further demineralization of enamel.
    - It thus contains pores accounting for 2 – 4 % of enamel volume. Some of these pores are so small that they are called micropores.
    - Molecules of Canada balsam or quinoline are too large that they are unable to fill these micropores thus this zone appears dark.

- It is thought that micropores result from remineralization of the larger pores in the periods in which acid production is not active.

3. Body of the lesion
   - It lies under the surface zone and constitutes the largest area in the carious lesion.
   - Polarized light examination revealed presence of pores accounting for 5 % at the periphery and 25 % at the center of the zone.
   - This zone is due to advanced demineralization.
   - This zone appears translucent.
   - Accentuated brown stria of Retzus appears in this zone.

4. Surface zone
   - One of the characteristic features of enamel caries is that the greatest degree of demineralization occurs at a subsurface level.
   - This zone although not intact, yet it appears more radiopaque and harder than the deeper zones. This may be due to:
     (a) Continuous remineralization from saliva
     (b) It contains much fluoride
     (c) It contains greater amounts of insoluble proteins
     (d) The usual presence of prismless enamel in this zone may delay diffusion of acids

Phase of bacterial invasion

Bacteria begin to invade enamel when sufficient spaces are created by the action of acids.

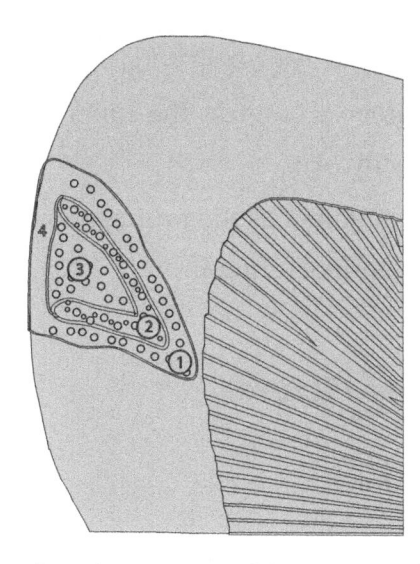

Figure 4.4: A diagram showing zones of initiation phase of enamel caries. zone (1) is the translucent zone, (2) is the dark zone, (3) is the body of the lesion and (4) is the surface. zone

Phase of destruction

In this phase proteolytic bacteria begin to act on the organic matrix of enamel leading to complete destruction of the area.

Phase of secondary enamel caries

Occurs when acids and bacteria reach the ADJ, they spread laterally along it and begin to invade enamel from beneath leading to its undermining.

4.6 Pathology of dentin Caries

4.6.1 Macroscopic Picture

- The outline of lesion is cone shape with the base toward the DEJ and the apex toward the pulp.

- Dentin appears to be brownish and is soft to the probe.
- As the caries process progress the superficial layers of dentin become more soft and jelly-like.
- This outline is acquired as the propagation of acids flows along the direction of the dentinal tubules.

4.6.2 Microscopic Picture

Initial uninfected lesions

Occurs prior to cavitation of enamel. The changes in this phase are due to the action of acids and not due to bacterial invasion of dentin. Acids reaching the DEJ will lead to the formation of the following zones:

1. Zone of reactionary (reparative dentin) (zone 1)

    This is a pulpal reaction against the attacking acid. The new dentin is formed at the pulpal end of the lesion.

2. Zone of sclerotic (translucent dentin) (zone 2)

    This zone occurs at the sides and the pulpal end of the caries lesion. In this zone deposition of calcium salts occurs along the inner wall of the dentinal tubules leading to their progressive narrowing and obstruction. Translucent dentin is considered as a defensive mechanism against the spread of acids.

3. Body of the lesion (zone 3)

    The body of the lesion is characterized by the presence of dead tracts. Dead tracts are dentinal tubules in which their odontoblastic processes and their related odontoblasts have degenerated and died. Dead tracts appear dark with transmitted light due to their high content of organic material .The superficial part of these dead tracts (near to the source of the acid) show decalcification.

Infected lesion

- This develops after bacterial invasion of enamel and formation of an enamel cavity. The dentinal tubules provide a pathway for invasion of dentin by bacteria. These organisms form two waves of invasion:
- The pioneer organisms: Are found at the front of the lesion and consists of acidogenic bacteria. They decalcify dentin leaving the organic matrix intact.
- The second wave: Consists of mixed infection containing proteolytic bacteria, which distort the matrix.
- The shape of the lesion remains conical with a broad base at the DEJ.
- The lesion consists of 4 zones which are:
    1. Zone 1: Mild pulpal inflammation
    2. Zone 2: Reparative or reactionary dentin
    3. Zone 3: Sclerotic dentin
    4. Zone 4: Body of the lesion. Body of the lesion consists of the following zones:
        (a) Decalcified uninfected zone

        Is the deepest zone showing decalcification but without the presence of bacteria.

        (b) Decalcified infected zone

        This shows the following zones:

         i. Pioneer bacteria: Which are usually cocci
         ii. Beading: Which is the lateral distension of the dentinal tubules by the action of the proliferating microorganisms
         iii. Liquefaction foci: Which is the coalescence of neighboring beads
         iv. Transverse clefts: Which is a liquefaction focus occurring at right angle to the direction of dentinal tubules because

Chapter 4. Dental Caries

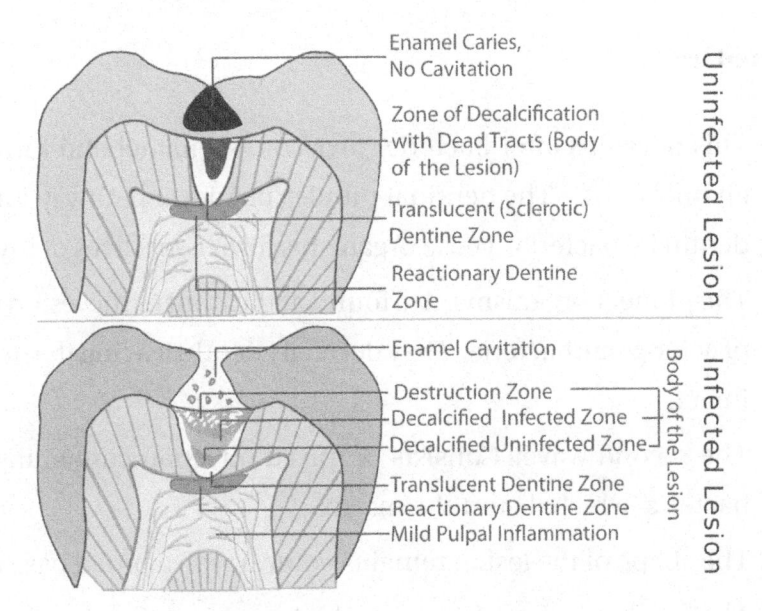

Figure 4.5: A diagram showing zones of uninfected (upper) and infected dentin caries (lower).

of their existence on a lateral branch of a dentinal tubule or along one of the incremental lines of dentin.

(c) Area of destruction

This zone results from destruction of the organic matrix after removal of dentin minerals

See figure (4.5) which illustrates diagrammatically the different zones of uninfected and infected dentin caries.

4.7 Immunology of Dental Caries

- Unfortunately, dental caries primarily affects enamel which is avascular tissue to which the body immunological reactions can not access effectively.
- Tissue-mediated immune response can not access enamel. Also the antibody-mediated immune reaction can not play its role in defensing

enamel as the later is avascular and being not in direct contact with blood.

- The only way by which antibodies can reach enamel is via saliva.
- As bacteria are a major factor contributing to poor oral health, there is currently research to find a vaccine for dental caries. As of 2018, such a vaccine has been successfully tested on animals, and is in clinical trials for humans.

CHAPTER 5
PERIODONTAL DISEASES

Periodontal diseases are the second most common diseases affecting the oral cavity, the first being dental caries. They are one of the major causes of tooth loss. Therefore, every effort should be made for early detection of periodontal disease

5.1 Back to Basics

- Periodontal diseases are a group of conditions which affect the supporting structures of the teeth, known as the periodontium. The periodontium consists of:
    - ★ The gingivae (gums)
    - ★ The periodontal ligament
    - ★ The alveolar bone
    - ★ Cementum
- Periodontal disease is the main cause of tooth loss in adults.
- Periodontal disease is the second commonest disease affecting the oral cavity, the first being dental caries.

5.2 Periodontium in health

- Teeth are embedded in sockets of alveolar bone, which surrounds the roots of all teeth.
- Tooth attached to bone by the fibers of the periodontal ligament, running from bone to cementum.
- Bone and periodontal ligament are covered by the mucous membrane of the gingivae lining the alveolar ridges.
- Gingivae is attached to neck of tooth at a specialized site called the junctional epithelium.
- In health, a gingival crevice no deeper than 2 mm exists, to form a "gutter" around each tooth. This gingival crevice is also termed gingival sulcus in some textbooks.
- Other periodontal ligament fibers run from the bone crest to the neck of the tooth, and from the neck of the tooth into the gingival papilla.
- Appearance of healthy periodontium thus is:
    * Pink color, often stippled like orange peel
    * Tight gingival cuff around tooth
    * Gingival crevice present, not deeper than 2 mm
    * No bleeding occurs when crevice is gently probed during dental examination
    * Knife-edge gingival papillae between teeth
    * Subgingivally, periodontal ligament and alveolar bone are intact
    * No alveolar bone loss in the radiographs
    * The periodontium in health is shown in Fig.(5.1).

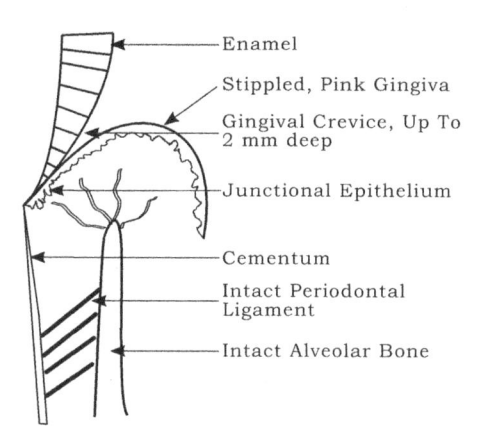

```
                    Enamel
                    Stippled, Pink Gingiva
                    Gingival Crevice, Up To
                    2 mm deep
                    Junctional Epithelium
                    Cementum
                    Intact Periodontal
                    Ligament
                    Intact Alveolar Bone
```

Figure 5.1: The Periodontium in Health

5.3 Etiology of Periodontal Diseases

- Periodontal diseases are ***multifactorial*** in nature
- The most important cause of periodontal disease is the presence and accumulation of ***dental plaque*** around the gingival margins of the teeth.
- Dental plaque is a combination of saliva, oral bacteria and bacterial products, which form a sticky film on the tooth surface and allows food debris to become incorporated into its structure. It tends to form initially at the gingival margin because this area is not easily self-cleansed by salivary flow, or by the tongue and soft tissue movements.
- Dental plaque is also involved in the causation of dental caries. Whether plaque causes periodontal disease or caries, depends mostly on the bacterial population of the plaque.

5.3.1 Host-Bacterial Balance

- In healthy periodontium, there is an equilibrium between the aggressiveness of bacterial plaque and the host tissue response. This equilibrium could be broken by an increased quantity or virulence of bacteria or decreased defensive capacity of the tissue.

- Host mechanisms that maintain such equilibrium are:
    1. The washing effect of the saliva and the gingival crevicular fluid (GCF)
    2. The regular shedding of epithelial cells.
    3. The presence of salivary antibodies.
    4. The presence of salivary anti-microbial substances such as lactoferrin, peroxidases and other similar agents.
    5. The phagocytic action of neutrophils that migrate continuously through the junctional epithelium into the gingival sulcus/pocket.
- Plaque biofilm is a climax community (Biofilm)
- A climax community is a steady-state community in which microorganisms, plants, or animals acquire a stabilized and balanced condition. This condition remains stable until a strong disturbing factor occurs. Examples of disturbing elements are fire and mechanical events.
- A biofilm is a group of microorganisms in which cells adhere to each other and also to a surface and are embedded within an extracellular matrix. This matrix is composed of extracellular polymeric substances (EPS). Because biofilm has a three-dimensional structure and represents a community-style for microorganisms, they have been metaphorically described as "cities for microbes". Mature biofilm represents a climax community as it reaches a steady-state condition.
- The oral flora develops through childhood to reach a climax community stage at puberty and serves as a defense barrier against the establishment of more pathogenic species.

5.3.2 Dental Plaque: Formation and Mechanism of Action

Refer to the chapter "Dental Caries", page (99).

5.4 Sequence of events leading to gingivitis

1. Bacteria in the dental plaque produce toxic byproducts as they utilize food debris
2. These toxic by-products irritate the gingivae in direct contact, and cause inflammation (chronic gingivitis)
3. The inflamed gingivae swell, and form false pockets around the necks of the teeth
4. False pockets allow more plaque to develop as self-cleansing becomes impossible, and the plaque then extends below the gingival margin
5. The continued action of saliva on plaque allows inorganic ions to be incorporated into the plaque, and thus *dental calculus* (tartar) forms.
6. Calculus formation can occur above the gingival margin, and is called supra-gingival calculus which is yellow in color
7. It can also occur below the gingival margin, and is then called sub-gingival calculus, which is brown/black in color owing to the incorporation of blood pigments
8. The calculus has a rough surface, allowing more plaque to form over it, and also irritating the gingivae further
9. The abrasion of the calculus and the chemical action of the toxins causes painless micro-ulceration of the gingivae, and they will then bleed on touching or dental probing
10. The visible appearance and bleeding on probing of the gingivae are the classic diagnostic signs of chronic gingivitis (Fig.(5.2))

Chapter 5. Periodontal Diseases

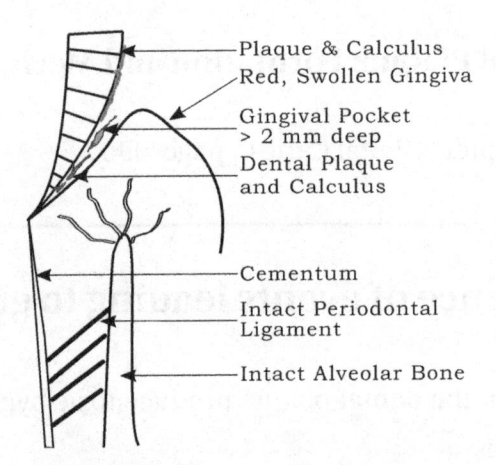

Figure 5.2: Chronic Gingivitis

11. Plaque deposits becoming calcified and form calculus (tarter)

5.5 Sequence of events leading to periodontitis

Lack of treatment of chronic gingivitis allows the toxins to build up and eventually enter the underlying gingival tissues through the micro-ulcerated areas and further events start:

- The toxins then gradually destroy the periodontal ligament so that a true pocket forms, as the periodontal attachment to the tooth is lost from the neck of the tooth and down the side of the root
- Further plaque develops and becomes mineralized, causing further irritation and more toxin infiltration
- The toxins eventually begin destroying the alveolar bone, and the tooth loosens in its socket and is eventually lost (Fig.(5.3))

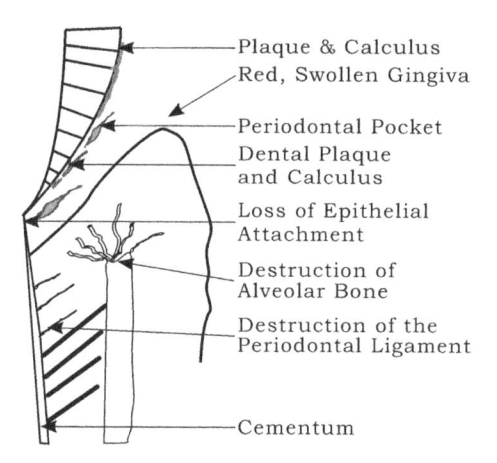

Figure 5.3: Chronic Periodontitis

Gingivitis can begin in childhood, but periodontitis can take many years to result in tooth loss. It is usually painless and therefore can be present undetected for years by the patient unless it is diagnosed by a dentist.

Periodontal disease also tends to have active phases, where much tissue destruction occurs, and quiescent phases with little destructive activity.

5.6 Diagnosis of periodontal disease

1. Medical history
2. Dental history
3. Clinical examinations

5.6.1 Chronic gingivitis

Early onset:

- Gingivae bleed on brushing
- Gingivae red and swollen (hyperplastic)

- Plaque visible at gingival margins
- Also detected by use of disclosing solution
- Halitosis (bad breath)

Established:

- Pus can be expressed from gingival crevice

5.6.2 Chronic periodontitis

- Periodontal probing detects pockets deeper than 2 mm
- Presence of supra- and subgingival calculus
- Radiographic evidence of alveolar bone loss, and deeper periodontal pockets
- Mobility of teeth

The periodontal pockets can be probed by several types of graduated instrument, to record the depth in millimeters of any pockets present. Usual instrument types include:

- CPITN probe (Community Periodontal Index of Treatment Need)
- WHO probe (World Health Organization)
- Pocket measuring probe (Fig.(5.4))

5.7 Non-surgical treatment of periodontal disease

- Prevention is always better than cure.

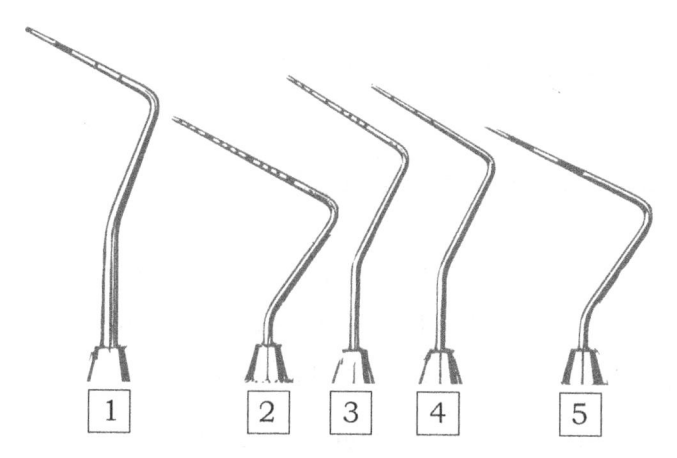

Figure 5.4: Types of periodontal probes. #1, WHO (World Health Organization) probe, which has a 0.5 mm small ball at the tip and millimeter markings at 3.5, 8.5, and 11.5 mm and color coding from 3.5 to 5.5 mm. #2, Marquis color-coded probe. Calibrations are in 3-mm sections. #3, University of North Carolina-15 probe, a 15-mm long probe with millimeter markings at each millimeter and color coding at the fifth, tenth, and fifteenth millimeters. #4, University of Michigan "O" probe, with Williams markings (at 1, 2, 3, 5, 7, 8, 9, and 10 mm). #5, Michigan "O" probe with markings at 3, 6, and 8 mm.

- Plaque suppressants are available, the commonest being chlorhexidene, but its use is advised only on a short-term basis owing to its staining capabilities.
- With chronic gingivitis, the removal of all plaque and the re-inforcement of oral hygiene instructions should bring about a complete resolution of the problem.
- The oral health message needs to be reinforced regularly if problems persist, and the advice given will be different for different age groups.

5.7.1 Supra-gingival calculus

If calculus is present, it needs to be professionally removed by either the dentist or the hygienist to allow healing of the periodontium. This is achieved for supragingival calculus by scaling and polishing.

A variety of hand scaling instruments are in use to remove supragingival calculus:

- Sickle scaler
- Cushing's push scaler
- Jaquette scaler (Fig.(5.5))

Ultrasonic scalers are also available with differing tips.

All these instruments are used to dislodge calculus from the tooth surface. Scaling by hand is tiring for the operator but gives superb tactile sensation, so specks of residual calculus are detectable.

The use of an ultrasonic scaler is less tiring and faster, but the cold water spray required for its action can be uncomfortable for patients with sensitive teeth.

Sickle

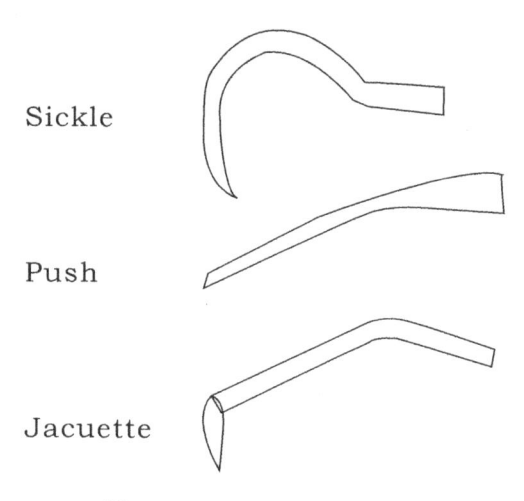

Push

Jacuette

Figure 5.5: Hand Scalers

Once all the calculus has been removed, the teeth are polished with prophylactic paste and a rubber polishing cup in the slow handpiece. This gives a smooth tooth surface and therefore slows down further plaque accumulation.

5.7.2 Subgingival calculus

With chronic periodontitis, any bone loss is permanent, but if subgingival calculus is removed thoroughly and good oral hygiene is then maintained, there is a chance that the periodontal ligament will reattach and periodontal pockets will heal.

Again, several instruments are available for subgingival calculus removal:

- Subgingival curette
- Periodontal hoe
- Ultrasonic scaler (Fig.(5.6))

The shanks of the curettes and hoes are long enough to pass deep into periodontal pockets and reach the subgingival calculus. This and the contami-

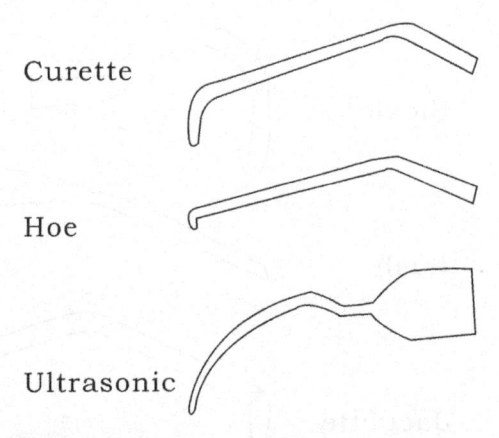

Figure 5.6: Subgingival Instruments

nated layer of cementum beneath are then scraped off and removed from the pockets by both aspiration and irrigation. This is called subgingival debridement. Healing of the periodontium can then occur, with reattachment of the junctional epithelium and the elimination of periodontal pockets.

Scaling subgingivally sometimes has to be carried out under local anesthesia, as the procedure can be quite painful for some patients.

Continued periodontal health is dependent to a large degree on the cooperation and motivation of the patient to maintain a good standard of oral hygiene. Of all the exacerbating factors, smoking plays the largest part in the failure of periodontal treatment and the ultimate loss of teeth.

5.8 Surgical treatment of periodontal disease

5.8.1 Gingivectomy

Sometimes, successful treatment of periodontal disease is hindered by the failure of established false pockets to be eliminated. These can be surgically eliminated by cutting off the hyperplastic gingivae level with the point of epithelial reattachment, a procedure called gingivectomy (Fig.(5.7)).

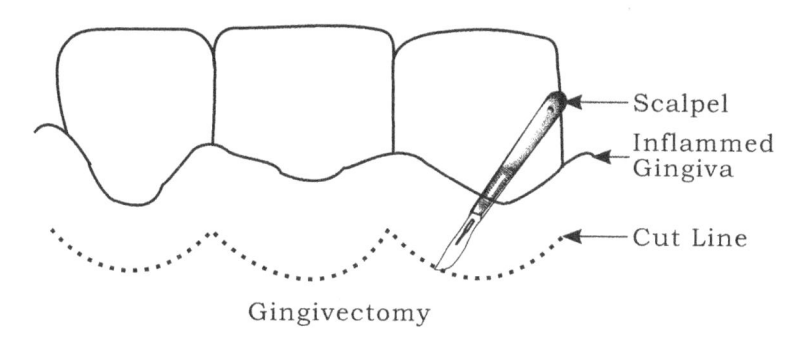

Figure 5.7: Gingivectomy

The point of reattachment is marked on the gingivae, then all hyperplastic tissue is removed with a Blake's knife or a specialized surgical lancet. This leaves a raw wound which is covered with a zinc oxide and eugenol dressing (such as Coepak®), to aid healing.

Gingivectomy allows thorough cleaning of the teeth surfaces once exposed, and thus prevents further plaque accumulation and calculus formation. The procedure is often carried out to remove drug-induced hyperplastic tissue too or hereditary gingival fibromatosis.

Surgical recontouring of the gingivae can also be carried out once periodontal health has been achieved, to aid thorough cleansing of the area. This is called gingivoplasty and is often carried out using an electrosurgery unit, which coagulates cut blood vessels at the same time.

5.8.2 Flap surgery

Often, only certain teeth are affected by periodontal disease, rather than the whole dentition. These localized areas of disease can be individually investigated by raising a part or full thickness surgical flap of mucoperiosteal tissue, to expose the persistent periodontal pockets to direct vision and clean-

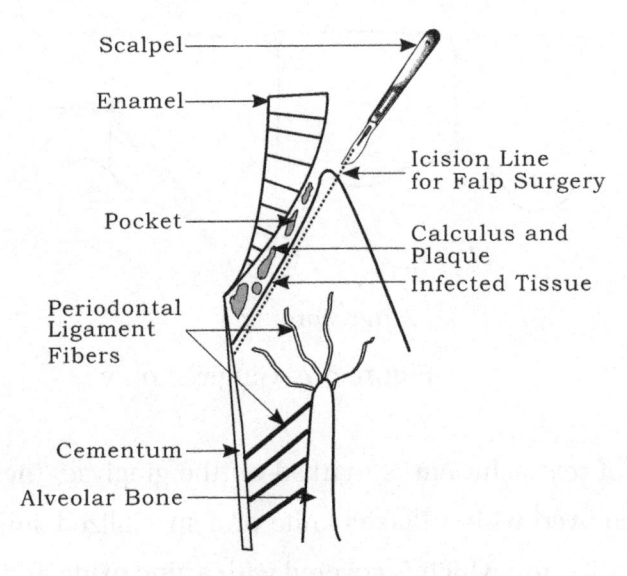

Figure 5.8: Flap Surgery

ing. Any granulation tissue present, due to the body's attempts to heal the area itself, is also removed.

Contaminated cementum, subgingival calculus and toxin-impregnated soft tissue are all removed before the flap is sutured back into place to allow full healing (Fig.(5.8)).

Some operators make use of local antibiotics in these areas to destroy bacteria and aid healing. These are available as gels (such as minocycline) which are packed into the pocket bases.

5.9 Other periodontal conditions

5.9.1 Acute necrotizing ulcerative gingivitis

See also chapter of "infections of the Oral and Para-Oral Tissues"

- Often occurs in teenagers, young adults and under stress conditions.
- Directly related to poor oral hygiene.
- Sudden onset.
- Very painful gingivitis.
- Ulceration of gingival papillae.
- Halitosis.
- Is a specific infection with either *Treponema Vincentii* combined *Busiform Bacilli*.
- Treated with the antibiotic metronidazole with penicillin.
- Followed by thorough scaling and oral hygiene instruction.
- Short course of chlorhexidene mouthwash.

5.9.2 Lateral periodontal abscess

- Acute abscess formation in an existing periodontal pocket.
- Occurs on the side of the root, that is laterally, of a vital tooth.
- Treated by draining the pus present.
- Thorough scaling of the area.
- Local administration of metronidazole into pocket.
- Oral hygiene instruction.

5.9.3 Pericoronitis

- Is the infection of the soft tissues surrounding the crown of a partially impacted tooth. In most cases, there is an operculum (gum tag) covering the involved tooth partially.
- Usually occurs with lower third molars.
- Food debris and bacteria accumulate under the operculum, causing inflammation and swelling of the tissues. The swollen tissue becomes

subjected to trauma by the opposing teeth thus aggravating the inflammatory process.
- Treated by irrigating food debris from under operculum.
- Oral hygiene instruction and advice on use of mouthwashes
- Broad spectrum antibiotics if patient has raised temperature
- Operculectomy if recurs (surgical removal of operculum)
- Extraction of the offending tooth, if there is no adequate space for its complete eruption
- Or extraction of the opposing tooth to prevent further soft tissue trauma.

Chapter 6
Diseases of Pulp and Periapical Tissues

The dental pulp is a small tissue but with a great issue.

6.1 Characteristics of Pulp Inflammation

- The most common pulp disease is the pulp inflammation. Pulp inflammation, if not treated promptly in its early stages will usually progress into periapical inflammation. Pulp inflammation possesses peculiar characThe pulp is a small tissue with a big issueteristics which are usually attributed to the anatomy and histology of the dental pulp.
- The dental pulp as a tissue is characterized by:
  1. Absence of collateral circulation.
  2. The constricted apical foramen presents a limitation to the pulp blood supply and venous return.
  3. The pulp is enclosed within a hard dentin chamber which will not allow the pulp to swell, thus edema will occur on the expense of the vascular channels leading to compression of the vessels. Hence pulp inflammation usually ends by pulp necrosis.
  4. Lack of proprioceptors, making pain localization to the correct tooth a diagnostic challenge.
  5. Moreover, pulps of individual teeth are not precisely represented on the sensory cortex. The pulp pain is therefore not only poorly

localized, but also may be felt in any of the teeth of the upper or lower jaw of the affected side. Rarely, pain may be referred to a more distant site such as the ear.

6.2 Etiology of pulp inflammation

1. Bacterial

    Bacteria can gain access to the pulp through one of the following:
    (a) Dental caries. This is the most common cause.
    (b) Fracture of the tooth exposing the pulp
    (c) Blood born infection (anachoresis) in which bacteria circulating in blood settle in the already slightly hyperemic pulp. Settlement of bacteria is facilitated by the stasis of blood stream caused by hyperemia and by the phenomenon that arteries of the pulp are end arteries.
    (d) Through a deep periodontal pocket via an accessory root canal (very rare).

2. Chemical
    (a) Free phosphoric acid in silicate or phosphate cements
    (b) Arsenic present in silicate cement.
    (c) Acrylic resin monomer.
    (d) Monomer present in composite restorations.
    (e) Sterilizing agents e.g. alcohol and tincture of iodine.

3. Physical
    (a) Thermal
        - Large metallic restorations without base.
        - Heat evolved during cavity, crown and bridge preparations.
        - Heat evolved during setting of some cements e.g. acrylic resin.

(b) Electric

Presence of two dissimilar metals (galvanism).

4. Mechanical

   (a) Trauma which may lead to crushing of blood supply of the pulp.

   (b) Cracked tooth syndrome. A tooth, particularly a premolar, may split, usually under masticatory stresses. These minute cracks are often invisible, but may allow organisms to get into the pulp chamber.

   (c) Abrasion

   (d) Lack of temporary coverage after crown and bridge preparation.

5. Barodontalgia (Aerodontalgia)

   Is a condition in which there is toothache in persons flying at high altitudes. It is usually associated with recently filled teeth or teeth affected by hyperemia. The pain is thought to be caused by a change in ambient pressure. The pain usually ceases at ground level. The condition can occur also in underwater divers because in deep dives pressures can increase by several atmospheres.

6.3 Classification of Pulpitis

Several detailed classifications of pulpitis based on histologic changes have been proposed. Most of these classifications are of little practical value because of the difficulties in correlating these changes with clinical features. Figure (6.1) shows a simplified classification that is helpful in diagnosis and treatment planning.

1. According to Type of Inflammation (chronicity)

   (a) Focal reversible Pulpitis (pulp hyperemia)

   (b) Acute Pulpitis

(c) Chronic Pulpitis
2. According to presence of absence of symptoms (clinical classification)
    (a) Symptomatic pulpitis
    (b) Asymptomatic pulpitis
3. According to Extent of Pulp Involvement
    (a) Partial Pulpitis (subtotal): the inflammatory process is confined to a portion of the pulp
    (b) Total Pulpitis: the entire pulp is involved.
4. According to the presence of communication between the pulp and the Oral Cavity
    (a) Closed Pulpitis: In which there is no direct communication between the pulp and the oral cavity.
    (b) Open Pulpitis: The pulp is partially or completely communicated with the oral cavity through a wide exposure area. In this condition the pain is usually less severe than that of closed pulpitis.
5. According to the presence or absence of infection
    (a) Septic Pulpitis (infective): Pulpitis is caused by bacteria gaining access to the pulp tissue.
    (b) Aseptic Pulpitis (sterile): Pulpitis caused by physical injury without bacterial involvement.

6.4 Correlation Between Clinical Signs and Histological Features

- Classic studies were performed in which the subjective and objective clinical findings related to carious teeth were recorded prior to tooth extraction and examining them histologically.

Oral Pathology for Dental Hygienists and Assistants

Always Remember

Pulpitis:
- Partial
- Total
- Septic
- Aspetic
- Acute Pulpitis
- Chronic Pulpitis
- Closed
- Open
- Reversible Pulpitis

Note

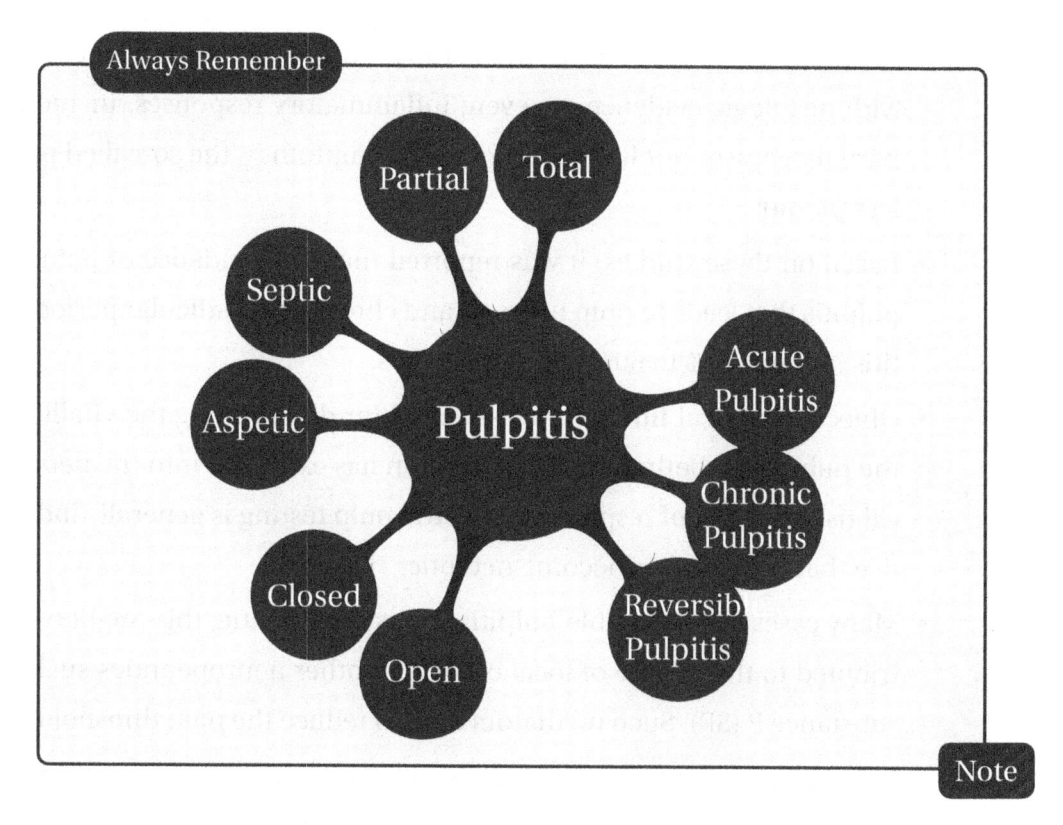

Figure 6.1: Classification of pulpitis.

- The underlying hypothesis in these studies was that the more severe the clinical symptoms, the more intense pulpal inflammation was evident histologically.
- The findings of these studies revealed that in the vital pulp, clinical symptoms generally did not correlate with gross histological findings.
- Furthermore, carious pulp exposure was associated with severe inflammatory response or liquefactive necrosis, regardless of symptoms. These histologic changes ranged in extent from being present only at the site of the exposure to deep into the root canals.
- In a few studies, prolonged or spontaneous severe symptoms were associated with chronic partial or total pulpitis or pulp necrosis.

- However, in these as well as other studies, it was common to find cases with histologic evidence of severe inflammatory responses, including partial necrosis, but little or no clinical symptoms – the so-called painless pulpitis.
- Based on these studies, it was reported that the incidence of painless pulpitis that leads to pulp necrosis and chronic periradicular periodontitis is about 40% to 60% of pulpitis cases.
- Objective clinical findings are essential for determining the vitality of the pulp and whether the inflammation has extended into the periapical tissues. Lack of response to electric pulp testing is generally indicative that the pulp has become necrotic.
- Many cases of irreversible pulpitis are asymptomatic, this might be attributed to the release of local opioids or other neuropeptides such as substance P (SP). Such mediators tend to reduce the pain threshold
- In apical periodontitis, there is also a weak correlation between the clinical symptoms and the histological feature. Some teeth with apical periodontitis are free of symptoms.
- Sensitivity to percussion is indicative for periapical inflammation.

6.5 Pulp Diseases

6.5.1 Focal Reversible Pulpitis (Pulp Hyperemia)

Definition

Is the active dilation of pulpal blood vessels representing the earliest stage of pulpitis. It is regarded as a reversible condition provided that the irritant is removed before the pulp is severely damaged.

Etiology

Any of the previously mentioned etiologic factors can cause pulp hyperemia

Clinically

- The tooth is sensitive to thermal changes particularly cold application.
- Pain is sharp shooting.
- Pain disappears rapidly on removal of the stimulus.
- Pain can not be localized.
- The tooth is more sensitive to electrical pulp tester.

Histologically

- Dilation of blood vessels.
- Edema in the connective tissue (fluid exudates).
- No extravasations of red blood cells.

Differential Diagnosis

Reversible pulpitis can be distinguished from irreversible pulpitis in two ways:

1. Reversible pulpitis causes a momentary painful response to thermal change that subsides as soon as the stimulus is removed while in irreversible pulpitis the pain persists for a while after removal of the stimulus.
2. Reversible pulpitis does not involve a complaint of spontaneous unprovoked pain while irreversible pulpitis commonly includes a complaint of spontaneous pain.
3. For further details about differential diagnosis of all types of pulp and periapical diseases, refer to table (6.1)

Treatment

Removal of the cause if possible.

Prognosis

The condition is reversible on removal of the irritant. Delayed or failure of treatment will results in progression for more severe forms of pulpitis. Sequelae of pulp inflammation are illustrated in figure (6.2)

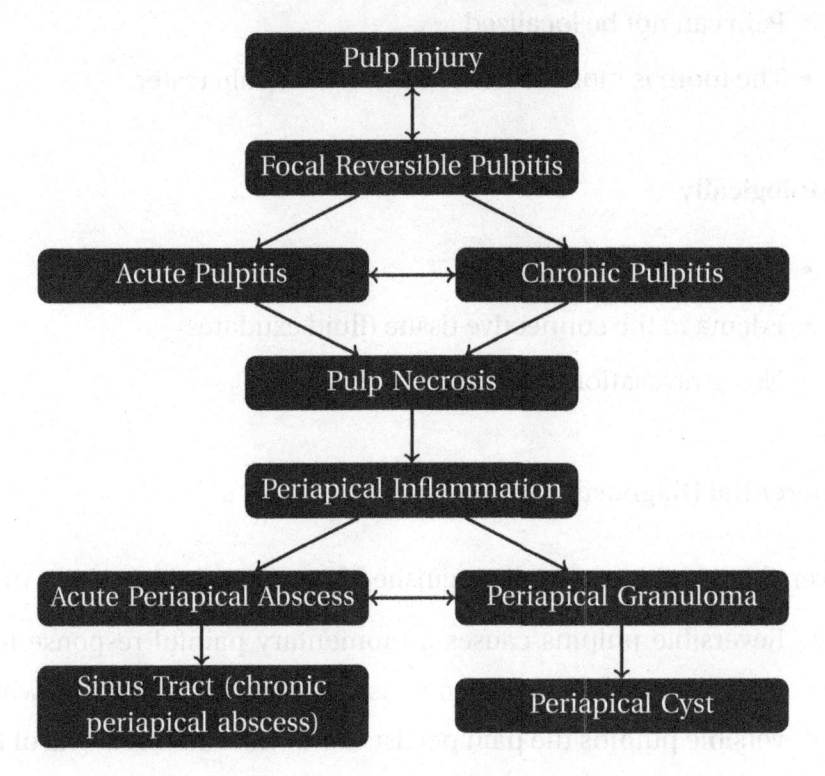

```
                    Pulp Injury
                         ↓
              Focal Reversible Pulpitis
              ↙                    ↘
      Acute Pulpitis  ←→  Chronic Pulpitis
              ↘                    ↙
                    Pulp Necrosis
                         ↓
              Periapical Inflammation
              ↙                    ↘
   Acute Periapical Abscess  ←→  Periapical Granuloma
              ↓                        ↓
      Sinus Tract (chronic        Periapical Cyst
       periapical abscess)
```

Figure 6.2: Sequelae of pulp inflammation.

6.5.2 Acute Pulpitis

Definition

Is an acute inflammation of dental pulp

Etiology

The condition may follow pulp hyperemia or exacerbation of chronic pulpitis. The previously mentioned etiologic factors can cause acute pulpitis.

Clinically

1. The tooth is sensitive to thermal changes particularly cold application.
2. Then the tooth becomes more sensitive to hot application.
3. Pain is sharp lancinating and persists for some time after removal of the stimulus.
4. In the later stages pain becomes spontaneous, often when the patient is trying to get to sleep.
5. Pain can not be localized.
6. The pain is due to pressure on the irritated nerve endings by the inflammatory exudates and also due to release of pain producing substances from damaged tissues.
7. The tooth is more sensitive to electric pulp tester.
8. The tooth is not sensitive to percussion.

Histologically

1. Destruction of the odontoblastic layer.
2. Dilation of blood vessels.

3. Edema in the connective tissue.
4. Acute inflammatory cell infiltration (polymorph nuclear leukocytes).
5. Focal areas of tissue destruction occurs leading to the formation of pus (pulp abscess). Pus consists of necrotic cells, dead and alive polymorphs and dead and alive bacteria.
6. Numerous abscesses appear. Finely fuse together and total liquefaction of pulp occurs and the condition is sometimes termed suppurative pulpitis.

Treatment

Acute pulpitis has no treatment except for extraction of the tooth or removal of the pulp by endodontic treatment.

6.5.3 Pulp necrosis

- Pulp necrosis may follow either pulpitis or a traumatic injury to the apical blood vessels cutting off the blood supply to the pulp. A coagulative type of necrosis is seen after ischemia, but if the necrosis follows pulpitis then breakdown of inflammatory cells may lead to a liquefactive type of necrosis which may become infected by putrefactive bacteria from caries. This gangrenous necrosis of the pulp is usually associated with a foul odor when such infected pulps are opened for endodontic treatment.
- Pulp necrosis has also been described in patients with sickle cell anemia, following blockage of the pulp microcirculation by sickled erythrocytes.

6.5.4 Chronic Pulpitis

Definition

Is a chronic inflammation of dental pulp. Chronic inflammation is defined as "the persistence of inflammation with continuous attempts of repair".

Etiology

- It may follow acute pulpitis or arises de novo.
- In case of de novo chronic pulpitis, the causative agents are usually of low virulence.
- The general etiologic factors for pulpitis can also cause chronic pulpitis.

Types

It may be total or partial, closed or open

Clinically

- Pain is not a feature, although the patient may complain of dull ache which is intermittent.
- The reaction to thermal changes and electric pulp tester is reduced.
- The tooth is not sensitive to percussion.

Histologically

Increased fibroblastic activity and the pulp becomes replaced by granulation tissue which consists of:

1. Proliferating capillaries

2. Proliferating fibroblasts
3. Delicate collagen fibrils.
4. Chronic inflammatory cell infiltration.

Treatment

As that of acute pulpitis.

Fate

If not treated, acute exacerbation will occur and pulp necrosis will follow after one of the acute episode.

Differential Diagnosis

The condition must be differentiated from acute pulpitis (see table (6.1) for further details)

6.5.5 Chronic Hyperplastic Pulpitis (Pulp Polyp)

Definition

This is a hyperplasia of chronically inflamed pulp.

Etiology

For pulp polyp to develop, 4 prerequisites should be fulfilled:

1. A good sheltered area for protection of the new tissue.
2. A wide apical foramen for good blood supply.

Table 6.1: Characteristics of pulpitis and periapical diseases

Characteristics of pulpitis and periapical diseases

Disease	Pain	Vitality Test	Percussion Test	Radiograph
Reversible pulpitis	Shooting	Reversible, sensitivity to cold	Not sensitive	No change
Acute pulpitis	Severe lancinating pain	Hyperresponse to no response	Not sensitive	No change
Chronic pulpitis	Mild, intermittent	Reduced response	Not sensitive	No change
Acute periapical abscess	Severe, pain on percussion	Severe response	Severe sensitivity	No change
Periapical granuloma	None to mild	No response	Mild sensitivity	Hazy radiolucency
Periapical cyst	None to mild	No response	None or mild sensitivity	Defined Radiolucency

3. A wide exposure to allow the new tissue to protrude from the pulp.
4. The patient should be young for the increased proliferative power in young age.

Clinically

- Usually affects children and young adults.
- Usually occurs in deciduous molars or the first permanent molar.
- There is a piece of tissue extruded from the pulp and present in a large carious lesion.
- The lesion is relatively insensitive to manipulation because it contains fewer nerve endings.

Differential Diagnosis

Should be differentiated from gingival polyp which is attached to the gingiva and is more sensitive to manipulation if compared to pulp polyp.

Histologically

- The lesion consists of granulation tissue with chronic inflammatory cells.
- This granulation tissue becomes epithelized later on. The source of epithelium may be:
    1. Desquamated epithelial cells found in saliva which become implanted on the surface of granulation tissue.
    2. Implantation of epithelial cells during rubbing of the cheek with granulation tissue.

Treatment

Extraction of the tooth or endodontic treatment.

6.5.6 Pulp Calcification

- Pulp calcification is a common phenomenon that occurs with increasing age for no apparent reason.
- Calcifications my be classified into:
    1. Linear or nodular:
        (a) Linear: Are typically found in the root canals and generally arc parallel to the blood vessels.
        (b) Nodular: Are often termed (pulp stones). usually found in the pulp chamber.
    2. Free or attached:

(a) Free: Free in the pulp and surrounded by the pulp tissue.

(b) Attached: Attached to the wall of the pulp chamber.

3. False or true:

   (a) True: Composed predominantly of dentin, they are referred to as true denticles. Denticles may form as a result of an epithelial mesenchymal interaction within the developing pulp through the entrapment of fragments of enamel organ or epithelial sheath of Hertwig into the pulp tissue with subsequent induction of odontoblastic differentiation.

   (b) False: Represents foci of dystrophic calcification, they are referred to as false denticles.

4. Coronal or radicular:

   (a) Coronal:

   (b) Radicular:

- Pulp stones increase in number and size with age and are apparently more numerous after operative procedures on the tooth.
- Pulp stones appear to have no clinical significance. They are not believed to be a source of pain and are not associated with any form of pulpitis. They may, however, be problematic during endodontic therapy.
- Pulp stones are commonly seen in dentinogenesis imperfecta, dentinal dysplasia, Ehlers-Danlos syndrome, pulpal dysplasia and end-stage renal disease[1].
- Radiographically, when they are large appear as radiopaque mass within the dental pulp. Diffuse calcifications are rarely detectable radiographically.
- See table (6.3) to view the various types of pulp stones.

---

[1] In end stage renal disease usually, there is hypercalcemia with increases the possibility of metastatic calcification.

- Some authors [2] proposed the following classification for pulp calcification:
    1. Pulp stones: Which are the dystrophic calcifications within the pulp and is usually nodular.
    2. Denticles: Which consists of tubular or rarely atubular dentin.
    3. Diffuse linear calcifications: Which are linear bodies often parallel the vasculature.

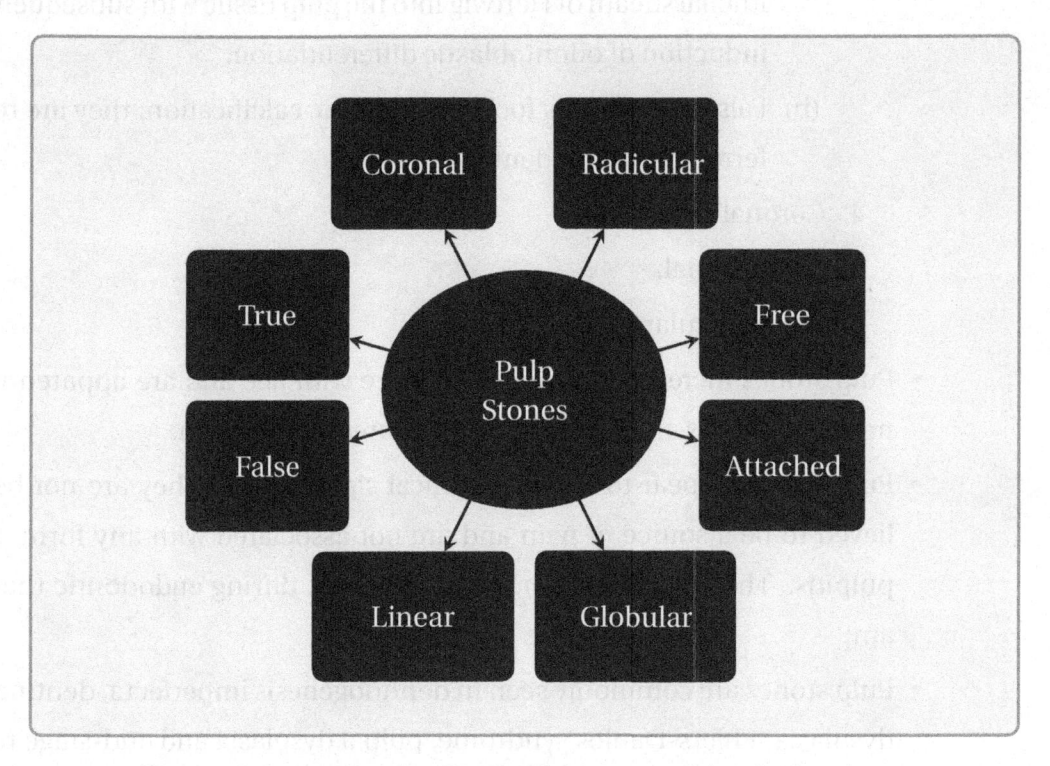

Figure 6.3: Various Types of Pulp Stones and Calcifications.

6.5.7 Calcific Metamorphosis

(Pulp Canal Obliteration, Dystrophic Calcification, Diffuse Calcification, Calcific Degeneration)

Definition

Calcific Metamorphosis is defined by the American Association of Endodontists as "A pulpal response to trauma characterized by rapid deposition of hard tissue within the canal space."

The condition is not the same as false pulp stones. True denticles (true pulp stones) are made of dentin which is lined by odontoblasts, whereas false pulp stones are formed by mineralization of pulp cells that have degenerated.

Etiology

- Dental trauma to the permanent dentition (concussion or subluxation injuries)
- Dentinal dysplasia
- Dentinogenesis imperfecta, mainly type 2
- Teeth which have been rigidly splinted.

Pathogenesis

- Is initiated by stimulation of odontoblastic activity.
- The mechanism is not known but may be due to injury to the neurovascular supply of the pulp.
- Another theory suggests that the bleeding in the canal and blood clot could be a focal point for calcification in case the pulp remains vital following trauma.
- Hence, traumatic injury to the apical blood vessels, which may not be sufficient to cause pulpal necrosis and the pulp remains vital, could lead to this condition.

Histologically

- A mixture of secondary and tertiary dentin is usually found. refer to page (208) to know the differences between types of dentin.
- Osteodentin could be observed in some cases.

Clinically

- Generally asymptomatic.
- The patients present with yellow coloration of the affected tooth crown. This discoloration is due to a greater thickness of dentin deposition.
- Not all teeth will undergo a color change.
- More common in the anterior teeth.
- May be recognized as early as 3 months after injury although it may not be detected up to 1 year.
- The incidence of pulp canal obliteration following dental trauma has been reported to be approximately 4–24%.
- Vital pulp testing may be unreliable (false negative) despite the presence of a vital pulp due to the increased thickness of dentin.

X-Ray

- Reveals partial or total obliteration of pulp space with absence of the pulp chamber.
- Unless there is evidence of apical involvement of bone, the lamina dura will be intact with no widening of the periodontal membrane space.

Treatment

- Endodontic therapy should be performed only if periapical pathosis or negative vitality testing is present.
- Because of the reduced canal space, location of the pulp canal can be difficult, and care must be exercised during access preparation to prevent perforation.
- If endodontic therapy is unsuccessful, then periapical surgery can be performed in those cases with evidence of periapical inflammatory disease.
- To improve aesthetics, full coverage is recommended for discolored anterior teeth with large restorations.

6.5.8 Internal Resorption

Refer to chapter "Physical, Chemical & Idiopathic Pathology of Teeth", page (214)

6.6 Periapical Diseases

6.6.1 Periapical Granuloma

(*Chronic Apical Periodontitis*)

Definition

Is a localized mass of granulation tissue related to the apex of a tooth. Periapical granuloma represents a state of chronically inflamed tissues around the apex of a tooth.

Etiology

- Results from extension of low grade infection from pulp tissue.
- May follow acute periapical abscess that has been inadequately drained and incompletely treated.
- Infection of the periapical area will produce inflammation with activation of osteoclasts to produce bone resorption and replacement of bone with granulation tissue.

Clinically

- Usually related to non-vital tooth.
- The patient may feel that the tooth is slightly extruded form the socket.
- No pain or slight discomfort on biting or chewing.
- The tooth is slightly sensitive to percussion.

X-Ray

- Hazy or ill defined radiolucent area related to the apex.
- In the long standing lesions with the reduction of the inflammatory response, the granuloma may appear as a well defined radiolucent area.

Differential Diagnosis

- It is difficult to differentiate radiographically between periapical granuloma and small radicular cysts.
- Data indicate that one cannot rely on the size of the lesion to establish a diagnosis except where the radiographic lesion is 2 cm in diameter or larger [3].

Histologically

1. Fibrous connective tissue capsule.
2. Granulation tissue.
3. Chronic inflammatory cells (plasma cells, lymphocytes, macrophages and less frequently neutrophils and mast cells.
4. Cholesterol clefts may be found. These clefts are potential spaces between collagen fibers that were occupied by cholesterol crystals. Cholesterol crystals may result from tissue breakdown due to chronic long standing inflammation or be of hematogenous origin. Cholesterol then dissolves in xylol during preparation of the histopathologic slides leaving a needle like spaces or clefts. Cholesterol crystals are rhomboid in shape resembling a detached stamp envelope.
5. Macrophages may accumulate to phagocytose cholesterol (foreign material), and thus termed foam cells.
6. Sometimes, foreign body giant cells could be seen.
7. When numerous plasma cells are present, scattered eosinophilic globules of gamma globulin (*Russell bodies*) may be seen. In addition, clusters of lightly basophilic particles (*pyronine bodies*) also may be present. Both of these plasma cell products are not specific for the periapical granuloma and may be found within any accumulation of plasma cells.
8. Sometimes epithelial cells are seen. These are usually epithelial rests of Mallassez. They play a role in changing granuloma into cyst later on.

Treatment

3 Lines of treatment may be followed according to the case:

1. Extraction of the involved tooth.
2. Endodontic treatment.

3. Endodontic treatment with apicectomy and curettage of the granuloma.

Fate of Granuloma

- With effective endodontic treatment or tooth extraction, granuloma heals. Healing occurs by fibrosis and scarring of granuloma with disappearance of inflammatory cells, bacteria and decrease of vascularity. Periapical scar may persist for months or years and appears in apical radiographs as a well-defined small radiolucency. Later on, calcification or ossification of the scar occurs.
- Without treatment, granuloma may progress into radicular cyst or undergoes acute exacerbation into acute periapical abscess.

6.6.2 Periapical Abscess

Traditionally, Many authors classify periapical abscesses into acute and chronic. However, these are misnomers because both types represent acute inflammation. Periapical abscesses should be designated as symptomatic or asymptomatic on the basis of their clinical manifestations.

Figure (6.4) illustrates the main differences between acute, chronic periapical abscess and periapical granuloma.

6.6.3 Acute Periapical Abscess

Definition

- Is a localized suppurative inflammation in the periapical area.
- In the earliest stage, the periapical periodontal ligament may exhibit acute inflammation with no frank abscess formation. This localized al-

Acute Periapical Abscess   Chronic Periapical Abscess   Periapical Granuloma

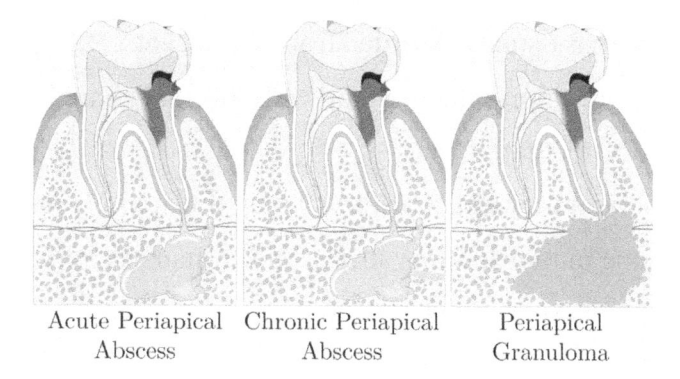

Figure 6.4: Diagrammatic illustration of periapical infections. Left panel is an acute periapical abscess with pus formation, middle panel shows chronic periapical abscess opening by a sinus tract to discharge pus, and the right panel shows periapical granuloma.

teration, best termed acute apical periodontitis, may or may not proceed to abscess formation.

- Although, acute periapical abscess often occurs in association with a non-vital tooth, acute apical periodontitis may present in vital teeth secondary to trauma, high occlusal contacts, or wedging by a foreign object.

Etiology

- Extension of infection from pulp tissue.
- May follow faulty endodontic treatment
- May result form acute exacerbation of periapical granuloma
- The causative organisms are pyogenic bacteria.

Clinically

- Severe throbbing pain.
- The tooth is extremely painful even to touch.

- The tooth is usually extruded from the socket.
- The tooth is non-vital, no pain with thermal changes and no response with electric pulp tester.
- The patient may give a history of pain due to previous pulpitis
- Systemic manifestations such as fever, malaise, leukocytosis and lymphadenitis could also be noted.
- With progression, the abscess spreads along the path of least resistance. The pus may spread through the medullary spaces away from the apical area, resulting in osteomyelitis, or it may perforate the cortex and spread diffusely through the overlying soft tissue (as cellulitis).
- Once an abscess is in soft tissue, it can cause cellulitis, spread to fascial spaces or may escape through the overlying soft tissue forming a sinus. The inflamed granulation tissue surrounding the orifice of the sinus tract is termed parulis (gum boil).

X-Ray

- In the early stages, no changes can be seen because there is insufficient time for bone changes to develop.
- Shortly after this stage, the lamina dura becomes hazy with widening of the periodontal membranes space.
- When acute periapical abscess is due to acute exacerbation of chronic infection (periapical granuloma), the original lesion appears as hazy or ill defined radiolucent area.

Histologically

- In the early stages, there is intense inflammation in the immediate vicinity of the apex (acute apical periodontitis)
- If not immediately treated, definite abscess is formed which consists of:

1. Central area containing pus.
2. Surrounded by pyogenic membrane which is a layer of fibrin heavily infiltrated with polymorph nuclear leukocytes.
3. The surrounding tissues show dilation of blood vessels, edema and infiltration with inflammatory cells.

Microbiology

Bacteria commonly isolated from acute periapical abscesses are:

1. Facultative anaerobes
   - Streptococcus milled
   - Streptococcus sanguis
   - Actinomyces spp.
2. Obligate anaerobes
   - Peptostreptococcus spp.
   - Porphyromonas gingivalis
   - Prevotella intermedia
   - Prevotella melaninogenica
   - Fusobacterium nucleatum

Treatment

- Early stages (acute apical periodontitis) could be treated by removal of the initiating cause such as premature contact.
- Acute periapical abscess is treated by extraction of the tooth or drainage of pus through the root canal followed by endodontic treatment if the tooth is to be preserved.
- The use of Antibiotic is controversial.

Prognosis and Sequelae

Under lack of treatment, once pus formation occurs, it may remain localized at the root apex and develop into:

1. Chronic abscess draining through a sinus tract giving immediate relief of symptoms.
2. Develop into a focal osteomyelitis

Spread into the surrounding tissues (Fig.6.5).

1. Direct spread
   (a) Spread into the superficial soft tissues may:
      - localize as a soft-tissue abscess (Fig.6.6)
      - extend through the overlying oral mucosa or skin, producing a sinus linking the main abscess cavity with the mouth or skin
      - extend through the soft tissue to produce a cellulitis.
   (b) Spread may occur into the adjacent fascial spaces, following the path of least resistance; such spread is dependent on the anatomical relation of the original abscess to the adjacent tissues. Infection via fascial planes often spreads rapidly and for some distance from the original abscess site, and occasionally may cause severe respiratory distress as a result of occlusion of the airway by edema (e.g. Ludwig's angina).
   (c) Infection may extend into the deeper medullary spaces of alveolar bone, producing a spreading osteomyelitis; this may occur in compromised patients.
   (d) In maxillary teeth, odontogenic infection may directly spread into the maxillary sinus, especially if the sinus lining and the tooth apex are subjacent, leading to acute or chronic secondary maxillary sinusitis (as opposed to primary sinusitis due to direct sinus infection). Such infection, if not arrested, may rarely spread to

the central nervous system, causing serious complications such as subdural empyema, brain abscesses or meningitis.

2. Indirect spread

   Indirect spread through lymphatics or blood stream:

   (a) Lymphatic spread, to regional nodes in the head and neck region (submental, submandibular, deep cervical, parotid and occipital). Usually the involved nodes are tender, swollen and painful, and rarely may suppurate, requiring drainage

   (b) Hematogenous routes: to other organs such as the lung, cavernus sinus or brain (rare)

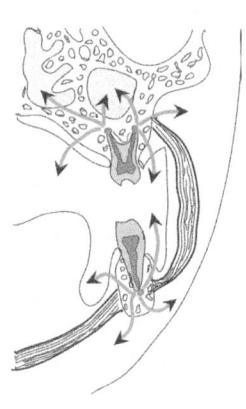

Figure 6.5: Possible pathways for the spread of pus from an acute periapical abscess

6.6.4 Chronic Periapical Abscess

- Although the term "chronic abscess" is not strictly accurate, if an acute periapical abscess achieves drainage through a sinus tract, the condition becomes asymptomatic due to lack of accumulation of pus within the alveolus. Such a condition is known as chronic periapical abscess or given an obsolete term *periapical phlegmon.*

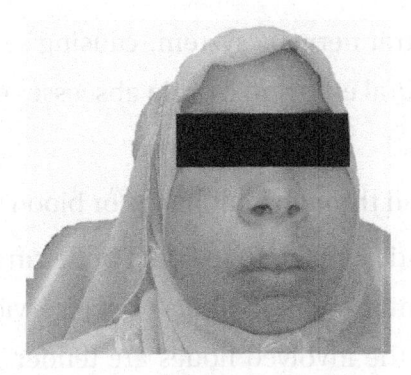

Figure 6.6: Young female with a combined buccal and infraorbtial spaces infection

- At the intraoral opening of the sinus tract, a mass of inflamed granulation tissue often is found, known as a parulis (gum boil).
- The parulis should be differentiated from gingival and periodontal abscesses.

6.6.5 Periapical Cemental Dysplasia and True Cementoma

Are lesions which occur at the apices of teeth, for further details, see chapter "Benign Odontogenic Tumors" on page 376.

6.6.6 Hypercementosis

A condition characterized by the deposition of excessive amounts of cementum on the root surface, for further details, see chapter "Physical, Chemical & Idiopathic Pathology of Teeth" on page 217.

Chapter 7
Cysts and Cyst-like Lesions

Cysts, cyst-like, and cystic tumors are common pathologies of the jaws and soft tissues surrounding the jaws. They usually appear as painless swellings that could be mistaken for tumors; however, they are not neoplastic in nature.

7.1 Introduction

7.1.1 Definition

A cyst by definition is a pathological cavity lined by epithelium and containing a fluid or a semifluid material. Cysts not lined by epithelium are called psuedocysts.

7.1.2 Histogenesis of Epithelial Lining

True cysts are lined by epithelium and the origin of the epithelial lining of cysts varies. In odontogenic cysts, the epithelium is supposed to be of odontogenic origin while in non-odontogenic cysts, the epithelium may be derived from remnants of embryonic tracts, vestiges or from epithelium entrapped at the line of fusion of embryonic processes (fissural cysts). The nature of the epithelial lining of cysts is used as the primary criteria in classification of cysts.

7.1.3 Pathogenesis of Cysts

- The epithelium present in the future cystic area undergoes hyperplasia and proliferates in a form of masses. As these masses enlarge, their central cells become away from the source of nutrition and thus they degenerate and liquefy forming microcysts. The microcysts enlarge and finely fuse together forming one large macrocyst.
- It is also postulated that the epithelium can proliferate in a form of strands or cords enclosing areas of connective tissue in between, later on breakdown of the inner strands occurs and the cyst is thus formed.

7.1.4 Mechanism of Cyst Enlargement

- The cyst enlarges due to presence of high intracystic pressure. This pressure results from the high osmotic pressure which is maintained by the persistent breakdown of the continuously shedding epithelial cells into the cavity of the cyst. There is some controversy whether the cyst lining acts as a perfect semipermeable membrane. The intracystic hydrostatic pressure is about 70 cm/ water and therefore higher than the capillary blood pressure.
- It is also postulated that some cyst linings can produce some inflammatory mediators (prostaglandins E2, E3, and interlukins-1) which can assist in the process of bone resorption. Also, collagenases are present in the wall of odontogenic keratocysts and some cases of dentigerous cysts, but their contribution to the growth of cysts is unclear.

7.1.5 Complications of Cysts

(Rationale for the treatment of cysts)

1. Infection: Cysts are liable to be infected at any time and can cause osteomyelitis, facial cellulitis, etc.
2. Pathological fracture of bone.
3. Disfigurement of face.
4. Squamous cell carcinoma or other malignancy may arise from the epithelial lining of cysts.
5. Ameloblastoma may arise from the wall of dentigerous cysts.
6. Some cysts e.g. dentigerous cysts may prevent the eruption of the involved tooth.
7. Large mandibular cysts produce paresthesia or anesthesia of the lower lip due to compression on the neurovascular bundle.
8. Any cyst may cause displacement of adjacent teeth.

7.1.6 Classification of Cysts

No satisfactory classification exists; however, the following classification which is based primarily on the origin of the epithelial lining is a workable one. It is to be noted that some cysts occupy more than one position in the classification, reflecting some controversy regarding their nature.

1. Odontogenic cysts:
    (a) Inflammatory odontogenic cysts
        i. Inflammatory apical cyst (periapical, radicular)
        ii. Inflammatory lateral cyst
        iii. Residual cyst
        iv. Paradental cyst
        v. Mandibular Infected Buccal Cyst (Buccal bifurcation cyst)
    (b) Developmental odontogenic cysts
        i. Developmental periodontal cysts

Chapter 7. Cysts & Cyst-Like Lesions

        A. Lateral cyst

        B. Botryoid odontogenic cyst

        C. Glandular odontogenic cyst

        D. Gingival cyst of newborn

        E. Eruption cyst

        F. Gingival cyst of adult

        G. Paradental

    ii. Dentigerous cyst

        A. Central

        B. Lateral

        C. Circumferential

        D. Paradental

        E. Eruption cysts (considered by some authorities)

    iii. Primordial cyst

    iv. Odontogenic keratocyst

    v. Calcifying epithelial odontogenic cyst (Gorlin cyst)

2. Non-odontogenic cysts:

    (a) Fissural cysts (obsolete terminology by many authors)

        i. Median alveolar cyst

        ii. Median palatal cyst

        iii. Median mandibular cyst

        iv. Globulomaxillary cystGorlin

        v. Nasolabial cyst

        vi. Dermoid cyst (considered by some authorities)

    (b) Cysts arising from embryonic vestiges or tracts

        i. Nasopalatine duct cysts

            A. Incisive canal cyst

                B. Palatine papilla cyst
            ii. Thyroglossal tract cyst
    (c) Cyst like lesions
            i. Aneurysmal bone cyst
            ii. Traumatic bone cyst
            iii. Latent bone cyst
    (d) Cysts of salivary glands:
            i. Mucous retention cyst
            ii. Mucous extravasation cyst
            iii. Ranula
    (e) Other soft tissue cysts:
        Lymphoepithelial cysts
            i. Oral lymphoepithelial cyst
            ii. Cervical lymphoepithelial cyst (branchial cleft cyst)
    (f) Cysts of the maxillary antrum
            i. Mucocele of the maxillary antrum
            ii. Retention cyst of the maxillary antrum
            iii. Pseudocyst of the maxillary antrum
            iv. Postoperative maxillary cyst

7.2 Odontogenic cysts

7.2.1 Inflammatory Odontogenic Cysts

Inflammatory Apical Cyst

(Radicular cyst, periapical cyst)

Chapter 7. Cysts & Cyst-Like Lesions

Definition

This is an inflammatory odontogenic cyst which occurs in the periodontium of a tooth. It is the most common odontogenic cyst of the oral cavity.

Histogenesis

The cyst arises from the epithelial rests of Malassez.

Histologically

1. **Epithelial wall:**
    - In newly formed cyst the epithelial wall is stratified squamous epithelium showing signs of inflammatory hyperplasia i.e. thick and long rete pegs.
    - In fully formed cyst the epithelium is stratified squamous epithelium, thin regular and flattened.
2. **Connective tissue wall (capsule):**
    - In newly formed cyst is fibrous connective tissue infiltrated with chronic inflammatory cells, cholesterol clefts, foam cells and sometimes multinucleated giant cells.
    - In fully formed cyst, chronic inflammatory cells disappear or become minimal in amounts.
3. **Variations in cyst wall:**
    (a) Sometimes the epithelial wall may be respiratory i.e. psuedostratified columnar cilliated or not cilliated epithelium, particularly if the cyst approaches the maxillary sinus or the nose.
    (b) Goblet cells may be found in some cysts.
    (c) Sometimes the epithelium may be embryonic or undifferentiated.

(d) Hyaline eosinophilic bodies may be present in the superficial layers of the epithelium. They are termed **Rushton bodies**. Their nature is controversial. It is postulated that Rushton bodies are keratinous structures or enameloid matrix as they are found only in odontogenic cysts.

(e) **Russell bodies** may be seen in some cysts. They are eosinophilic masses found usually in the connective tissue wall. They represents ageing plasma cells.

(f) Dystrophic calcific bodies may be seen. These are basophilic bodies found usually in the connective tissue wall.

(g) **Cholesterol clefts** may be found within the connective tissue wall. They are fine needle-like spaces left by dissolution of cholesterol during preparation for sectioning. The cholesterol is derived from breakdown of blood cells. Other view is that cholesterol may result from tissue breakdown as a consequence of long standing inflammation. Clefts are usually surrounded by foam cells and multinucleated giant cells. Clefts may be seen extending into the cystic lumen as they shed from the cyst wall.

4. **Contents:**
   - The cystic fluid is essentially an inflammatory exudate with some modifications.
   - Low molecular weight proteins are present in similar concentrations to those in the plasma but there are smaller amounts of high molecular weight proteins.
   - The cystic fluid is a yellowish transparent fluid and is sterile unless the cyst is infected.
   - The fluid contains albumin, globulin, nucleoprotiens and cholesterol. Cholesterol gives the fluid a metallic sheen if examined in fresh state. Cholesterol crystals are rhomboidal in shape if exam-

ined in fresh smear. Cholesterol crystals are not specific for radicular cysts as they can be found in other odontogenic and non-odontogenic cysts.

Clinically

1. **Incidence:**
    - Is the most common cyst in the oral cavity.
    - The most common site is the anterior upper region.
    - Is always associated with a non-vital tooth.
2. **Signs:**
    - When small, nothing could be detected clinically.
    - When the cyst enlarges a slight bony expansion may be present, then the bone becomes thin, egg shell crackling could be elicited on pressure.
    - When bone is completely resorbed, fluctuation could be detected.
    - Aspiration biopsy reveals presence of a fluid and is a valuable aid in differentiating cysts from tumors, see table (7.1).
3. **Symptoms:**
    Symptomless unless infected, if infected it will behave as an abscess. If the cyst enlarges and presses on the inferior alveolar nerve, numbness of the lower lip will occur.

X-Ray

The cyst appears in X-ray films as a well defined radiolucent area surrounded by a radiopaque margin. If the cyst becomes infected, it will appear as a hazy radiolucent area without the characteristic radiopaque margin.

Table 7.1: Aspiration Biopsy

Aspiration Biopsy

- Aspiration biopsy is an important aid in discriminating cysts from tumors or maxillary sinus.
- A wide bore needle should be used for the procedure, which may be done under local anaesthesia.
- A diagnosis of a cyst can be confirmed if aspirate is light straw coloured fluid containing cholesterol crystals. These crystals appear shining when the fluid is taken on a dry swab.
- In odontogenic keratocysts, the colour and consistency of fluid vary depending on the concentration of keratin.
- When infected, the fluid becomes turbid and yellow.
- Aspiration of pure blood raises the possibility of central haemangioma or aneurysmal bone cyst.
- Aspiration of air shows that needles may be in maxillary sinus. It can be confirmed by injection of 20 ml of sterile water, which would come at through the nostrils.
- There is a risk of introducing infection during aspiration and ideally this should be performed under antibiotic cover.

Note

Treatment

If small enucleation is performed and if large marsupialization is preferred to avoid injury to the adjacent structures e.g. the inferior alveolar nerve.

Inflammatory Lateral Periodontal Cyst

This is essentially an inflammatory odontogenic cyst occurring on the lateral surface of a root of a non-vital tooth, possibly related to an accessory root canal. It is rare and should be differentiated form the developmental lateral periodontal cyst.

Inflammatory Residual Periodontal Cyst

(Residual Cyst)

This is a radicular cyst persisting after extraction of the causative tooth. Residual cysts are a common cause of swelling of the edentulous jaw in older persons.

Paradental Cyst

Paradental cysts are small cysts related to the distal surface of vital partially erupted teeth, particularly the lower third molars. Great controversy exists regarding their nature. Three postulates have been proposed:

1. That these cysts are merely inflammatory cysts resulting from pericoronitis affecting partially erupting third molars. This is supported by the frequent presence of inflammatory cells in its wall and its histologic similarity to inflammatory radicular cysts.
2. A type of developmental lateral periodontal cyst occurring distal to third molars
3. A type of dentigerous cyst (lateral dentigerous cyst)

Mandibular Infected Buccal Cyst

- The mandibular infected buccal cyst (MIBC) also called buccal bifurcation cyst, is another inflammatory cyst which in many ways is similar to the paradental cyst.
- MIBC is seen almost exclusively associated to the buccal aspect of the first mandibular molar in children.
- The reason for being considered a unique entity is based on its particular location and age preference. The pathogenesis of this cyst may be related to an inflammatory pathology at the level of the root furcation.
- The treatment of MIBC is surgical enucleation without tooth extraction.

7.2.2 Developmental odontogenic cysts

Developmental Periodontal Cysts

Developmental Lateral Periodontal Cyst

- This is a developmental intraosseous cyst related to the lateral surface of a root of a vital tooth.
- The epithelial lining is thought to be derived from the epithelial rests of Malassez.
- Origin from epithelial rests of Serres was also proposed.
- Radiographically, the cyst usually appears as a small, well defined radiolucency located between the roots of vital teeth
- Clinically, the cyst is usually less than 1 cm in diameter and usually is symptomless unless infected.
- Histologically, the lining is non-keratinized or orthokeratinized squamous or cuboidal epithelium, frequently only one or two cells thick but

sometimes with focal thickening. Some of the cells may show clear cytoplasm and resemble cells of the dental lamina.
- Treatment is by enucleation and the related tooth can be retained if healthy.

Botryoid odontogenic cyst

- Botryoid odontogenic cyst is probably a variant of the developmental lateral periodontal cyst occurring in the same location.
- It typically affects the mandibular premolar region in adults over 50 years of age
- Histologically, it is typically multicystic with fine fibrous septa. The lining consists of flattened non-keratinized epithelium with bud-like proliferation protruding into the cystic lumen. Most of the cells are clear and filled with glycogen. The bud-like proliferation give the cyst its peculiar name (Botryoid means a form similar to a bunch of grape).
- Radiographically, appears as a small usually multilocular radiolucency related to the lateral surface of a tooth.
- Treatment is by excision as it has a strong tendency to recur.

Glandular odontogenic cyst

(Sialo-odontogenic cyst)

- Glandular odontogenic cyst is probably a variant of botryoid odontogenic cyst occurring in the same location and characterized by presence of mucin and mucous secreting cells within the epithelial lining.
- It is frequently multilocular and has a strong tendency to recur.

Gingival cyst of newborn

(Bohn's nodule)

- These are small whitish swellings occurring on the alveolar crest of newly born infants. They are small cysts thought to arise from cystic degeneration of remnants of the dental lamina. If a gingival cyst of newborn persists till the time of eruption of teeth and interferes with the process of eruption, then it may be termed eruption cyst or eruption hematoma.
- Eruption cyst is considered by some authors to be a type of dentigerous cysts.
- Histopathology, the cyst is usually lined by stratified squamous epithelium, which may show some degree of keratinization.
- Epstein's pearls should not be confuses with Bohn's nodules. They are small whitish swellings found on the soft tissues of the midpalatine raphe of newly born infants. It is postulated that Epstein's pearls arise due to cystic degeneration of the non-odontogenic epithelium entrapped at the line of fusion of the two palatine processes.

Eruption cyst

(eruption hematoma)

- Eruption cyst is a soft tissue cyst occurring over the crown of an erupting tooth and can interfere with the process of eruption.
- Eruption cyst is thought to arise form cystic degeneration of the remnants of the dental lamina or from the reduced dental epithelium after enamel formation is complete.
- It appears as a reddish or bluish dome-shaped mass on the crest of the alveolar ridge.
- Eruption cyst is considered as a superficial dentigerous cyst.

Gingival cyst of adult

- This is a developmental soft tissue cyst that occurs in the free or attached gingiva of adults and should be differentiated from gingival cyst of newborn (*(Bohn's nodule)*) which occurs only on the alveolar crest of the newborn. Gingival cyst of adult should be also differentiated from the developmental lateral periodontal cyst, which is an intra-bony cyst with a positive X-ray picture. The gingival cyst of adult arises as a result of cystic degeneration of the remnants of the dental lamina or the remnants of epithelial rests of Malassez.
- Clinically, the cyst appears as a small, painless and fluctuant swelling in the free gingiva, attached gingiva or sometimes in the interdental papilla. Its size rarely exceeds 1 cm in diameter and may resemble a superficial mucocele.
- X-ray picture, the cyst is a soft tissue cyst and does not manifest itself in X-ray films.
- Histologically, the cyst is lined by stratified squamous epithelium, which may show some degree of keratinization.

Paradental cyst

Was discussed before

Dentigerous Cyst (follicular cyst)

Definition

This is a developmental cyst which encloses the crown or part of a crown of an unerupted tooth.

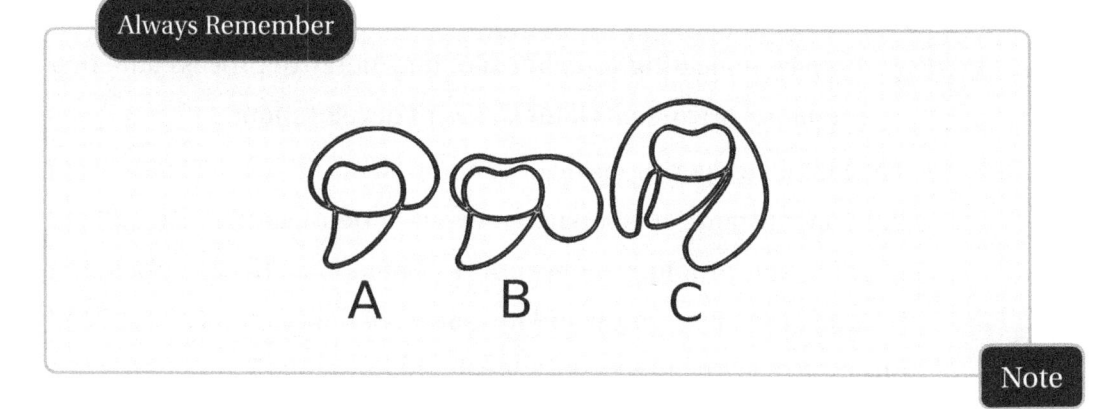

> **Always Remember**
>
> [Diagram showing three teeth labeled A, B, C illustrating types of dentigerous cysts]
>
> **Note**

Figure 7.1: Types of Dentigerous Cysts: (A) is the central, (B), is the lateral and (C) is the circumferential.

Types

- Central: The cyst encloses the whole crown.
- Lateral: Related to the lateral surface of the crown.
- Circumferential: The cyst surrounds the crown circumferentially.
- Paradental: Could be considered as a type of dentigerous cyst.
- Eruption cyst: Could be considered as a type of dentigerous cyst
- See figure (7.1)

Histogenesis

- The cyst arises from the reduced dental epithelium i.e. from the enamel organ after enamel formation is complete. In support for this postulate:
    1. The epithelial lining is attached at the amelocemental junction.
    2. Cystic fluid sometimes accumulates between the outer and the inner enamel epithelium and the latter remains attached to the surface of enamel.

3. Enamel hypoplasia is sometimes noted in teeth with dentigerous cysts, indicating some form of degenerative process affecting the enamel organ in its later stages of development.

- The factors triggering cystic degeneration of the reduced dental epithelium are obscure. It is unknown whether dentigerous cyst is the cause or the result of failure of eruption. There is a strong association between failure of eruption and formation of dentigerous cysts. Dentigerous cysts usually affect teeth which are particularly prone to failure of eruption, namely, maxillary canines and mandibular third molars.

Clinically

- Common in males than females (2 to 1).
- Most often found between the ages of 20 and 50 and being rare in children.
- Usually affects mandibular third molars and maxillary canines.
- The cyst is typically associated with an unerupted tooth.
- Uncomplicated dentigerous cysts cause no symptoms until the swelling becomes large enough.
- Infection of dentigerous cyst causes the usual symptoms of pain and accelerated swelling.

Radiographically

- A well defined radiolucent area surrounded by a radiopaque border which encloses the crown or part of a crown of unerupted tooth.
- The unerupted tooth is usually displaced from its normal position. A third molar may be pushed to the lower border of the mandible.

Histologically

- Dentigerous cyst is lined by a uniform layer of non-keratinized, stratified squamous epithelium measuring two to ten cells in thickness.
- The epithelium may sometimes be keratinized.
- Mucous cells are occasionally seen in the epithelial lining of this cyst. This finding has been described as mucus cell metaplasia.
- The epithelial lining may show dysplastic (premalignant) changes.
- A feature in common with radicular cyst, cholesterol clefts, hemosidrin deposits, and hyaline (Rushton) bodies are sometimes detected.
- The fibrous wall is similar to that of radicular cysts, but inflammatory changes are typically absent.

Differential Diagnosis

From dilated dental follicle, the pericoronal width is less than 3–4 mm.

Complications

In addition to the common complications of cysts, dentigerous cysts possess the increased risk of the following additional complications:

1. Development of ameloblastoma (mural ameloblastoma).
2. The dysplastic changes can progress into squamous cell carcinoma
3. Mucous cells can give rise to mucoepidermoid carcinoma.

Treatment

The cyst responds to enucleation or marsupialization and do not recur after treatment

Primordial Cyst

Definition

- This is an *obsolete* term describing a developmental cyst arising from the tooth primordium being characterized by presence of an absent tooth and non-keratinized or orthokeratinized epithelial lining.
- The involved tooth fails to form.
- Most new texts consider this cyst as odontogenic keratocyst. Other texts consider that most if not all primordial cysts are keratocysts histologically.
- Therefore, most "primordial cysts" are actually keratocyst odontogenic tumors (keratocysts).
- Until now, there is much debate regarding the term "primordial cyst". For further details, see reference [4].

Histogenesis

- The cyst arises from the enamel organ before amelogenesis.
- However, it is difficult to reconcile such origin with the appearance of primordial cysts in middle age and its relative rapid growth. The etiology of primordial cysts is therefore speculative.

Clinically

- The most common site is the mandibular third molar area and ascending ramus.
- Usually affects middle age (20 – 40 years).
- Associated with missed tooth.

- Like other jaw cysts primordial cysts remain symptomless until they enlarge or become infected.

Radiographically

- Appears as a well-defined unilocular or multilocular radiolucency in place of a tooth.
- The cyst tends to eccentrically expand into the ramus.

Histologically

- The epithelial lining usually consists of non-keratinized or orthokeratinized stratified squamous epithelium.
- In other instances, the morphology suggests odontogenic epithelium with columnar basal cell layer, and "stellate reticulum" type looseness of the cells.
- Other characteristics of primordial cyst, the linings may include microcysts.

Treatment

- Simple surgical enucleation or marsupialization.
- Recurrence is common.

Odontogenic Keratocyst

(Keratocystic Odontogenic Tumor)

Chapter 7. Cysts & Cyst-Like Lesions

Definition

- The term odontogenic keratocyst has caused a great deal of confusion as it was originally applied to any cyst of the jaw which shows keratinization of the epithelial lining.
- Recently, there is a general agreement that odontogenic keratocyts are special type of dentigerous or primordial cysts characterized by specific histopathologic features.
- About 10% of dentigerous and almost 30% of primordial cysts can undergo keratinization.
- It is not known why the lining of some dentigerous and primordial cysts keratinize.
- Similarly, it is not known why keratinization makes these cysts more aggressive than their non-keratinizing counterparts.
- It should be emphasized that other non-odontogenic keratininizing cysts are not as aggressive as odontogenic keratocysts.
- Two types of odontogenic keratocysts are recognized. The first type is parakeratinized variant and the second is the orthokeratinized variant. They have slightly different demographic characters, but the more important difference is that parakeratinized type is far more likely to recur than the orthokeratinized one. The parakeratinized type is much more common (88%) than the orthokeratinized one (12%). The issue of considering orthokeratinized keratocysts as separate entity is still controversial; these cysts might represent primordial cysts.
- OKs cannot be differentiated on the radiographs from nonkeratinizing dentigerous or primordial cysts.
- Odontogenic keratocysts are the most aggressive of all jaw cysts, may become large and often recur after enucleation.

- Recurrence rates of over 25% were reported; dentists should become alert to the special treatment considerations these cysts require.
- Recently it is named Odontogenic Keratocystic Tumor (KCOT) in the WHO Classification of Head and Neck Tumors, 2005.

Histogenesis

- OKs can arise from the enamel organ before amelogenesis or from the reduced dental epithelium. It was also postulated that OKs can arise form the dental lamina or its remnants.
- However, it is difficult to reconcile such origin with the appearance of OKs in middle age and their relative rapid growth. The etiology of OKs are therefore speculative.

Clinically

- Peak incidence between the ages 20 to 40 years.
- The most common site is the mandibular molar area particularly at the angle of the mandible tending to expand forward into the body of the mandible and upwards into the ramus.
- Similar to other jaw cysts, OKs are symptomless until they become large enough or they become infected.

Radiographically

- Well defined unilocular or multilocular radiolucent area surrounded by a radiopaque margin.
- It may be associated with missed or unerupted tooth.

Histologically

The epithelial lining of OKs is characteristic:

1. Thin, regular, and uniform.
2. Flat rete pegs.
3. Palisaded layer of columnar or cuboidal basal cells.
4. A corrugated layer of parakeratin.
5. Folded, due to the greater growth of the wall which exceeds expansion of the cyst.
6. Epithelial lining is weakly attached to the fibrous wall.
7. Inflammatory cells typically absent or scanty.

Treatment

- Complete enucleation trying to be certain that every fragment of the lining has been removed. Enucleation alone is likely to lead to a recurrence rate of up to 60%.
- Resection provides the lowest recurrence rate but at the expense of normal tissues.
- There is no absolute certainty of a cure, and patients should be followed up with regular radiographic examinations.
- Possible reasons for recurrence of keratocysts are:
    1. Thin fragile linings, difficult to enucleate intact.
    2. Finger-like or bud-like extensions into the cancellous bone.
    3. Daughter cysts sometimes present in the wall.
    4. More rapid proliferation of keratocyst epithelium.

Nevoid basal cell carcinoma syndrome

(Gorlin-Goltz syndrome, Gorlin syndrome, Basal cell nevus, jaw cysts, bifid rib syndrome)

- Autosomal dominantly inherited disease.
- Characterized by a triad of:
    1. Multiple basal cell carcinomas
    2. Multiple keratocysts
    3. Skeletal abnormalities usually bifid ribs
- The basic defect is caused by mutations in the patched (PTCH) tumor suppressor gene. This gene is important for the normal function of the cell cycle.
- The mutation was mapped to the chromosome 9q.
- The mutation was also found in non-syndromal tumors and cysts such as basal cell carcinoma, trichoepithelioma, medulloblastoma and sporadic keratocysts.

Calcifying epithelial odontogenic cyst

(Gorlin cyst)

Discussed in the chapter "Benign Odontogenic Tumors, page 369"

7.3 Non-odontogenic cysts

7.3.1 Fissural cysts

Fissural cysts are cysts occurring at the line of fusion of embryonic processes. The concept that face development occurs by fusion of embryonic processes

Chapter 7. Cysts & Cyst-Like Lesions

is no longer accepted by many researchers. The current concept is that what is known as embryonic processes are merely swellings rather than actual processes and their merging occurs by elimination of the furrows lying in between them. Hence the existence of the so-called fissural cysts is denied by many authors. However, the pathogenesis of some puzzling cysts can only be interpreted on the basis of fusion of embryonic processes and hence are considered as true fissural cysts.

Median Alveolar Cyst

The existence of the so-called median alveolar cyst as a fissural cyst is denied by many authors. This is because there is no line of fusion between the upper two centrals. The current view is that these cysts are either developmental lateral periodontal cysts or primordial cysts arising from the enamel organ of a supernumerary tooth.

Median Palatal Cyst

- Median palatal cysts are probably true fissural cysts arising from the epithelium entrapped at the line of fusion of the two palatine processes.
- They are presented as a small intrabony swelling in the midline of the palate.
- Care should be taken not to confuse this cyst with the incisive canal cyst which occurs at a much anterior position.
- The epithelial lining is either stratified squamous epithelium or respiratory epithelium.
- The cyst appears radiographically as a rounded well defined radiolucent area surrounded by a radiopaque margin.

- Epstein's pearls are multiple small whitish swellings found on the soft tissues of the midpalatine raphe of newly born infants (see chapter "Developmental Disturbances of Oral & Para-Oral Tissues, page (92")).

Median Mandibular Cyst

The existence of the so-called median mandibular cyst as a fissural cyst occurring between the roots of the lower centrals is also denied by many authors. The current view is that this cyst is an odontogenic cyst most probably a developmental lateral cyst which is related to one of the two mandibular central incisors.

Globulomaxillary Cyst

This cyst was traditionally described as a fissural cyst resulting from entrapped epithelium at the line of fusion of the maxillary and globular processes and occurring between the roots of the upper canine and lateral incisor. The current view is that this cyst is an odontogenic cyst most probably a developmental lateral type. There is no evidence that epithelium become entrapped at this site of fusion. The cyst was also described as being inverted pear shaped in X-ray films.

Nasolabial Cyst

- Nasolabial cysts are small soft tissue cysts occurring at the ala of the nose deep in the nasolabial fold.
- It is thought that this cyst results form the epithelium entrapped at the line of fusion of the maxillary, globular and lateral nasal processes.
- Other view is that the cyst results form cystic degeneration of the remnants of the nasolacrimal duct.

- The cyst, if allowed to grow sufficiently, will produce swelling of the upper lip and distorts the nostrils.
- The cyst is negative in X-ray films as it is a soft tissue cyst.
- The epithelial lining is usually stratified squamous epithelium, respiratory epithelium or a mixture of the two.
- Treatment is usually by surgical excision with no recurrence.

Dermoid cyst (Sublingual dermoid)

- Dermoid cysts are considered by some authors as fissural cysts arising from the ectoderm entrapped at the line of fusion of first and second branchial arches. However, this view is only speculative since the fissure between the two arches is closed by filling of mesoderm (elimination of furrow) rather than by actual fusion.
- The cyst occurs between the hyoid bone and the jaw in the floor of the mouth usually below the mylohyoid muscle. However, cysts occurring above the mylohyoid muscle have been described in the literature.
- They are filled with desquamated keratin and sebaceous material giving a cheesy consistency to its content.
- Dermoid cyst is more deeply situated than a ranula; the later is more superficial, having a thin wall and a bluish appearance.
- The cyst can interfere with speech and eating.
- The epithelial lining is keratinized stratified squamous epithelium. Respiratory epithelium (ciliated columnar) could be found in some cysts.
- Skin appendages such as hair follicles, sweat glands and sebaceous glands could be found in the connective tissue wall of the cyst.
- The epidermoid cyst closely resembles a dermoid cyst except that the former exhibits no dermal appendages. They are lined by orthokera-

tinized squamous epithelium and exhibit a lumen that is generally filled with desquamated keratin.

7.3.2 Cysts arising from embryonic vestiges (tracts)

Nasopalatine duct cysts

Nasopalatine duct cysts are cysts derived from remnants of the nasopalatine duct. These cysts may be situated inside the incisive canal as an intrabony cyst, or be situated in the soft tissue covering the incisive canal, namely the palatine papilla.

Incisive canal cyst

- Incisive canal cyst is a variant of the nasopalatine duct cyst occurring in the incisive canal.
- The cyst arises from remnants of the nasopalatine duct.
- The cyst is an intrabony cyst and presents in the X-ray films as a well defined heart shaped radiolucent area due to superimposition of the anterior nasal spine. The lower portion of the incisive canal (anterior palatine fossa) should be differentially diagnosed from the incisive canal cyst. The maximum size of the fossa is up to 6 or 7 mm.
- Occasionally, the cyst cause intermitted discharge with a salty taste.
- The epithelial lining is usually either stratified squamous epithelium or ciliated columnar (respiratory) or both.
- Mucous glands and neurovascular bundle are sometimes present in the connective tissue wall. These are the long sphenopalatine nerve and vessels which pass through the incisive canal and are often removed with the cyst.
- Treatment is by enucleation and recurrence is rare.

Palatine papilla cyst

- This is the soft tissue counterpart of the incisive canal cyst.
- The cyst appears as a small soft tissue swelling of the palatine papilla.
- A salty discharge can be felt by some patients.
- The cyst is negative in X-ray
- Treated by excision with no recurrence.

Thyroglossal tract cyst

Discussed in the chapter of "Developmental Disturbances of Oral & Para-Oral Tissues", page (88)

Cyst-like lesions

Aneurysmal bone cyst

- Aneurysmal bone cysts are lesions of unknown nature most probably representing vascular malformations of bone or unusual reaction of bone against unknown injury or irritant.
- Clinically, most patients are between 10 and 20 years of age and usually affecting the mandibular molar area with possibility of extension into the angle and the ramus. Lesions usually appear as painless slowly growing swellings. However, 50% of patients may experience pain, discomfort or tenderness.
- Characterized by profuse bleeding at surgery and the lesion appears as a blood-soaked sponge.
- **Radiographically**, the lesion usually appears as multilocular radiolucent area soap bubble or honey comb in appearance.
- **Histopathology**, ABC consists of large blood-filled spaces separated by fibrous septa. The septa are composed of connective tissue containing

osteoid deposits, spicules of woven bone, and deposits of hemosidrin. Varying numbers of multinucleated giant cells may be observed. The picture is typically similar to other giant cell lesions.
- **Treatment**, ABC is usually treated by curettage.

Traumatic bone cyst

(Solitary bone cyst, Simple bone cyst, Hemorrhagic bone cyst, Idiopathic bone cyst)

- A condition of unknown nature consisting of an intrabony empty cavity.
- It is postulated that the cyst results from trauma followed by intrabony hemorrhage followed by failure of organization and repair of bone.
- However, there is little evidence to support this theory as blood filled spaces are formed in the jaws as a consequence of enucleation of true cysts, but solitary bone cysts do not arise as a result. Furthermore, a common form of treatment of solitary bone cysts is to open the cysts to allow bleeding into the cavity and normal healing then follows.
- **Clinically**, the predominant site of occurrence is the molar/premolar region of the mandible. Most lesions occur in patients under 20 years of age. A slight female predilection has been reported. Lesions are asymptomatic and are generally discovered during routine radiographic examination. Surgical exploration of the lesion reveals a cavity that may be empty or contains a small amount of straw colored fluid.
- **Radiographically**, traumatic bone cyst appears as a well-circumscribed, solitary radiolucency of variable size. Larger lesions frequently extend between the roots of the associated teeth to produce a scalloped appearance that is characteristic of this lesion. Although buccal or lingual cortical expansion of the mandible is usually absent, it has been reported in some cases.

- **Histopathology**, tissue obtained from the wall of the lesion reveals a thin layer of loose and delicate connective tissue overlying a zone of reactive bone.
- **Treatment**, surgical hemorrhage induced during diagnostic exploration and curettage of the cavity is usually all that is required to achieve complete resolution of the lesion. Spontaneous resolution was reported in some cases.

Latent bone cyst

Discussed in the chapter "Developmental Disturbances of Oral & Para-Oral Tissues", page (90).

7.3.3 Cysts of salivary glands:

Discussed in the chapter of "Diseases of Salivary Glands", page (416)

7.3.4 Other soft tissue cysts

Lymphoepithelial cysts

Lymphoepithelial cysts are cysts characterized by presence of normal lymphoid follicles in their connective tissue wall. They occur in several areas of the head and neck. That occurring in the oral cavity are termed oral lymphoepithelial cysts and those occurring on the lateral aspect of the neck are termed cervical lymphoepithelial cysts. Although lymphoepithelial cysts of the oral cavity are smaller than those on the neck, their histologic features are the same.

Oral lymphoepithelial cyst

- A soft tissue cyst which appears as a symptomless, small yellow to white submucosal mass usually measuring less than 1 cm in diameter.

- It develops where extratonsillar lymphoid tissue is found. Therefore, the most common site is the floor of the mouth, the posterior lateral border of the tongue, undersurface of the tongue, oropharynx and soft palate.

- Their origin is unclear; it may result from entrapment of epithelial invaginations (crypts) into the lymphoid tissue. In support for this postulate, is the occasional presence of a small pore or crypt that communicates the cystic cavity with the oral mucosa. The presence of bacteria within the cystic cavity is further evidence that communication with the oral cavity is present.

- **Histologically**, the cyst consists of:
    1. A small, keratin-filled cavity.
    2. Lined by keratinized squamous epithelium.
    3. A layer of lymphoid tissue with germinal centers which partially or completely surrounds the cyst.

- This cyst is thought to be a miniature variety of the larger branchial cleft cyst (cervical lymphoepithelial cyst) that occurs in the neck anterior to the sternocleidomastoid muscle from the ear to the clavicle.

Cervical lymphoepithelial cyst

(Branchial cleft cyst, Benign cystic lymph node)

- This is a developmental cyst occurring on the side of the neck anterior to the sternocleidomastoid muscle.

- It is thought to be derived from epithelium entrapped within lymphoid tissues of the neck during embryologic development of the cervical sinuses or the second branchial clefts or pouches. The cervical sinus is a primitive structure found in young mammalian embryos as a depression in the nuchal region (back of the neck) caudal to the hyoid arch; normally it is obliterated after the second month, but occasionally cervical fistulae persist as vestiges of it.
- **Clinically**, the cyst becomes apparent in late childhood or adulthood as a painless swelling on the lateral aspect of the neck anterior to the sternomastoid muscle. A draining fistula that communicates between the cyst and the overlying skin surface occasionally develops.
- **Histopathology**, the cyst lumen is usually lined with a thinned, stratified squamous epithelium and contains desquamated orthokeratin. The connective tissue contains large numbers of well-formed lymphoid follicles.
- **Treatment**, the cyst is treated by conservative surgical excision; recurrence is rare.

7.3.5 Cysts of the Maxillary Antrum

Figure (7.2) illustrates the different types of maxillary sinus cysts.

Pseudocysts of the maxillary sinus

The only example is the Antral Pseudocyst

Antral pseudocyst

- This condition continues to be inappropriately termed sinus mucocele or sinus retention cyst by many clinicians.

- The lesion appears as a dome-shaped, faintly radiopaque lesion often arising from the floor of the maxillary sinus.
- The antral pseudocyst develops due to an accumulation of an inflammatory exudate (serum, not mucus) under the maxillary sinus mucosa, causing a sessile elevation. It must be stressed that the edematous fluid is in the stroma underneath the epithelium, not surrounded by it.

True cysts of the sinus

Antral cyst (antral mucocele)

- This type of cysts results from an obstruction of the *sinus ostium*, thus blocking normal drainage. This blocked sinus then acts like a separate cyst-like structure lined by epithelium and filled with mucus.
- Sinus mucoceles enlarge in size as the intraluminal pressure increases and can distend the walls of the sinus and erode through bone; they often clinically mimic malignancy of sinus origin.
- Sinus mucocele is a distinct, separate pathologic entity that is unrelated to the common mucocele of minor salivary gland origin

Surgical ciliated cyst (traumatic ciliated cyst, or postoperative maxillary cyst)

- A portion of the sinus lining becomes separated from the main body of the sinus and forms an epithelium-lined cavity into which mucus is secreted.
- The cyst most frequently originates after a Caldwell-Luc operation but may arise from difficult extraction of a maxillary tooth in which the floor of the maxillary sinus is damaged.

Chapter 7. Cysts & Cyst-Like Lesions

Always Remember

Cysts of the Maxillary Sinus
- Pseudocyst
  - Antral Pseudocyst
- True cysts
  - Aantral mucocele (Antral cyst)
  - Surgical ciliated cyst
  - Retention Cyst of the Maxillary Sinus

Note

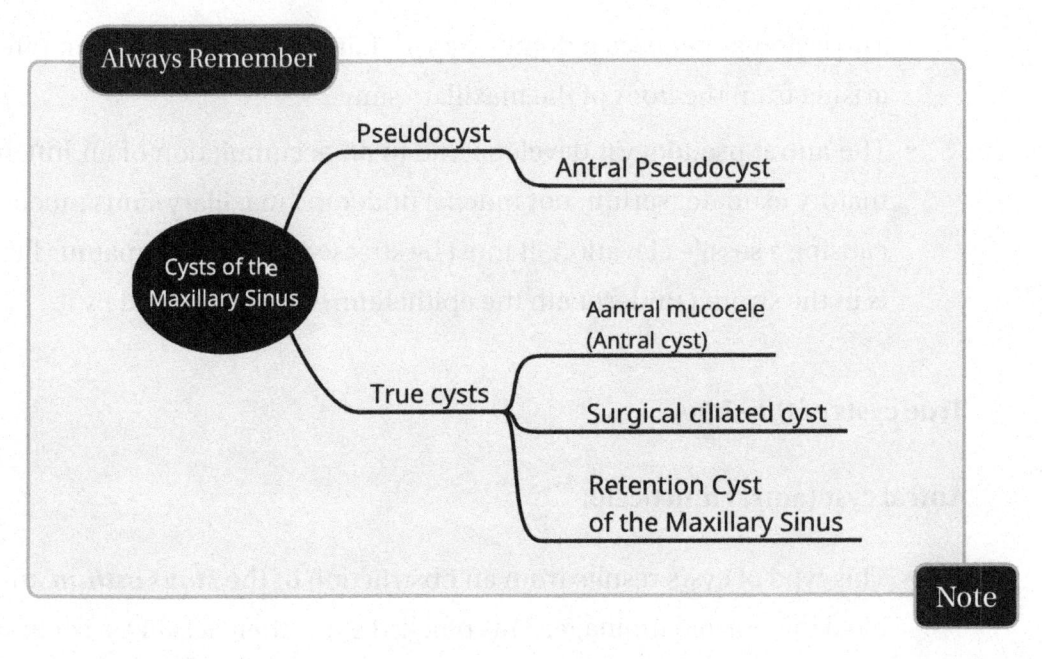

Figure 7.2: Proposed classification for cysts of the maxillary sinus.

- In addition, sinus or nasal epithelium rarely can be transplanted accidentally to the mandible during genioplasty or chin augmentation procedures and lead to formation of ciliated cysts in ectopic locations

Retention Cyst of the Maxillary Sinus

- These lesions result from the partial blockage of a seromucous gland duct within the sinus wall, or from an invagination of the respiratory epithelium.
- Most retention cysts are located around the ostium or within antral polyps.
- The majority of retention cysts are small, not evident clinically, and discovered during histopathologic examination of antral polyps.

CHAPTER 8
PHYSICAL, CHEMICAL AND IDIOPATHIC PATHOLOGY OF TEETH

Pathological changes in the dental tissues that include a variety of alterations, which are neither inflammatory nor developmental, have been traditionally described in older literature as "***regressive alterations of teeth***". Some of these lesions may be associated with the general aging process, while others arise because of injury to the dental tissues or other obscure causes.

8.1 Attrition

Definition

- It is defined as the increased *physiologic* mechanical wearing down of the teeth due to tooth-to-tooth contact.
- The condition is not pathologic and not related to dental caries. Attrition is severe on teeth of patients who habitually clench and grind their teeth (bruxism).

Clinically

Age Old age. Occasionally, children may suffer from attrition if dentinogenesis or amelogenesis imperfecta are present.

Sex Males are affected more than females, probably because of the greater masticatory forces.

Site Occlusal, incisal and proximal surfaces are the only surfaces affected. With malocclusion other surfaces can be affected.

Shape

1. At first, attrition appears as a small polished area on the cusp tips, or as slight flattening of the incisal edge.
2. As the person becomes older and the wear continues, there is gradual reduction in the cusp height and flattening of the occlusal surfaces.
3. Advanced attrition may cause wearing down of the full thickness of enamel with yellowish or brownish coloration of the exposed dentin. Since the process is slow, attrition leads to progressive secondary dentin formation. In rare cases, severe attrition in old persons might result in teeth worn down to the gingival margins.

The amount of attrition is dependent upon:

1. Age, the older the person the more attrition is expected
2. Sex, males being affected more than females
3. Consistency of diet. Persons usually eating coarse diet suffer more attrition
4. Habits such as chewing tobacco or *bruxism* (grinding of teeth) may predispose to more rapid attrition
5. Structure of the teeth (degree of mineralization)
6. Extraction of a number of teeth will increase the load of mastication on the reminder

Bruxism

Bruxism is the term given to periodic repetitive clenching or rhythmic forceful grinding of the teeth. Some 10–20% of the population report the habit but the incidence rises to 90% when mild subconscious grinding is included.

8.2 Abrasion

Definition

Is the *pathological* mechanical wearing away of the tooth substance due to vigorous mechanical processes.

Clinically:

- Vigorous (forceful) use of a hard tooth brush in a horizontal direction. The areas most severely affected are the labial or buccal surfaces of the necks of the teeth. The lesion appears as a v-shaped or wedge-shaped ditch on the root side of the cemento-enamel junction. In a right-handed person the left canine and premolars are usually most severely affected.
- With abrasion, the gingival margin recess exposing the coronal part of the root. Cementum and then dentin become exposed and eventually grooves are worn into the neck of the teeth. The gingival recession although severe but usually accompanied with healthy gingiva, because the vigorous tooth brushing remove plaque from around the teeth and leaves the gingiva pale, firm and tightly attached.
- Certain habits or occupations that involve biting or habitual placement of foreign objects between the teeth might cause abrasion. For example,

opening of hair pins with the teeth might cause notching in the incisal edge. Also, carpenters who hold nails or pins between their teeth.

8.3 Erosion

Definition

Is the pathologic loss (dissolution) of tooth substance by chemicals, usually non-bacterial acids.

Clinically

The lesion appears as a shallow, broad, smooth area not chalky in appearance occurring on the enamel surface of the cemento-enamel junction.

Causes

The cause of erosion might be:

1. Exposure to acids from an external source such as:
    - Occupational (battery manufactures) where there is exposure to acid fumes
    - Habitual ingestion of large amounts of citrus fruits or apples. In such case the gingival one third of the labial surfaces of several anterior teeth are affected
2. Exposure to acids from an internal source. This occurs in patients suffering from chronic *regurgitation* of the gastric contents (acids) as a result of chronic vomiting. The pattern of erosion in such case is usually generalized affecting both the buccal and lingual surfaces of the teeth.

8.4 Abfraction

Definition

Loss of tooth surface at the cervical areas of teeth during tooth flexure (bending).

Causes

The exact etiology is controversial. But the condition appears to results from excessive tensile and compressive forces on the tooth causing the enamel to "pop" off starting at the base of the tooth.

Clinically

- Abfraction represents cervical erosions that can not be attributed to any particular cause.
- Appears as a wedge-shaped notching at cervical areas of involved teeth.

Treatment

- Consists of the application of composite resin or glass-ionomer cement restorations
- Removal of the cause, if possible (correction of malocclusion).

8.5 Dentinal Sclerosis

(*Transparent Dentin, Translucent Dentin, Sclerotic Dentin*)

Chapter 8. Physical, Chemical & Idiopathic Pathology of Teeth

Definition

This is defined as the over calcification of dentin through the deposition of calcium salts on the internal wall of the dentinal tubules.

Causes

Dentinal sclerosis occurs as a result of the following:

1. As an age change in dentin.
2. As a result of injury to the dentin by caries or abrasion. This represents a defense reaction of the dentin against the penetrating acid or the irritation.

   The increased mineralization or sclerosis of the dentinal tubules decreases the conductivity of dentin.

8.6 Secondary dentin and Tertiary dentin

dentin is formed either under physiologic or pathologic conditions.

1. Secondary dentin, termed in the old literature as "physiologic secondary dentin", which starts to form just after complete root formation and is considered as an age change in dentin. The secondary dentin formed is usually similar in appearance to the primary dentin, but with fewer tubules.

2. Tertiary dentin, termed also in the old literature as, "pathologic secondary dentin" is formed as a result of stimulation of the exposed dentinal tubules and odontoblastic processes by irritation from caries, attrition, abrasion, erosion, and fracture or cavity preparation. The formed tertiary dentin is usually irregular in nature and is composed of fewer dentinal tubules having a tortuous course. Sometimes the odontoblasts

become completely entrapped in the rapidly formed dentin, which thus resembles bone and is therefore called osteodentin. For further details, see tables (8.1), (8.2) and figure ((8.1)).

Table 8.1: Types of Dentin

Main Types of Dentin

1. Primary dentin forms most of the tooth. It is the dentin which forms during tooth development and ends when roots are completely formed. The outer layer closest to enamel is known as mantle dentin.
2. Secondary dentin develops after root formation is complete and forms much slower than primary dentin
3. Tertiary dentin forms as a biological response to stimuli such as caries. Tertiary dentin is only formed by cells directly affected by stimulus, therefore the architecture and structure depends on the intensity and duration of the stimulus. Tertiary dentin is of two types:
   (a) Reactionary, where dentin is formed from a pre-existing odontoblast
   (b) Reparative, where dentin is formed from newly differentiated odontoblast-like cells that develop from a pulpal progenitor cell due death of the original odontoblasts.

8.7 Pulp Calcification

Refer to chapter "(6)", page (154)

8.8 Resorption of Teeth

Resorption of the roots of the deciduous teeth is a physiologic process where pressure from the underlying successors causes progressive root resorption

Table 8.2: Predentin

> **What is Predentin**
> - Newly secreted dentin is unmineralized and is called predentin.
> - It is easily identified in haematoxylin and eosin stained section since it stains less intensely then dentin.
> - It is usually 10–47 micrometer and lines the innermost region of the dentin.
> - It is unmineralized and consists of collagen, glycoproteins and proteoglycans. It is similar to osteoid in bone and is thickest when dentinogenesis is occurring.

and ultimate loosening and shedding. Resorption may also affect the permanent teeth and is then regarded as a pathological condition. The mechanism remains the same, i.e. osteoclastic activity, but the stimulus is abnormal. Whenever resorption takes place, there is virtually always some attempt at repair by apposition of cementum or bone; resorption and cementosis must be regarded as closely associated processes.

There are two types of pathological resorption:

1. External resorption, this occurs on the external surface of the root or the crown and extends inwards into the pulp. It is the result of a tissue reaction in the periodontal or pericoronal tissue respectively.
2. Internal resorption, this occurs on the inside of the tooth and extends outwards in a uniform pattern towards the tooth surface. It results from a pulpal tissue reaction.

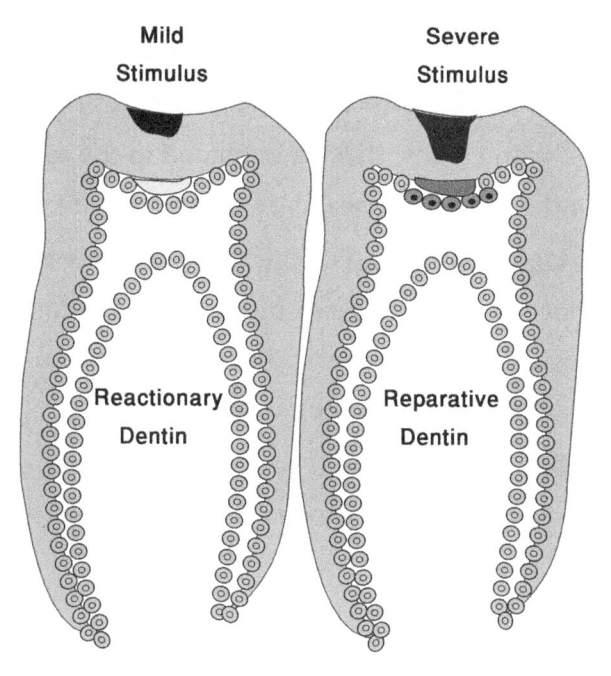

Figure 8.1: Reactionary dentin vs reparative dentin. Left panel shows reactionary dentin in which dentin matrix is secreted by surviving post-mitotic odontoblasts in response to mild stimulus. The right panel shows reparative dentin in which the matrix is secreted by a new generation of odontoblast-like cells in response to severe stimulus, after the death of the original post-mitotic odontoblasts.

8.8.1 External Resorption

Definition

This is the resorption of teeth from external surfaces, usually affecting roots.

Causes

1. **Chronic inflammatory lesions (Inflammatory Resorption)**
    - Inflammatory resorption typically involves the apical portion of the root, as a result of periapical inflammation following pulp necro-

Chapter 8. Physical, Chemical & Idiopathic Pathology of Teeth

sis or trauma, and is associated with a periapical radiolucency on a radiograph. However, there is no ankylosis.

- The pathogenesis has been related to the release of chemical mediators, increased vascularity, and pressure.
- Periapical granuloma, which is a highly vascular mass of granulation tissue usually causing bone resorption and less commonly causing root resorption. This root resorption appears in the X-ray as slight blunting in the root apex.
- Endodontically treated teeth, in which periapical inflammation persists may occur leaving the filling projecting out of the shortened root.

2. **Cysts**
   - Cysts can also cause root resorption by pressure, which stimulates the differentiation of osteoclasts.
   - The periodontal cyst is the most common cyst causing resorption.

3. **Benign tumors and malignant neoplasms.**
   - Both benign and malignant tumors produce root resorption through the pressure they create.
   - However, benign lesions are more likely to produce displacement rather than actual destruction of the tooth.

4. **Trauma, excessive mechanical or occlusal forces**
   - Trauma that causes injury to or necrosis of the periodontal ligament may initiate resorption of tooth roots. This trauma may be from a single event, from malocclusion, or from excessive orthodontic forces. Trauma causing injury to the periodontal ligament may initiate resorption of the tooth root.
   - Root resorption associated with pressure/mechanical stimulation may be seen in patients undergoing orthodontic treatment and can be caused by the application of excessive force. It occurs in

the apical region and the resorbed area undergoes repair and remodeling when the cause is removed.

- It is possible that excess force could cause an aseptic necrosis of the periodontal ligament, followed by inflammation.

5. **Reimplantation or transplantation of teeth**
   - Reimplanted teeth, whether root canal filled or not, are non-vital tissues that usually undergo resorption.
   - The resorbed area is replaced by bone and can produce ankylosis.

6. **Impactions**
   - Impacted teeth, when they impinge or exert pressure on adjacent teeth, may cause root resorption of the otherwise normally erupted tooth.
   - The crown of the impacted tooth usually remains intact; this is because the tissue most resorbed is cementum, while enamel is the most resistant.
   - Impacted teeth themselves may occasionally undergo resorption. The cause of this phenomenon is unknown, although it is believed to be related to a partial loss of the protective effect of the periodontal ligament or reduced enamel epithelium, allowing the connective tissue to come in contact with the crown or root and thus initiating the resorptive process.

7. **Idiopathic external resorption**
   - A rare type of resorption affecting multiple teeth is seen in young women.
   - Any tooth may be involved, although molars are least likely to be affected.
   - Idiopathic resorption is particularly frustrating for both patients and practitioners because there is no plausible or evident explanation for the condition and no effective treatment.

- The cervical portions of the roots resorb, leaving only unsupported crowns that must then be extracted.
- The cause of this resorption is unknown, thus the name idiopathic external resorption.

Histologically

- Microscopic areas of superficial (surface) resorption of the roots of permanent teeth are common but are transient and are repaired by the apposition of cementum or of a bone-like tissue. Such microscopic foci are of no clinical consequence. In contrast, resorption sufficient to be diagnosed radiologically is always pathological.
- Pathological resorption start from the root surface, osteoclast-like giant cells (sometimes called odontoclasts) sitting in resorption lacunae are seen on actively resorbing surfaces. However, as resorption is not a continuous process the osteoclast-like cells are not always present and in this case some resorption lacunae may show attempts at repair.

Treatment

- Removal of the cause, if possible
- Hopeless teeth are extracted

8.8.2 Internal Resorption

(Chronic Proliferating Pulp Hyperplasia - Pink Spot)

- This is a form of tooth resorption in which the dentin is resorbed from within the pulp. This condition might affect the pulp chamber or root canal.

Table 8.3: Principle Causes of External Resorption of Teeth

> **External Resorption**
>
> 1. Chronic inflammatory lesions (Inflammatory Resorption) Cysts
> 2. Benign and malignant neoplasms.
> 3. Trauma, excessive mechanical or occlusal forces
> 4. Reimplantation or transplantation of teeth
> 5. Impactions
> 6. Idiopathic external resorption

- The resorption occurs as a result of the activation of osteoclast or dentinoclasts on internal surfaces of the root or crown. In time, the root or crown is perforated by the process, making the tooth useless.

Causes

- Exactly unknown but it is suggested that it may results from a low-grade pulpal inflammation.
- However some cases are completely idiopathic and occur without apparent cause.

Clinically

- Usually a single tooth is affected, although rarely, may affect more than one tooth.
- Usually localized giving the characteristic sign of a well-defined rounded area of radiolucency in the tooth.

- Internal resorption in the crown appears as a pink area because of the proximity of pulp tissue to the tooth surface and the condition may be termed *"pink spot"*.
- Internal resorption in the root usually causes no signs or symptoms until the root fractures.

Histologically

1. Vascular granulation tissue, whcih replaces the pulp tissue with osteoclasts (odontoclasts) bordering the affected dentin or enamel.
2. Chronic inflammatory cell infiltrate and increased vascularity of the pulp tissue.
3. Reversal lines may also be found in the adjacent hard tissue, indicating attempts at repair.
4. Areas of irregular bone formation may be seen.

Treatment

- If a pink-spot in an incisor tooth is noticed at an early stage, pulp extirpation and root canal treatment are indicated before the pulp becomes exposed.
- In case of root internal resorption, once there is communication between pulp and periodontal ligament, the prognosis for saving the tooth is very poor.
- The process occasionally may spontaneously stop for no apparent reason.

8.9 Hypercementosis (Cementum Hyperplasia)

Definition

- A condition characterized by the deposition of excessive amounts of cementum on the root surface
- It may affect one or several teeth and may be associated with root ankylosis, when cementum is directly continuous with the alveolar bone.
- Hypercementosis may be idiopathic or the result of local or general disorders.

Causes

1. **Periapical Inflammation**

   Although resorption of cementum may occur close to the center of the inflammatory focus, apposition of cementum may be stimulated a little further away. This produces a generalized thickening of the cementum or a localized knob-like enlargement.

2. **Mechanical Stimulation**

   Excessive forces applied to a tooth may produce resorption, but mechanical stimulation below a certain threshold may stimulate apposition of cementum.

3. **Functionless and Unerupted Teeth**

   Such teeth may show areas of cementum resorption, but excessive apposition of cementum may also occur. In unerupted teeth the cementum may even extend over the surface of the enamel if the reduced enamel epithelium is lost.

4. **Accelerated elongation of a tooth**

Loss of a tooth may be followed by elongation of its antagonist accompanied by hyperplasia of the cementum to maintain the normal width of the periodontal ligament.

5. **Root repair**

   In cases of root fracture, healing is through the deposition of new cementum growing into and filling the fractured area.

6. **Paget's Disease of Bone**

   Hypercementosis is often seen in teeth of patients with Paget's disease, the thickened cementum showing a mosaic appearance analogous to that seen in the bone. The cementum forms irregular masses and ankylosis of the tooth is common.

7. **Idiopathic**

   Some cases occur without apparent cause.

8.10   Hypocementosis

- Hypoplasia and aplasia of cementum are rare.
- In cleidocranial dysplasia there is a lack of cellular cementum following the deposition of acellular cementum.
- Aplasia of cementum is seen in hypophosphatasia: a recessive autosomal disease, characterized by a reduced serum alkaline phosphatase level and skeletal abnormalities. Premature loss of some or all deciduous and permanent teeth is seen.

8.11   Tooth Ankylosis

- Is the fusion of the cementum or dentin to the surrounding bone after loss of the intervening periodontal ligament.

- This will result in cessation of eruption. Normally, eruption continues after the emergence of the teeth to compensate for masticatory wear and the growth of the jaws
- Other terms for this process within the literature include infraocclusion, secondary retention, submergence, reimpaction, and reinclusion
- The periodontal ligament (PDL) might act as a barrier that prevents osteoblasts from applying bone directly onto cementum
- The pathogenesis of ankylosis is not exactly known and may be secondary to trauma or local inflammatory process
- Chronic or acute trauma, either of which can cause inflammation and destruction of the periodontal ligament. Autoimplanted or reimplanted avulsed teeth in which the periodontal membrane has been destroyed usually undergo some degree of ankylosis if they are not lost by external resorption. In general, nearly any factor that can cause external root resorption has the potential to result in ankylosis. This includes rapid orthodontic movement, periapical infections, and occlusal traumatism.
- On rare occasions, long-standing impacted teeth will become ankylosed. Often the impacted tooth is not completely ankylosed but fused only in one or two areas.
- The most common example of ankylosis is the submerged (retained) deciduous molar, usually located in the second mandibular premolar location. The submerged appearance occurs because the occlusal table of the retained smaller deciduous molar is located below the rest of the teeth in the arch. In many cases it is merely a deciduous tooth that has not yet undergone normal root resorption, allowing it to be shed in the proper time. In such situations if an underlying premolar is present, it will either remain impacted or will eventually erupt buccally or lingually in the arch, resulting in local malocclusion.

- Several authors believe genetic predisposition has a significant influence and point to monozygotic twins who demonstrate strikingly similar patterns of ankylosis to support this hypothesis
- Ankylosis may occur at any age; however, clinically the condition is most obvious if the fusion develops during the first two decades of life.
- Although any tooth may be affected, the most commonly involved teeth is in the following order of frequency are the mandibular primary first molar, the mandibular primary second molar, the maxillary primary first molar, and the maxillary primary second molar. Ankylosis of permanent teeth is rare. In the deciduous dentition, mandibular teeth are affected 10 times as often as the maxillary dentition.
- The occlusal plane of the involved tooth is below that of the adjacent dentition (infraocclusion).
- A sharp, solid sound may be noted on percussion of the involved tooth but can be detected only when more than 20% of the root is fused to the bone.
- Radiographically, absence of the PDL space may be noted; however, the area of fusion is often in the bifurcation and interradicular root surface, making radiographic detection most difficult.
- Ankylosed teeth that are allowed to remain in position can lead to a number of dental problems. The adjacent teeth often incline toward the affected tooth. In addition, the opposing teeth often exhibit over-eruption. Occasionally, the ankylosed tooth leads to a localized deficiency of the alveolar ridge or impaction of the underlying permanent tooth.
- Because they are fused to the adjacent bone, ankylosed teeth fail to respond to normal orthodontic forces, with attempts to move the ankylosed tooth occasionally resulting in movement of the anchor teeth.

- Making an accurate assessment that a tooth may be ankylosed is very important, when extraction by luxation is performed. Failure to do so usually results in root breakage and fracture of the surrounding alveolar bone. The most effective aid to diagnosis is the availability of periapical radiographs that demonstrate the presence or absence of a uniform periodontal space.

- Recommended treatment for ankylosis of primary molars is variable and often is determined by the severity and timing of the process. When an underlying permanent successor is present, extraction of the ankylosed primary molar should not be performed until it becomes obvious that exfoliation is not proceeding normally or adverse occlusal changes are developing. After extraction of an ankylosed molar, the permanent tooth will erupt spontaneously in the majority of cases. In permanent teeth or primary teeth without underlying successors are treated best by distraction osteogenesis.

8.12 Tooth Concussion

- No displacement or loosening.
- Crushing injury to adjoining areas and blood vessels.
- Early radiographic changes may be minimal.
- Widened widened periodontal ligament spaces: few days to weeks.
- Long term effects: pulpal sclerosis, necrosis, periapical lesions.

8.13 Tooth Luxation

- Dislocation of teeth: Intrusion, extrusion, lateral, lingual or buccal.
- Early radiographic observation: Widened periodontal ligament spaces.

- Long term effect: Pulpal sclerosis, necrosis, periapical lesion.

8.14 Tooth Avulsion

- Loss of tooth.
- Socket outline in radiographic picture.
- Fracture of alveolar bone.
- Possibility of reimplantation.

Chapter 9
Spread of Dental Infection

Dental infection, if not treated properly, will not remain localized and can spread locally and systemically to affect other tissues.

9.1 Basic Definitions

Abscess Versus Cellulitis

Cellulitis is a diffuse infection of the soft tissues with no localized area of pus susceptible to drainage. The affected area is described as indurated, warm, red, and swollen. It is also painful. A component of lymphangitis (infection involving the lymphatics) is indicated by red lines, progressing from the affected area.

An ***abscess*** is a localized collection of pus, often with an area of surrounding cellulitis. One sign of an abscess is that it is fluctuant i.e. when you apply gentle digital pressure over the area, you can push and feel a "give," indicating the presence of fluid underneath. Another sign is that an abscess often seems to "point;" that is, the skin starts to thin from the pressure of the fluid underneath. The distinction between cellullitis and abscess is important. The main treatment for an abscess is incision and drainage (cutting into the abscess and widely opening the abscess cavity). Cellulitis does not need this intervention.

In cellulitis and abscess the causative organisms are usually streptococcus and staphylococcus are the most frequent aerobic bacterial, whereas bacteroids sp. is the predominant anaerobic pathogen.

9.2 Introduction to Dental Infections

- Odontogenic Infections are one of the most common causes of sever infectious swellings in the head and neck region.
- Examples of odontogenic infections include:
    1. Periapical Abscesses
    2. Pericoronitis
    3. Suppurative Osteomyelitis
    4. An infection in the Socket Following Extraction
    5. Alveolar Osteitis

9.3 Methods of Spread of Odontogenic infections

Infections usually tend to spread From Local areas related to the infected tooth to remote areas through the following routes:

1. Local Spread:

    Infections spread locally through tissue fluids.

2. Lymphatic Spread:

    Odontogenic infections are drained by lymphatic vessels to the regional lymph nodes (e.g. submental and submandibular lymph nodes). This usually leads to the Inflammation of the lymph node (lymphadenitis).

3. Hematological Spread:

Pathogenic bacteria invade the blood through the injured blood vessels and may be carried to remote areas of the body. These microorganisms may cause the inflammation of the walls of veins (thrombophlebitis); Producing thrombi and septic emboli in the systemic circulation resulting in bacteremia, pyemia or septicemia.

Unlike the other veins of the human body, veins of the head and neck region are *valveless*, where it is allowed for blood to move in both directions, but in fact, gravity causes blood to move towards the heart. Subsequently pathogenic bacteria in veins of the head and neck region could move in either direction.

- Role of Emissary Veins in the Spread of Odontogenic Infections:
  * Emissary Veins are those veins that pass through the Skull foramina to connect intracranial veins (dural venous Sinuses) with extra cranial veins. There are nine emissary veins (2 from Superior Sagittal sinus, 3 from sigmoid sinus and 4 from Cavernous sinus).
  * In odontogenic infections, bacteria in the extra cranial emissary veins can gain access to the intracranial veins leading to cavernous Sinus thrombosis (see later on this chapter).

4. Spread along the fascial spaces:
   - Dental infections usually spread through the fascial spaces (discussed Later on this chapter).

9.4 Factors governing the spread of dental infection

Three factors govern the spread of dental infection namely: microbial factors, host physiological factors and host anatomical factors.

9.4.1 Microbial Factors:

Streptococci and *Staphylococci* seem to be accused of exerting a considerable influence on the fate and pathogenesis of the infection and probably their rate of spreading infection.

It has been evident that not only does the type of bacteria or its virulence factors play an important role in dental infections, but also the number of microorganisms invading the tissues.

9.4.2 Host Factors:

Host Physiological Factors:

1. The nutritional status of the patient: Maxillofacial infections may affect the nutritional status of the patient through interfering with food intake caused by trismus or dysphagia, helping in the loss of fluids and electrolytes due to fever and the increased demand for cellular energy. Thus it is clear that infections worsen the nutritional status of the patient, which itself may aggravate the infectious process.

2. The immunological mechanism and state: The immune system plays an important role in limiting the infectious process as well as eliminating the invading microorganism. Consequently Patients with compromised health or those with immunodeficiency diseases might experience more severe forms of maxillofacial infections.

Host Anatomical Factors:

Anatomical Factors play a great role in the spread of dental infections to the maxillofacial region. The position of teeth in alveolus and their relation to the surrounding tissues and structures determine in which path the infection would be expected to spread.

1. Position of the tooth in the Alveolus
   - Maxillary teeth: vary in their position in the alveolus. Infection will go through the areas of least resistance. Maxillary central incisors, canines and buccal roots of the premolars and molars are covered by thin plate of bone, so infection is seen buccally. Whereas the maxillary lateral incisor and the palatal roots of the premolars and molars are much closer to the palatal cortical plate, Therefore infection will be seen palatally.
   - Mandibular teeth: In mandibular incisors and premolars, Infections tend to be labially. On the other hand the lower first and second molar is centrally localized in the alveolus thus infection may be buccally or lingually.
2. Relation of the tooth apex to the surrounding muscles attachments
   - The relation of the tooth apex to muscle attachments plays a great role in the determination of the destination where the infection might spread into.
   - It is worthy to mention the differences in the anatomical positions of teeth and their surroundings among individuals, which will shape the diverse clinical appearances of odontogenic infections among the different patients.

9.5 Complications associated with the spread of dental infection

- Odontogenic infections are among the most frequently infections in man. In the vast majority of patients. these infections are minor and resolve either by spontaneous drainage through the gingival tissues, oral mucosa or by extraction of the offending tooth.

- Removal of the offending tooth almost always results in rapid resolution of the infection, even without antibiotic therapy.
- Unfortunately, these minor tooth-related infections occasionally become serious and life-threatening.

9.5.1 Ludwig's Angina

Definition

- This is a severe cellulitis of the submental, sublingual and submandibular spaces bilaterally. It is a serious, potentially life-threatening cellulitis.
- Thus in this disease, five spaces are affected: The bilateral Submandibular spaces, the bilateral sublingual spaces, and the Submental space.

Predisposing causes

Include lowered resistance of the general health plus bad oral hygiene.

Exciting cause

Passage of bacteria and their toxins through the mandibular root into the surgical spaces. Tonsillitis and sialadenitis may start the condition.

Responsible teeth

Usually the lower second and third molars are responsible because of:

1. Their apices are nearer to the lingual plate of bone.
2. Their apices lie below the level of attachment of the mylohyoid muscle so pus will reach the spaces instead of opening into the oral cavity.

Paths of spread

After infecting the sublingual spaces, infection passes:

1. To the submandibular space.
2. To sublingual spaces of the other side
3. To the lateral pharyngeal space, into the pharyngeal muscle and to the glottis.

Bacteriology

Responsible bacteria are *Streptococci* (hemolytic, non-hemolytic and viridance), *Staphylococci* (aureus and albus), *Spirochetes* and *Fusiform Bacilli*.

Clinically

There is rapid swelling in the sublingual and submandibular regions, edema and inflammatory exudate are observed. Pain is severe; the tongue is raised causing difficulty in swallowing and in respiration. If the glottis becomes edematous, suffocation and death result. Headache, temperature and rigors are present.

Complications:

Ludwig's angina may spread to include:

1. The glottis causing suffocation
2. The lateral pharyngeal space causing phlebitis of the internal jugular
3. The mediastinal spaces by spreading downwards
4. The pterygopalatine fossa with passage of infection through emissary veins to the cavernous sinus inside the skull causing its thrombosis, and starting a dangerous form of meningitis

5. The lungs causing pneumonia
6. The blood stream causing septicemia

Treatment

- Maintain the airway either by tubing or by tracheostomy.
- Antibiotics, given intravenous until symptoms subside followed by oral doses till complete recovery.
- Dental treatment may be needed to treat tooth infections that caused Ludwig's angina.
- Incision and drainage may be needed to drain pus.

9.5.2 Cavernous Sinus Thrombosis

- Cavernous sinus thrombosis is the formation of a blood clot within the cavernous sinus, a cavity at the base of the brain which drains deoxygenated blood from the brain back to the heart.
- The cause is usually from a spreading infection in the nose, sinuses, ears, or teeth. Staphylococcus aureus and Streptococcus are often the associated bacteria.
- Cavernous sinus thrombosis symptoms include: decrease or loss of vision, chemosis[1], exophthalmos (bulging eyes), headaches, and paralysis of the cranial nerves which course through the cavernous sinus.
- This infection is life-threatening and requires immediate treatment, usually includes antibiotics and sometimes surgical drainage.

9.5.3 Bacteremia

- Is the presence of bacteria circulating in the blood.

---

[1] edema of the mucous membrane of the eyeball and eyelid lining

- Sometimes the bacterial burden in blood is very low and in this case it is clinically insignificant – i.e. bacteremia is asymptomatic.
- Slight bacteremia could be produced simply by brushing of teeth or chewing, especially in the presence of periodontitis.

9.5.4 Septicemia

- Is the presence of bacteria with their toxins in the blood.
- Seen when large numbers of organisms enter and/or actively multiply and persist in the blood stream, producing clinical signs and symptoms such as hypotension, fever and rigors.

9.5.5 Septicemia and sepsis syndrome

Etiology

- Infected wounds, burns
- Osteomyelitis
- Pneumonia
- Intravascular devices
- Food poisoning e.g. *Salmonella spp.*

Pathogenesis

Once the blood stream is invaded by bacteria, the host responds by activating its immune mechanisms, leading to the production of inflammatory cytokines (e.g. interleukin-1, tumor necrosis factor).

Generally, these cytokines are beneficial in eliminating the organisms, but ***excessive production*** may lead to organ dysfunction and circulatory septic shock – the sepsis syndrome.

Clinical features

Hypotension, fever, rigors, oliguria and renal failure.

Diagnosis

Blood should be cultured for a diagnosis of septicemia and antibiotic sensitivity test should be performed.

Treatment

The principles of therapy are:

- Potent bactericidal (rather than bacteriostatic) intravenous antibiotic therapy in adequate dosage.
- Stabilization of the hemodynamic status (e.g. intravenous fluids, cardiogenic drugs, oxygen)
- Removal of the focus of infection (e.g. removal of a foreign body, surgical intervention by draining an abscess).

Chapter 10
Oral Tumors and Tumor-Like Lesions: Preamble

Many tumors and tumor-like lesions occur in the oral cavity. In this chapter, you will be familiar with some terms such as tumor, neoplasia and hyperplasia and how to differentiate between them.

10.1 Overview

10.1.1 Definitions

Tumor

The word tumor means literally an abnormal swelling and because almost all neoplasms appear in a form of swellings, the term tumor became synonymous with neoplasm in modern medicine.

Neoplasm

- A neoplasm, by definition, is a new growth, which is self-autonomous, progressive and persists after withdrawal of the initiating cause.
- Tumors can result from the neoplastic transformation of any nucleated cell in the body, although some cell types are prone to tumor formation than others; the transformed cells are called neoplastic cells.

- By transformation involving a series of genetic alternations, cells escape permanently from the normal growth regulatory mechanisms.
- Neoplastic cells grow to form abnormal swellings, but this is not the only cause of abnormal swellings. Swellings can also result form inflammation, cysts, hypertrophy or hyperplasia. In this chapter, lesions, which are not strictly neoplasms, are also described, merely because most of them appear clinically as tumors (swellings). In fact the majority of these lesions are developmental disturbances or of still debatable etiology.

Hyperplasia

Is the increase in number of cells, which is usually due to definite cause and there is always a relationship between the degree of hyperplasia and the degree of the stimulus. Hyperplasic growths are not, in general, self-autonomous.

10.1.2 Structure of Tumors

- Tumors consist of neoplastic cells and stroma.
- The neoplastic cell population give the tumor its characteristic behavior and morphology.
- Depending on its functional resemblance to the mother tissue, the neoplastic cells secrete cell products such as collagen, mucin or keratin; these substances accumulate within the tumor where they are recognizable histologically.
- Other cell products are secreted into the blood where they can be detected by other methods. Pathologists usually depend on such cell products in the process of tumor diagnosis.

- The neoplastic cell population is embedded in a connective tissue framework called the *stroma* (from the Greek word meaning a matrix), which provides mechanical support and nutrition to the neoplastic cells.
- The process of stroma formation is thought to be due to induction of connective tissue proliferation induced by the neoplastic cells via the production of growth factors. Induction of blood vessels formation (a process called *angiogenesis*) is essential for tumor growth and in fact the growth of the tumor is dependent upon its ability to induce blood vessels to perfuse it.
- The stroma often contains a lymphocytic infiltrate of variable density; this may reflect a host immune reaction to the tumor, a hypothesis supported by the observation that patients whose tumors are densely infiltrated by lymphocytes tend to have a better prognosis.

10.1.3 Differentiation

- The term differentiation – in pathology – means the degree of similarity of the tumor cells to their mother cell (i.e. the cell of origin).
- Tumor differentiation determines the tumor grade. Highly undifferentiated tumors are of grave prognosis if compared to the well-differentiated tumors.
- Benign tumors are not further classified in this way because they nearly always well differentiated.

10.1.4 Classification of Tumors

Precise classification of tumors is essential for proper treatment planning.

According to Histogenesis

1. Epithelial tumors
2. Connective tissue tumors
3. Mixed tumors (arising from epithelium and connective tissue simultaneously and they are rare e.g. ameloblastic fibroma)
4. Tumors of debatable origin

According to the Clinical Behavior

1. Benign
2. Malignant
3. Intermediate behavior. (Some tumors defy precise behavioral classification because their behavior is intermediate between that associated with benign and malignant tumors; these are referred to as "borderline" tumors). Main differences between benign and malignant tumors are summarized in table (10.1):

10.1.5 Nomenclature of Tumors

- All tumors have the suffix "-**oma**"
- Benign epithelial tumors are papillomas or adenomas.
- Benign connective tissue tumors have a prefix denoting the cell of origin e.g. fibr-oma, lip-oma, oste-oma, etc.
- Malignant epithelial tumors are carcinomas.
- Malignant connective tissue tumors are sarcomas.
- Some tumors have inherited the name of the person who first recognized the lesion e.g. Burkitt's lymphoma, Ewing's sarcoma and Kaposi's sarcoma.

Table 10.1: Main differences between benign and malignant tumors

Always Remember

Feature	Benign	Malignant
Mode of growth	Mainly expansion	Invasion & expansion
Rate of growth	Slow	Rapid
Metastasis	No	Usually metastasize
Cellular differentiation	Well differentiated	Varying degrees of differentiation
Roots	Short + conical	Nearly normal
Mitosis	Little, normal mitosis	Abnormal mitosis
Hyperchromatism	Normal nuclei	Hyperchromatic nuclei
Capsulation	Ususally capsulated	Not capsulated

- Other tumors have inherited a descriptive name which may describe a feature of the neoplastic cell e.g. granular cell myoblastoma, or describes the supposed origin of the neoplastic cell e.g. ameloblastoma. Such descriptive terms particularly those pertaining to the histogenesis are sometimes incorrect and many of them are obsolete. Remember that in pathology, *old terms die slowly* or never die. See table (10.2)

10.1.6 Biology of Tumor Cells

- Tumor cells are genetically unstable.
- This will result in the phenomenon that while most tumors start from a monoclonal cell, they end with the formation of a polyclonal mass of cells showing divergent properties.
- This is often reflected in the histology. Some areas of the tumor may appear better differentiated than others. The most obvious biological characteristics of tumors could be summarized in the following items:

Chapter 10. Oral Tumors and Tumor-Like Lesions: Preamble

Table 10.2: Naming of Some Tumors

Tissue Origin	Bengin	Maignant
Epithelium		
Squamous cells	Papillom	Squamous cell carcinoma
Basal cells	-	Basal cell carcinoma
Glandular epithelium	Adenoma	Adenocarcinoma
Neuroectoderm		
Melanocyte	Nevus	Melanoma
Connective tissue		
Fibrous tissue	Fibroma	Fibrosarcoma
Cartilage	Chondrom	Chondrosarcoma
Bone	Osteoma	Osteosarcoma
Fat	Lipoma	Liposarcoma
Endothelium		
Blood vessels	Hemangioma	Angiosarcoma
Lymphatic vessels	Lymphangioma	Lymphangiosarcoma
Muscle		
Smooth muscle	Leiomyoma	Leiomyosarcoma
Striated muscle	Rhabdomyoma	Rhabdomyosarcoma

1. **Cellular immortalization**

   Neoplastic cells show features of immortalization especially when studied in cultures.

2. **DNA of tumor cells**

   Tumor cells have abnormal nuclear DNA. The total amount of DNA per cell commonly exceeds that of the normal diploid (2N) population. This is evident in histological sections as nuclear hyperchromatism.

   The amount of DNA may appear to increase in exact multiples of the diploid state (*polyploidy*) such as teraploid (4N) and octaploid (8N); also, there may be *aneuploidy*, the presence of *inexact* multiples of DNA per cell.

3. **Mitotic and apoptotic activity**

   Malignant tumors frequently appear to exhibit more mitotic activity than normal cell population. In histological sections, mitoses are abundant, and mitotic figures are often grossly abnormal showing tripolar and other bizarre arrangements.

4. **Cell surface properties**

   The surface of tumor cells is abnormal. Tumor cells have a greater negative surface charge than do normal cells, and are also less cohesive. In epithelial neoplasms, poor cellular cohesion is also due to a reduction in specialized intercellular junctions such as desmosomes. These changes may explain the ease with which malignant tumor cells spread through tissues and detach themselves to populate distant organs.

5. **Metabolic abnormalities**

   Tumor cells may retain the capacity to synthesize and secrete products characteristic of the normal cell type from which they are derived, often doing so in an excessive and uncontrolled manner.

10.2 Carcinogenesis

Malignant tumors of the oral tissues constitute about 6% of all malignant neoplasms in men and about 2% of those in women. Over 90% of these tumors are squamous cell carcinoma. The other forms of carcinoma together with sarcomas account for the remaining 10%.

10.3 Basic Concepts of Carcinogenesis

- There is overwhelming evidence that gene mutations can cause cancer. In this context, mutations are defined broadly to include any change in the genome such as point mutation, deletion, insertion, translocation or amplification.
- Carcinogenesis results from non-lethal genetic damage of cells. Such damage may be acquired by environmental factors such as viruses, chemicals or radiation. The genetic hypothesis of cancer implies that a tumor mass results from the clonal expansion of a single progenitor cell that has acquired the genetic damage i.e. tumors, with very few exceptions (as in field cancerization), are monoclonal.
- Carcinogenesis is a multistep process. The formation of a tumor mass by the clonal descendants of a transformed cell is a complex process requiring sequential acquisition of more than one genetic mutation. This scenario is termed "multiple hits".
- Genes that act as the primary targets for genetic damage during carcinogenesis are of 4 classes:

1. **The growth promoting protooncogenes.**

   Protooncogenes are normal cellular genes that encode proteins that promote cell growth. Oncogenes, or cancer producing genes, are mutated genes derived from the normal cellular protooncogenes. Mutant alleles of protooncogenes are considered dominant because they can transform cells despite the presence of their normal counterpart. Oncogenes encode proteins called oncoproteins. Thus, oncogenes and oncoproteins are altered versions of their normal counterparts. The mechanisms by which protooncogenes are transformed into oncogenes could be one of two broad categories of changes:

- Changes in the structure of the gene, resulting in the synthesis of an abnormal gene product (oncoprotein) having an aberrant function.
- Changes in regulation of gene expression, resulting in enhanced production of the structurally normal growth-promoting protein.

These changes in the structure and/or gene expression may be mediated by any of the following:

(a) Point Mutation.

Irradiation and chemical carcinogen can cause point mutation.

(b) Chromosomal Rearrangement.

Which result in movement of the gene to a location other than that it normally occupies e.g. in Burkitt's lymphoma.

(c) Gene Amplification.

In which there are several copies of the gene.

(d) Viral Insertion.

Result from retroviral infection in animals other than man.

Oncogenes and oncoproteins might be classified on the basis of their role in the signal transduction cascade and cell cycle regulation into:

(a) Growth Factors

(b) Growth Factor Receptors

(c) Signal Transducing Proteins

(d) Nuclear Regulatory Proteins and transcriptional activators

(e) Cell Cycle Regulators

2. **The growth inhibiting or tumor suppressor genes (antioncogenes).**

   While protooncogenes encode proteins that promote cell growth, the products of tumor suppressor genes apply brakes to cell proliferation. Mutant alleles of tumor suppressor genes are considered recessive because both alleles should be damaged before transformation can occur. Tumor suppressor genes become inactivated in human cancer. Generally, inactivation occurs through genetic mechanisms that disrupt gene structure or gene expression. The retinoblastoma gene (RB), the p53 gene, BRCA1, BRCA2, NF-1, NF-2, APC, and PACH are examples of tumor suppressor genes (see later for detailed discussion on the hereditary factors and cancer).

3. **Genes that regulate programmed cell death (apoptosis).**

   A large family of genes that regulate apoptosis has been identified. They could be classified into two classes, the first is the antiapoptotic genes e.g. (bcl-2 and bcl-xL) and the second class is the apoptosis favoring genes (protoapoptotic genes) e.g. (bax, bad and bcl-xS). Apoptosis regulating genes may be dominant or recessive. Overexpression of the bcl-2 gene product is involved in 85% of B-cell lymphomas of the follicular type. Bcl-2 proteins protect lymphocytes from apoptosis and allow them to survive for long periods; thus there is steady accumulation of B-lymphocytes, resulting in lymphadenopathy and marrow infiltration.

4. **Genes that regulate repair of damaged DNA.**

   These genes can affect cell proliferation indirectly by affecting the ability of the organism to repair non-lethal damage in other genes including protooncogenes, tumor suppressor genes and genes that regulate apoptosis. Both alleles of DNA repair genes must be inactivated to induce such genomic instability and hence they are considered recessive.

In the sense that DNA repair genes can prevent cancer transformation, they may be regarded as tumor suppressor genes. Xeroderma pigmentosa, ataxia telangiectasia and Fanconi's syndrome are diseases characterized by mutation in the DNA repair genes.

10.4 Etiologic Factors of Malignancy

- The etiology of malignancy is not fully understood, however the condition is thought to be multifactorial.
- Many recent studies have assessed in the identification of factors that can lead to genetic defects which in turn can result in the development of malignancy.
- The main factors that seem to play a role in the etiology of malignancy are classified into essential and modifying factors.

10.4.1 Essential factors in carcinogenesis

Oncogenic Viruses

Viruses that can cause tumors in man are called "oncogenic viruses". An essential step in malignant transformation of normal cells by most oncogenic viruses is the integration of all or part of the viral DNA (or DNA copy of retroviral RNA) into the host cell genome. Integration of viral DNA could be the cause of mutation of certain cellular genes related to malignancy. Oncogenic viruses are either DNA or RNA-containing viruses.

Chapter 10. Oral Tumors and Tumor-Like Lesions: Preamble

A- DNA oncogenic viruses, these include:

1. Human papova virus: These are both polyoma viruses which usually affect mice, and Papilloma virus that causes either skin wart or carcinoma of the genitourinary tract

2. Adeno virus: upper respiratory tract infections

3. Hepatitis B virus: hepatocellular carcinoma.

4. Herpes virus, this includes:

    (a) Herpes simplex virus type-2 (HSV-2): Primary infection with this virus usually causes a subclinical infection or rarely a severe herpetic infection. Recurrent infection with this virus causes either recurrent herpetic infection or cervical carcinoma

    (b) Epstein-Barr virus (EBV): Primary infection with this virus usually causes subclinical illness in children. In the adults infection with this virus results in infectious mononucleosis. Recurrent infection causes Burkitt's lymphoma or nasopharyngeal carcinoma.

    (c) Cytomegalovirus (CMV): Primary infection with this virus in the fetus usually causes congenital abnormalities. After birth, infection with this virus usually causes a subclinical illness or might cause an infection similar to infectious mononucleosis. Recurrent infection causes either wide spread infection or Kaposi's sarcoma.

B- RNA oncogenic viruses (also called retroviruses), these include:

1. Human immunodeficiency virus (HIV): infection with this virus is recognized widely as the causative agent of Acquired Immunodeficiency Syndrome (AIDS) leading to immunosuppression and opportunistic infections. HIV infection predisposes to several neoplastic conditions, especially lymphoma, Kaposi's sarcoma or cervical carcinoma. The role

of HIV in malignancy is probably linked to its immunosuppressive effect.
2. Human T-cell leukemia Virus (HTLV): this virus is the causative agent of adult T-cell leukemia.
3. Human B-type particle (Bittner milk factor): leading to breast cancer.

Chemical Carcinogens

- Chemical carcinogenesis is a multistep process, divided into three stages: (1) initiation, (2) promotion, and (3) progression.
- Initiation: an initiated cell is one in which, a chemical carcinogen has interacted with DNA to produce a mutation in the genome. Initiation is irreversible, but not all initiated cells will go on to establish a tumor, since many cells will die through the normal process of programmed cell death, or apoptosis. An initiated cell is not a tumor cell, since it has not acquired any autonomy of growth.
- Promotion: tumor promoters usually influence the proliferation of the preneoplastic cells and the formation of nodules or polyps. Unlike initiators, most promoters do not bind covalently to DNA and usually do not cause mutation.
- Progression: during progression the cells gain additional genetic changes resulting in karyotype instability. Mutation in oncogenes and/or tumor suppressor genes is a break point in progression. The tumor cells acquire the ability to grow, invade local tissue, and establish distant metastases.
- Chemical carcinogens can include the flowing examples:
    1. Polycyclic hydrocarbons: these are not directly carcinogenic; they are procarcinogens as they are metabolized locally in most types of cells to form carcinogenic compounds. Thus they are locally acting

2. Aromatic amins and related compounds will cause liver cancer because the liver is the site of their conversion to an ultimate carcinogen
3. Alkylating agents: such as Procarbazine and Nitrosourea
4. Arsenical compounds
5. Non-genotoxic Carcinogens: The actions previously described are those of agents which react with cellular DNA and cause genomic alterations. As more and more chemicals are tested for carcinogenicity, a number are now being recognized as "non-genotoxic". These chemicals do not form stable covalent bonds with cellular DNA or other macromolecules. Solid state materials (asbestos) are an example. The mode of action of non-genotoxic carcinogens is not known. Asbestos is synergistic with cigarette smoking in inducing bronchial carcinoma. Some metals such as nickel acts as non-genotoxic carcinogen.

- Chemical carcinogens are either locally acting e.g. polycyclic hydrocarbons or remotely acting e.g. Aromatic amines.
- The chemical carcinogens modify the genome of the cells either through direct action on the DNA or through modification of transfer RNA (tRNA) followed by the production of mutant DNA by reverse transcription.

Irradiation

- These are either:
    1. Ionizing radiation
    2. Ultraviolet radiation causes squamous cell carcinoma, basal cell carcinoma and malignant melanoma.
- The initial step in radiation transformation is the induction of DNA damage leading to genetic instability. The majority of genetic damage to DNA caused by radiation is deletion, inversion or chromosomal

translocation. This in turn might lead to mutation of genes related to malignancy.

10.4.2 Modifying factors in carcinogenesis

Immunological factors (immunosurveillance)

This represents the immunological reaction against cancer. It is thought that cancer develops only if there is a breach in the immune system of the patient. This concept is known as immunosurveillance. Evidences of immunity against cancer are:

- Cancer is common in old age than young age due to decreased immunity by aging.
- Rare cases of cancer regress spontaneously.
- Increased incidence of Kaposi's sarcoma, squamous cell carcinoma and hairy leukoplakia in AIDS patients.

On the other hand, most cancers occur in individuals who do not suffer from any obvious immunodeficiency. If immunosurveillance exists, how do cancers evade the immune system in apparently immunocompetent individuals? Several escape mechanisms have been proposed:

1. Selective outgrowth of antigen-negative tumor cells

    During tumor progression, strongly immunogenic subclones may be eliminated.

2. Loss of reduced expression of major histocompatibility complexes

    Tumor cells may fail to express normal levels of human leukocyte antigen (HLA) class I, thus escaping attack by cytotoxic T cells. Such cells however may trigger NK cells

3. Lack of costimulation

Sensitization of T-cells requires two signals, one by foreign peptide presented by MHC and the other by costimulatory molecules. Although, tumor cells may express peptide antigens with class I molecules, they often do not express co stimulatory molecules such as B7-1. This is not only prevents sensitization but also may render T-cells anergic or cause them to undergo apoptosis.

4. Immunosuppression

- Many oncogenic agents (e.g. chemicals and ionizing radiation) suppress host immune responses.
- Also some tumor products are immunosuppressive. For example, transforming growth factor (TGF-β) secreted in large quantities by many tumors is a potent immunosuppressant.
- Another clever mechanism used by some tumors is to express Fas ligand (FasL), which engages Fas on the surface of T-cells and sends a death signal to the immune cells.

Hereditary factors (Hereditary and Cancer)

It is now established that some families have high incidence of certain types of cancer. This finding is based on the belief that tumor suppressor genes act in a recessive manner, thus mutations of one allele of the gene may be inherited from one family to another without a clinically obvious disease. A second mutation of the other copy (allele) of the same tumor suppressor gene will result in complete loss of the tumor suppressor function and malignancy will develop. Thus, tumor suppressor genes figure prominently in the development of familial cancers. Examples of such inherited mutations include:

- Mutations in the retinoblastoma gene (Rb) in children with retinoblastoma.
- Mutations of the p53 gene in the Li-Fraumni syndrome (familial breast cancer in young women)

- Mutations in the BRCA1 and BRCA2 genes, which are associated with familial breast and ovarian cancer.
- Mutations in the neurofibromatosis 1 and neurofibromatosis 2 genes (NF-1 and NF-2) are associated with multiple neurofibromatosis.
- Mutations in the adenomatous polyposis coli gene (APC) is associated with familial adenomatous polyposis (Gardener syndrome).
- Mutations in the patched (PTCH) tumor suppressor gene which is associated with the basal cell carcinoma/jaw cysts syndrome (Gorlin-Goltz syndrome, Gorlin syndrome, Basal cell nevus, jaw cysts, bifid rib syndrome).

Age

Cancer in general is common in old age. It is believed that through out life abnormal mutant cells are produced during cell proliferation and these are destroyed by the immune system. In later life the recognition and destruction of mutant cells is less active and more mutant cells are produced. Thus the chance of developing malignancy is increased.

Sex

This affects the incidence of cancer in various organs. Cancer breast is common in females while squamous cell carcinoma and cancer bladder are common in males.

Race

Skin cancer is common in white race while ameloblastoma is common in black populations.

Chapter 10. Oral Tumors and Tumor-Like Lesions: Preamble

Geography

Means the variation of incidence of cancer in different parts of the world. This may be due to variation in activities, habits, diet, and pollution.

Hormones

Growth of some tumors depends on hormonal secretions. Cancer of breast and uterus in females depends on estrogen, while cancer prostate in males depends on testosterone

Chronic mechanical irritation

As sharp broken down teeth or prosthetic clasps.

Chronic diseases

Such as: (1) Syphilis causing syphilitic leukoplakia that might terminate by squamous cell carcinoma, (2) Chronic candidosis that might appear clinically as speckled leukoplakia.

CHAPTER 11

BENIGN NON-ODONTOGENIC TUMORS AND TUMOR-LIKE LESIONS

Benign tumors of the oral cavity are common; some of these tumors are not actual neoplasms but rather reactive lesions or developmental disturbances. They are mentioned here for the sake of simplicity.

11.1 Benign Epithelial Tumors

11.1.1 Squamous Cell Papilloma

Definition

Benign tumor of surface stratified squamous epithelium.

Clinically

- Age: No age predilection.
- Site: Palate is the most common site.
- Features: Squamous cell papilloma is an exophytic single or multiple cauliflower like mass. The lesion is either sessile or pedunculated, having a rough whitish surface that is hard if keratinized and soft if not.

Histologically

The tumor consists of:

1. Connective tissue core carrying blood vessels and lymphatics
2. Covered with stratified squamous epithelium, which shows Acanthosis and sometimes hyperkeratosis

11.1.2 Verruca Vulgaris (Common Wart)

Definition

- This is a viral infection of the skin, rare in the oral cavity.
- Warts are caused by human papilloma viruses (HPV). Currently, more than 150 types of HPV have been identified.
- Certain HPV types tend to occur at particular anatomic sites; however, warts of any HPV type may occur at any site.
- The primary clinical manifestations of HPV include:
    1. Common warts
    2. Genital warts
    3. Flat warts
    4. Deep palmoplantar warts (myrmecia)
    5. Focal epithelial hyperplasia (Heck's disease)

Etiology

- Infection with a DNA virus known as the human papilloma virus (HPV types 6, 11, 16, & 18). The disease usually results from autoinoculation from warts on hands.
- Warts can affect any area on the skin and mucous membranes.

- Infection is confined to the epithelium and does not result in systemic dissemination of the virus. Replication occurs in differentiated epithelial cells in the upper level of the epidermis; however, viral particles can be found in the basal layer.
- A small subset of HPV types is associated with the development of malignancies. Malignant transformation most commonly is seen in patients with genital warts and in immunocompromised patients.

Clinically

The clinical features of verruca vulgaris are similar to those of squamous cell papilloma. Oral warts are occasionally multiple but if numerous, immunodeficiency should be suspected.

Histopathology

Similar to squamous cell papilloma except for the occasional presence of intracellular inclusion bodies (viral bodies) in some of its cells.

Treatment

Treatment is by conservative surgical excision, laser ablation or cauterization.

11.1.3 Focal Epithelial Hyperplasia (Heck's Disease)

This is a term used to describe multiple lesions of verruca vulgaris (warts) occurring anywhere in the oral mucous membrane. It is caused by a different strain of the virus (HPV types 13 & 32) and shows the same histologic features. Lesions are small, discrete, often clustered and may have many papillary or cobblestone surface texture. Treatment is by conservative surgical excision.

11.1.4 Keratoacanthoma

(Self healing carcinoma, Molluscum sebaceum)

Definition

- A lesion of unknown nature, which was considered to be a benign lesion similar to squamous cell carcinoma both clinically and histologically.
- Although KAs were once considered benign based on behavior, it is now believed that they should be regarded as well-differentiated variants of SCC that are capable of spontaneous regression. Some KAs have displayed aggressive biologic behavior that has led to metastases and even death. Because of this potential for local recurrence and metastasis, treatment by wide excision is recommended.
- KAs can be difficult to distinguish histologically from conventional SCCs. This has caused some to consider KAs and SCCs to be the same. Clinically, they are differentiated by their history of rapid growth and their volcano shape, yet histologically, there are too many features that overlap with SCC to allow reliable separation.
- KA was reported to progresses, although rarely, to invasive or metastatic carcinoma; therefore, aggressive surgical treatment often is advocated. Whether these cases were SCC or KA, the reports highlight the difficulty of distinctly classifying individual cases.

Etiology

- The definitive cause of KA remains unclear
- Possible etiologic factors may be:
    - Sunlight
    - Chemical carcinogens

- ★ Trauma
- ★ Human papilloma virus
- ★ Genetic factors
- ★ Immunodeficiency
- ★ Recent work has identified that up to one third of keratoacanthomas harbor chromosomal aberrations.

Clinically

- Sex: Males are affected more than females (2:1)
- Age: 50 – 70 years of age
- Race: KA is less common in darker-skinned individuals
- Site: sun-exposed skin of the face is the most common site. The lesion is rare intraorally
- Features: The lesion appears clinically as an elevated nodule with depressed central core (Crater shaped)
- It reaches full size in: 4 – 8 weeks (proliferative phase)
- Remains static for: 4 – 8 weeks (maturation phase)
- And regress in: 4 – 8 weeks leaving a permanent scar in most cases (involution phase)

Histologically

1. Pseudoepitheliomatous hyperplasia i.e. hyperplasia of epithelium which mimics that of epithelioma but with pseudo invasion of the connective tissue, see figure (256).
2. Benign dyskeratosis (refer to the chapter "Premalignant Lesions of the Oral Cavity" page (291).
3. Hyperkeratosis.

4. The underlying connective tissue shows chronic inflammatory cell infiltration.

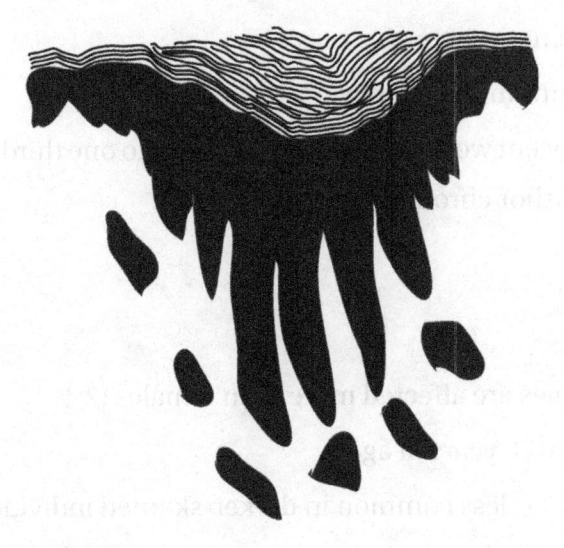

Figure 11.1: Diagrammatic representation of keratoacanthoma and pseudoepitheliomatous hyperplasia. When rete pegs are cut in cross sections they can look like invasion caused by squamous cell carcinoma.

Treatment

- The primary therapy for KA is surgical excision.
- Excise tumors with adequate margins (3–5 mm) and histopathologic evaluation to exclude invasive SCC.
- Since the biological behavior of an individual KA cannot be predicted, many consider surgical treatment of KA to be equivalent to treatment for SCC.
- KAs are radiosensitive and respond well to low doses of radiation.
- Radiation therapy may be useful in selected patients with large tumors in whom resection will result in cosmetic deformity or for tumors that have recurred following attempted excisional surgery.

- Both laser therapy and cryotherapy have been used successfully in small KAs, in KAs found in difficult to treat locations, and as an adjunct to surgical removal.
- Antineoplastic agents: Useful in patients with large or multiple tumors or tumors that are inoperable because of anatomic location or the patient's poor medical status. Agents (e.g. topical 5-fluorouracil, intralesional methotrexate, interferon α-2a, and bleomycin) also have been used with some success.

11.2 Benign Connective Tissue Tumors

11.2.1 Fibroma

Definition

Fibroma is a benign tumor of fibrous connective tissue. True neoplastic fibroma is thought to be rare in the oral cavity and most cases are thought to be hyperplastic growths.

Types

Fibromas could be classified in many different ways, but the following classification might be an appropriate one. The only type to be mentioned here is the peripheral non-odontogenic soft fibroma. The reader is advised to refer to other types of fibromas in their relevant chapters.

1. Peripheral
    (a) Hyperplastic:
        i. Soft with little collagen

ii. Firm (sometimes-called mature fibroma) with abundant collagen

  (b) Neoplastic:

    i. Soft with little collagen.

    ii. Firm (sometimes-called hard fibroma, which is a misleading term,) with abundant collagen.

2. Central

  (a) Odontogenic:

    i. Soft

    ii. Cementifying

  (b) Non-odontogenic:

    i. Soft

    ii. Ossifying

    iii. Calcifying

Clinically

The tumor appears as a mass which is usually sessile or pedunculated, of smooth surface and of normal color.

Histologically

1. Interlacing bundles of collagen fibers
2. Fibroblasts and fibrocytes
3. Small blood vessels

11.2.2 Frenal Tag

- A fibrous hyperplasia, which most frequently occurs on the maxillary labial frenum.
- Such lesions present as small, asymptomatic, exophytic growths attached to the thin frenum surface.
- A similar lesion may be found on the lingual frenum.
- No treatment is required.

11.2.3 Retrocuspid Papilla

- Is a normal variant of the oral mucosa that occurs on the gingiva lingual to the mandibular cuspid.
- It is frequently bilateral and appears as a small, pink papule that measures less than 5 mm in diameter.
- Retrocuspid papillae are quite common, having been reported in 25 % to 99 % of children and young adults. The prevalence in older adults drops to 6 % to 19 %, suggesting that the retrocuspid papilla represents a normal anatomic variation that disappears with age.
- Frenal tags and retrocuspid papillae are considered as tissue tags and considered by many authors as a normal variants of the oral mucosa.

11.2.4 Pyogenic Granuloma

(Lobular capillary hemangioma)

Definition

Traditionally, pyogenic granuloma was described as a hyperplastic growth due to low-grade pyogenic infection. However, recent views consider that the term pyogenic granuloma is misnomer, being neither pyogenic nor granuloma and hence considered as an acquired vascular tumor due to unknown cause.

Etiology

- The traditional view was that the causative organisms might be staphylococci and or streptococci
- However, recent literature deny this view considering the lesion to be a disorder of angiogenesis whose underlying etiology remains unknown
- Others view the lesion as a true neoplasm
- Suggested potential risk factors include pregnancy, birth control pills, bacterial and viral infections and chronic trauma, but no good evidence supports any of these as primary causative factors

Clinically

- The most common site for pyogenic granuloma is the gingiva typically the interdental papilla.
- More common in females
- It appears as a sessile or pedunculated mass deep red in color with ulcerations and bleeding.
- The lesion is usually less than 2 cm in diameter.
- Their occurrence on extragingival sites in the head and neck region is rare and often has atypical presentation.

Histologically

- Surface epithelium, which is thin and atrophied.
- The underlying mass resembles granulation tissue and consists of:

1. Delicate collagen fibrils
2. Proliferating fibroblasts
3. Proliferating capillaries
4. Chronic inflammatory cells

Differential diagnosis

- Bacillary angiomatosis:
  - An infectious disease characterized by proliferative vascular lesions; it mainly affects HIV-positive patients. Caused by infection with *Bartonella* species (gram negative bacilli)
  - Nuclear dust and granular material (bacteria) present
  - Bacteria detected by silver stain (Warthin-Starry silver staining)
- Capillary hemangioma
  - No inflammatory cells
  - History of long duration
- Kaposi's sarcoma
  - Usually multiple with skin involvement
  - Incompetent immune system

Fate

- It is thought that, if left untreated it will progress into fibroepithelial polyp.
- Rare cases can regress spontaneously.

11.2.5 Epulis Granulomatosa

- A term used to describe hyperplastic growth of granulation tissue that arise in healing extraction sockets.
- These lesions resemble pyogenic granulomas and usually represent a granulation tissue reaction to bony sequestra in the socket.

11.2.6 Pregnancy Tumor

(Granuloma gravidarum)

- A lesion, which is similar to pyogenic granuloma both clinically and histologically.
- The two lesions can only, be distinguished by the nature of the patient and the possibility of associated pregnancy gingivitis.
- Many cases may regress spontaneously after delivery.
- Many authors suppose that pregnancy tumor is nothing but a pyogenic granuloma modified by the hormonal status of pregnancy.

11.2.7 Fibroepithelial Polyp

(Epulis Fissuratum, Fibrous Epulis, Denture-induced granuloma, Denture Fissuratum, leaflike denture fibroma)

Definition

A hyperplastic growth due to chronic mechanical trauma. The term epulis means "upon the gum".

Etiology

Any chronic mechanical irritations e.g. ill-fitting denture, sharp broken down tooth or sharp clasp.

Clinically

Similar to fibroma.

Histologically

- Stratified squamous epithelium showing some inflammatory hyperplasia
- Connective tissue core consisting of collagen bundles, fibroblasts and blood vessels. Collagen bundles may be arranged in concentric manner in sessile lesions and fan shaped in pedunculated lesions. Chronic inflammatory cells may be seen.

11.2.8 Papillary Hyperplasia of the Palate

(Inflammatory Papillary Hyperplasia, Denture Papillomatosis)

- This is essentially multiple fibroepithelial polyps occurring under an ill-fitting upper denture.
- Some authors believe that candida albicans may play a role in the pathogenesis of papillary hyperplasia of the palate and the lesion is sometimes classified as a subtype of chronic hyperplastic candidiasis.
- Chronic candidosis is supposed to be the cause for the rare cases in which palatal papillary hyperplasia occurs in non-denture wearers.
- Inflammatory papillary hyperplasia is usually asymptomatic.
- The mucosa is erythematous and has a pebbly or papillary surface.

- **Histologically:** Hyperplastic, stratified squamous epithelium. In advanced cases, ***pseudoepitheliomatous hyperplasia*** may be seen and the pathologist should not mistake it for carcinoma. The connective tissue can vary from loose and edematous to densely collagenized. A chronic inflammatory cell infiltrate is usually seen. If underlying salivary glands are present, sclerosing sialadenitis may be seen.
- There is no justification for surgically stripping palatal papillary hyperplasia. Dentures should be corrected, kept clean and not worn overnight.
- Any superimposed candidal infections should be treated with an antifungal drug.

11.2.9 Peripheral Giant Cell Granuloma

(Giant Cell Epulis, Myeloid Epulis)

Definition

A lesion of unknown nature, it may represent an unusual reaction of tissues against an unknown irritant. The lesion should be differentiated from other giant cell lesions. The term myeloid epulis reflects the past view that the lesion might arise from bone marrow.

Clinically

A mass, sessile or pedunculated, soft usually found on the interdental papilla.

Histologically

1. The lesion is covered by stratified squamous epithelium.
2. There is a sub-epithelial giant cell free zone.

3. Loose vascular connective tissue rich in mononuclear cells thought to be fibroblasts.
4. Multinucleated giant cells, which are usually found around, blood vessels or areas of hemorrhage. These giant cells are thought to originate from histiocytes, osteoclasts or from stromal cells.
5. Sometimes trabeculae of bone or osteoid are found.

11.2.10 Myxoma

Definition

A tumor consists of tissues resembling primitive mesenchyme.

Types

1. Peripheral myxoma
2. Central myxoma.

Histogenesis

1. Some authors believe that peripheral myxomas are not a true tumor and they result from myxomatous degeneration affecting fibroma.
2. Others believe that myxoma arises from primitive fibroblasts, which are dormant in most tissues (more accepted).

Clinically

Peripheral myxoma is poorly circumscribed swelling which tends to infiltrates the surrounding tissues.

Histologically

1. Mucoid matrix rich in acid mucopolysaccharides
2. Spindle or stellate shaped cells
3. Delicate connective tissue fibers
4. The tumor is non-capsulated

11.2.11 Lipoma

Benign tumor of adipose tissue.

Clinically

A mass, soft, and of normal color.

Histologically

- Connective tissue capsule and connective tissue septa.
- Masses of rounded or polygonal cells with clear cytoplasm. The nucleus is compressed against one side of the cell membrane (signet ring appearance).

11.2.12 Chondroma

Definition

A benign tumor consists of cartilage.

Clinically

- Chondroma seldom occurs in membrane bones because no cartilaginous rests exist but the tumor can occurs in the mandible or maxilla as they contain such remnants in the following sites, see also figure (266):
- In the mandible:
    1. Mental region
    2. Molar region
    3. Coronoid process
    4. Condyle
- In the maxilla:
    1. Between upper centrals
    2. At the junction of malar bone
- Features: Swelling of the jaw, which can cause looseness of teeth.

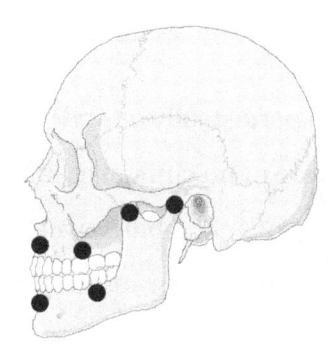

Figure 11.2: Typical sites for the incidence of chondroma

Histologically

- Connective tissue capsule and connective tissue septa.
- Hyaline cartilage showing areas of calcification or necrosis

X-Ray:

Radiolucency with central areas of radiopacities

Differential diagnosis:

From chondrosarcoma which represents a challenge.

11.2.13 Benign Tumors of Bone

Osteoma

Definition

Benign tumor characterized by proliferation of compact or cancellous bone.

Clinically

- The tumor may be periosteally or endosteally.
- Endosteal lesions are of no clinical manifestations.
- Periosteal lesions appear as a hard swelling.
- Soft tissue osteoma may occur in the tongue or buccal mucosa and is termed osteoma mucosae.

Histologically

- Compact osteoma consists of a dense mass of compact bone.
- Cancellous osteoma consists of a core of cancellous bone covered by a shell of compact bone.
- Sometimes foci of cartilage may be found and the lesion is termed osteochondroma.

X-Ray

The lesion appears as a well circumscribed radiopaque mass.

Osteoid Osteoma

Definition

A lesion of unknown etiology. Inflammatory or neoplastic nature have been proposed.

Etiology

Controversial, some authors believe that the lesion is a true neoplasm, others consider it to be an inflammatory condition.

Clinically

- Small size rarely exceeds 2 cm in diameter
- Painful and could be relieved by aspirin
- Second to third decade of life
- Male more than females in a ratio of 2:1 or 3:1

X-Ray

A radiolucent area surrounded by a radiopaque rim. However, a radiolucent nidus of osteoid osteoma is not always easily recognized on a radiograph because of superimposition of other bony structures or because it is often obscured by extremely dense sclerosis around it.

Histologically

- Central nidus of osteoid tissue interspersed with vascular connective tissue showing chronic inflammatory cells.
- Surrounded by new bone formation.

11.2.14 Benign Tumors of Muscles

Leiomyoma

Definition

- Leiomyoma is a benign tumor of smooth muscle.
- Smooth muscles are present in the wall of blood vessels, in the wall of viscera or in the dermis of the skin.
- In the oral cavity, leiomyoma arises from wall of blood vessels.

Clinically

Soft mass, painless and slowly growing.

Histologically

- Bundles of smooth muscle cells, the nuclei showing palisading appearance.
- Fibrous connective tissue stroma with no capsule.

Rhabdomyoma

Definition

Benign tumor of striated muscle. Striated muscles are all voluntary except:

- Upper third of the esophagus
- Pharynx.
- Spermatic cord.

Clinically

Similar to leiomyoma.

Histologically

Nests of striated muscle cells showing cross striations.

Granular Cell Tumor

(*granular cell myoblastoma*)

Definition

A Benign tumor of unknown nature.

Histogenesis

The tumor is thought to arise from either: Primitive muscle cell, striated muscle, histiocytes or schwann cell.

Clinically

The common age of this lesion is between 30-40 years of age. It appears as a mass, which is slowly growing and painless and usually affects the tongues.

Histologically

- Masses of polygonal cells showing granular cytoplasm.
- Fibrous connective tissue stroma.
- The overlying epithelium shows pseudoepitheliomatous hyperplasia, which can be mistaken for squamous cell carcinoma.

Congenital Epulis of Newborn

A lesion similar to granular cell myoblastoma being possibly of the same origin. The lesion differs from granular cell myoblastoma in the following aspects:

1. Occurs in newborn
2. Affects the gingiva
3. No pseudoepitheliomatous hyperplasia

11.3 Nevi

Introduction

- A nevus by definition is a developmental malformation of skin or mucous membrane arising from cells native to skin or mucous membrane and simulating a neoplasm although non neoplastic.
- A hamartoma by definition is a developmental malformation appearing in a tumor like condition due to presence of cells in normal site but in exaggerated amount. A nevus is considered to be a subtype of hamartoma.
- Nevi are of 3 types:
    1. Keratotic nevi: white spongy nevus

2. Vascular nevi: hemangioma and lymphangioma
3. Pigmented nevi: or melanotic nevi

11.3.1 Pigmented Nevus

(*Melanocytic Nevi, Nevocellular Nevus, Mole*)

Definition

A type of nevi, which arises from, altered melanocytes known as nevus cells. Nevus cells differ from their normal counterparts (melanocytes) in that they are usually smaller in size, without dendrites, and are less metabolically active.

Although, some of the pigmented nevi are congenital, many cases can evolve in early childhood and thus given the name "***Acquired Melanocytic Nevus***".

Pathogenesis

- Melanocytes originate from neural crest and migrate to the skin and mucous membrane along the course of peripheral nerves to reside between basal cells
- Melanocytes synthesize melanin from tyrosine by the action of tyrosinase enzyme. This melanin is synthesized in specialized granules known as the melanosomes. Melanocytes transfer melanin through their dendritic processes to the epithelial cells. Melanin forms a supranuclear halo to protect nuclei of epithelial cells from the damaging effect of actinic rays. There is approximately one melanocyte to 5-8 basal keratinocytes and this constitutes the epidermal (epithelial) melanocyte unit. In colored races, the number of melanocytes is similar to that in

whites but melanin is synthesized more rapidly and the granules are coarser. See figure (11.3)

- Melanocytes are DOPA positive because they contain tyrosinase. They stain black with DOPA.
- Melanophores are macrophages engulfing the extruded extra-cellular melanin. They are DOPA negative.
- The clinical types of nevi are believed to be stages in the evolution of the same pathological entity. This is not to say that any one lesion must pass through all of these changes, for their development may cease at any point.
- The pathogenesis of all pigmented nevi is practically similar. The only difference is the site on which the migrating melanocytes are arrested during their migration from the neural crest.
- Mutations of the BRAF gene were identified in approximately 80% of acquired melanocytic nevi. Such mutations also are common in cutaneous melanomas. BRAF is a protooncogene that encodes a protein of the family serine/threonine kinase involved in the mitogen-activated protein kinase (MAPK) signaling pathway, which mediates cell proliferation and differentiation.

Differential Diagnosis of Nevi

Nevi should be differentially diagnosed from oral melanotic macules, page (645) and freckles, page (643).

Treatment of Pigmented Nevi

- No treatment is required unless for cosmetic reasons.
- Nevi subjected to chronic mechanical irritation should be surgically removed.

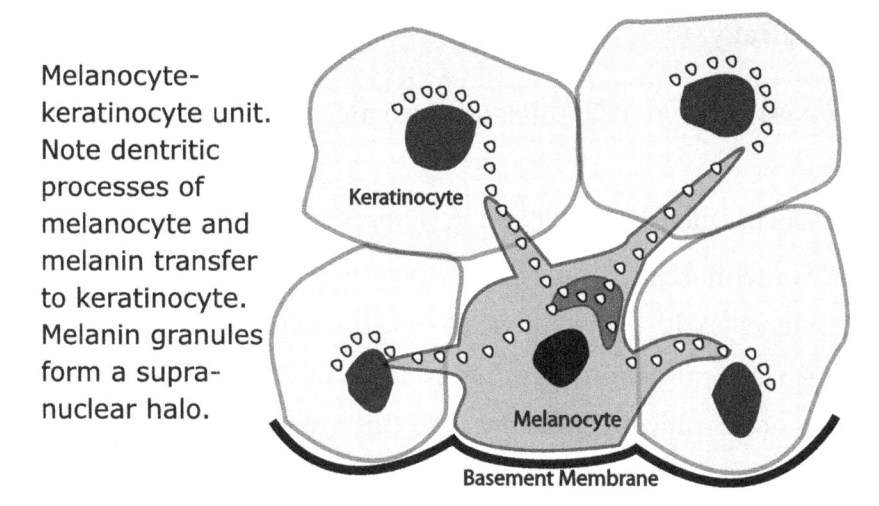

Melanocyte-keratinocyte unit. Note dentritic processes of melanocyte and melanin transfer to keratinocyte. Melanin granules form a supra-nuclear halo.

Figure 11.3: Melanocytes and their function

Types of Pigmented Nevi

1. Junctional nevus
2. Intradermal nevus
3. Compound nevus
4. Juvenile melanoma
5. Blue nevus

1- Junctional Nevus

Definition

A type of pigmented nevus in which nevus cells are present on the dermo-epidermal junction.

Clinically

- Occurs on the skin or mucous membrane
- Flat, pigmented lesion, devoid of hair

Histologically

- Nests of nevus cells (melanocytes) present at the dermo-epidermal junction.
- Nevus cells are epithelioid in shape.
- Sometimes junctional activity occurs, which means proliferation of nevus cells with some mitosis. Nevus cells will appear to be dropping from surface epithelium (dropping effect). Junctional activity below 17 years is not significant clinically, after this age it is of grave prognosis and denotes malignant transformation.

2- Intradermal Nevus

Definition

This is a type of pigmented nevus in which nevus cells are situated in the dermis.

Clinically

- Is the most common nevus
- It does not occur on the palms of hands, soles of feet or genital organs
- It is a flat or warty lesion, light to dark brown in color
- Sometimes hairy

Histologically

- Nests of nevus cells situated in the dermis
- Nevus cells are epithelioid or cuboidal in shape
- Nevus cells may fuse to form giant cells similar to Touton giant cells

- Sometimes nevus cells form neuroid figures similar to Wanger-Meissner corpuscles.

3- Compound Nevus

Definition

This is a type of pigmented nevus, which contains a junctional element and an intradermal element.

Clinically

Similar to intradermal nevus, but usually found at a younger age group. It is the junctional element of compound nevus, which renders them dangerous.

4- Juvenile Melanoma

Definition

A type of pigmented nevus found in children about puberty.

Clinically

- Occurs usually in the face, and rare in the oral cavity.
- It is pink rather than pigmented.

Histologically

- Nevus cells are arranged as in compound nevus i. e.:
    1. Junctional element consists of clear cuboidal nevus cells and showing junctional activity.

2. Intradermal element, consists of epithelioid or spindle shaped cells showing some mitosis and little melanin with dilated blood vessels.

- Juvenile melanoma is thus histologically malignant although clinically benign.

5- Blue Nevus

(*Dermal Melanocytoma*)

Definition

This is a type of pigmented nevus in which nevus cells are situated very deep in the dermis. Melanocytes fail to reach to the surface epithelium and are arrested very deep in the dermis during their migration from the neural crest.

Clinically

- Flat bluish lesion found on the skin.
- The cause for the blue color is postulated to result from Tyndall effect.
- Hairless.
- Mongolian spots are variants of blue nevus occurring in mongolism (Down's Syndrome).

Histologically

Spindle shaped nevus cells, which are present deep in the dermis.

Figure (11.4) illustrates the different types of pigmented nevi.

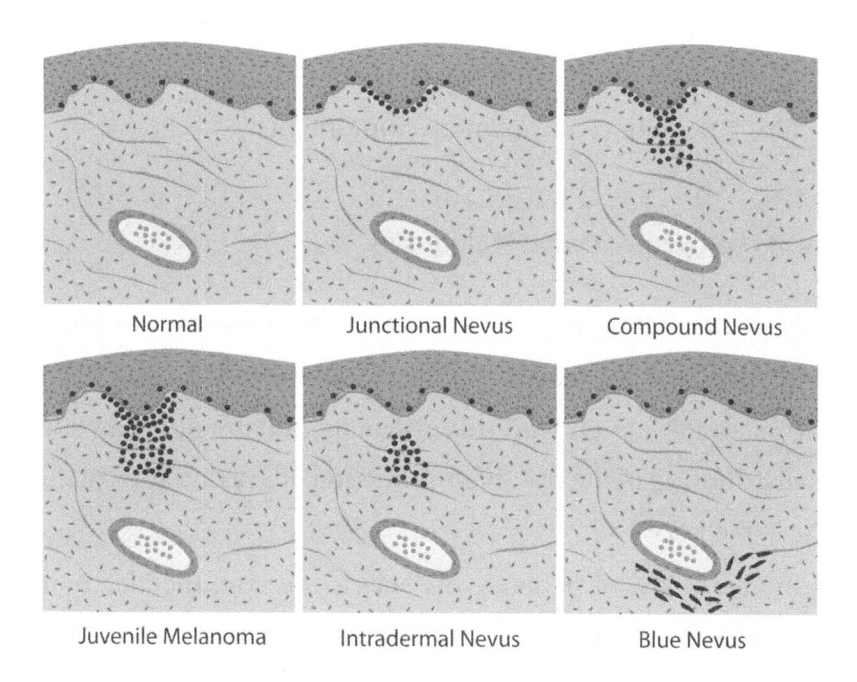

Figure 11.4: Types of pigmented nevi. Normal melanocytes occur within the basal cell layer (about one melanocyte to six basal cells). The various types of nevi appear to be stages in the evolution of the same pathological entity. Juvenile melanoma is histologically a compound nevus with junctional activity. In blue nevus, nevus cells are spindle shaped and situated deep in the dermis.

Variants of Pigmented Nevi

Halo Nevus (Sutton Nevus)

- Halo nevus is a type of pigmented nevi surrounded by a halo of depigmentation.
- The cause of pigmentation loss is unknown but postulated to be an immune reaction against melanocytes.
- This type of nevi may regress spontaneously.

Nevus of Ota (Oculodermal Melanosis)

- Naevus of Ota is not uncommon in the Japanese, but is only occasionally seen in Caucasians and Afro-Caribbeans.
- It is an ill-defined ***slate-blue***, usually unilateral, lesion situated in the distribution of the ophthalmic and maxillary divisions of the trigeminal cranial nerve.
- In about 60% of patients, the sclera and conjunctiva are involved; occasionally, the mucous membranes of the nose and oral cavity are also affected.
- Rarely, a similar discoloration involves the leptomeninges.
- Over 50% of these lesions are present at birth and most of the remainder appear at around puberty.
- In contrast to the Mongolian blue spot, the nevus of Ota is permanent.
- **Histopathology:**
    - The epidermis may show hyperpigmentation and increased numbers of melanocytes, but there is no junctional activity.
    - Situated within the upper and mid-dermis are collections of heavily pigmented, spindle-shaped, bipolar or dendritic melanocytes.

- ★ Most are orientated parallel to the skin surface, but they may sometimes be seen encircling epidermal appendages.
- Could be considered as a subtype of blue nevus?

11.3.2 Vascular Nevi

Are types of vascular tumors. Their neoplastic nature is still debatable and many authors consider vascular nevi as developmental malformations [5].

1- Hemangiomas

Types

1. Capillary hemangioma
2. Cavernus hemangioma
3. Venous hemangioma

A. Capillary Hemangioma

Definition   A type of vascular nevi in which there is aggregation of capillaries.

Clinically

- Appears as a pink or dark red lesion, which is leveled or slightly elevated above the surface.
- Capillary hemangioma is often described as "birthmarks".
- The "port wine stain" is a diffuse cutaneous angioma.
- The juvenile capillary hemangioma, the so-called strawberry nevus of infancy, often grows rapidly for some months then usually regresses completely by 5 years of age but some cases persist throughout life.

Histologically A network of capillaries lined by endothelial cells and containing red blood cells. Supported by delicate Connective tissue.

Treatment

- Should be considered only if there is significant or recurrent hemorrhage.
- Special precautions are needed to guard against excessive hemorrhage during the operation
- Cryotherapy, laser ablation or injection of sclerosing agents may give better cosmetic results than conventional surgery.

B. Cavernous Hemangioma

Definition A type of vascular nevi which consists of large blood filled spaces.

Clinically

- Peripheral hemangioma appears as a swelling, deep red in color usually affecting lip or tongue.
- Sometimes described as port-wine nevus or nevus flammeus
- Central hemangioma may occur in the mandible or maxilla and appears in x-ray as a multilocular radiolucent area. It leads to *fatal hemorrhage* after extraction of an involved tooth.
- Multiple hemangiomas form part of several syndromes. These include: von-Hippel Lindau disease, Osler Weber-Rendu disease and Sturge Weber syndrome.

Histologically Blood filled spaces lined by endothelial cells and supported by fibrous connective tissue.

Treatment   As capillary hemangioma.

2- Lymphangioma

Definition   A type of vascular nevi in which there are aggregations of lymphatics. Lymphangioma may be capillary of cavernous. Cystic hygroma is a large and cystic type of cavernous lymphangioma that is most commonly occurs in the neck.

Clinically

- When it is superficial, it appears as a swelling with a papillary surface of normal color or slightly deeper red.
- When deep, it appears as a diffuse nodular swelling of normal color.
- The lesion is usually found at birth or shortly after birth.

Histologically   Spaces lined by endothelial cells containing coagulated lymph or empty and supported by fibrous connective tissue.

11.4   Benign Tumors of Nerve Tissue

Back to Basics

To revise the normal structure of nerve tissues, see figure (11.5)

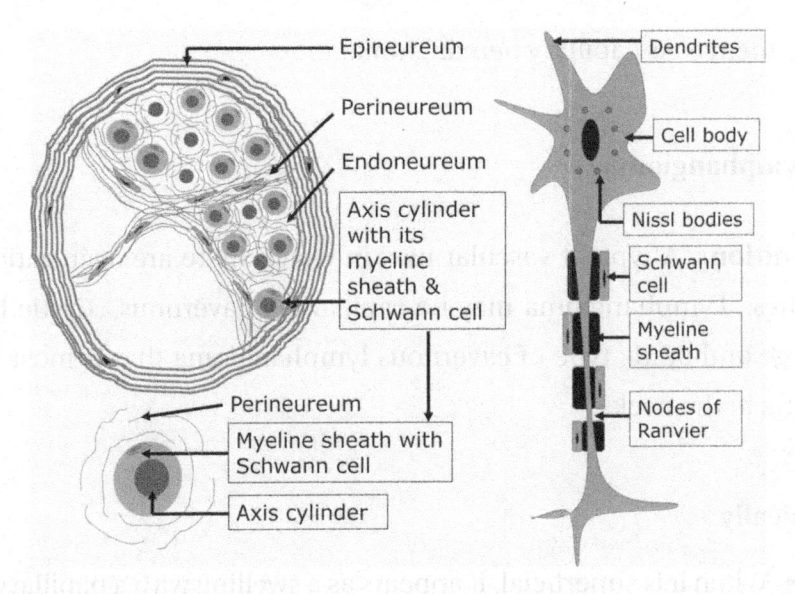

Figure 11.5: Diagrammatic structure of nerve trunk and nerve cell

11.4.1 Neurofibroma

Definition

Benign tumor arising from the fibrous connective tissue, which surrounds the axis cylinder (endoneurium, perineurium or epineurium).

Clinically

Two forms exist:

1. Solitary lesions: Which are true neoplasms, appearing clinically as fibroma.
2. Multiple lesions (Multiple Neurofibroma, Von Recklinghausen's disease of skin): This condition is considered to be a hamartoma and is characterized by (see later for details of neurofibromatosis):
    - Multiple neurofibromas on the skin and oral mucosa.
    - Cafe au lait pigmentation of the skin is also present.

Histologically

Consists of spindle shaped cells arranged in whorled pattern.

11.4.2 Multiple neurofibromatosis

The neurofibromatoses consist of at least two autosomal dominant disorders. They are referred to as neurofibromatosis type I (NF-1; also known as Von Recklinghausen disease of skin) and neurofibromatosis type II (NF-2; also known as bilateral acoustic neurofibromatosis or central neurofibromatosis). Although, neurogenic tumors are common to both types, they are clinically and genetically distinct. Type I is much more common than type II and constitutes around 90% of cases.

11.4.3 NF-1 (Von Recklinghausen disease of skin):

- Three major features:
    1. Multiple neurofibromas.
    2. Cafe au lait spots, sometimes patients with NF-1 have only the cafe au lait spots indicating variable expressivity of the genetic defect.
    3. Pigmented iris hamartomas, called Lisch nodules, do not present any clinical problem but are helpful in diagnosis.
- Multiple neurofibromatosis is a serious problem because in around 3% of patients, malignant transformation of neurofibromas into neurofibrosarcomas can occur. Also patients are at greater risk of developing other tumors.
- The NF-1 gene has been mapped to chromosome 17 and it encodes a protein (neurofibromin) that acts as a tumor suppressor gene product negatively regulating the RAS oncogene.

11.4.4 NF-2 (Bilateral acoustic neurofibromatosis)

(*Central neurofibromatosis*):

- Two major features:
    1. Bilateral acoustic schwannomas and multiple meningiomas.
    2. Cafe au lait spots on the skin.
- The gene for NF-2 has been mapped to chromosome 22 (22q21) and it encodes a protein (merlin). Like neurofibromin, it is also a tumor suppressor protein. Its mode of action is unknown.

11.4.5 Neurolemmoma (Schwannoma)

Definition

This is a benign tumor arising from Schwann cell.

Clinically

- The lesion appears as a round of ovoid mass similar to fibroma.
- Usually affect the tongue.
- Central cases are rare and usually occur in the mandible.
- They are considered to be arising from the inferior alveolar nerve.
- Central lesions occasionally may cause pain or numbness.
- They appear radiographically as a well defined radiolucent area.

Histologically

Two patterns may be seen:

1. Antoni type A:

   Rows of spindle shaped cells arranged in palisading manner. The intercellular collagen fibers are arranged in parallel manner between rows of cells. These rows are called **"nuclear rows of Verocay"**.

2. Antoni type B:
   - The cells are disposed haphazardly.
   - Small hyaline bodies may be seen (Verocay bodies).

11.4.6 Traumatic Neuroma (Amputation Neuroma)

Definition

This is a hyperplastic growth resulting from abortive attempt of repair of a peripheral nerve following trauma or transection.

Clinically

- Small tender nodule.
- Usually found at the area of previous surgery or trauma.
- Intraorally, the most common site is the area of the mental nerve following apicectomy or surgical removal of the lower premolars.

Histologically

- A haphazard proliferation of mature, myelinated and unmyelinated nerve bundles within a fibrous connective tissue stroma.
- An associated mild chronic inflammatory cell infiltrate may be present.
- When inflammation is present, the lesion is more likely to be painful than lesions without significant inflammation.

Treatment

Surgical excision, with a small portion of the involved proximal nerve bundle.

Chapter 12
Premalignant Lesions of the Oral Cavity

Premalignant or potentially malignant lesions and precancerous conditions are frequently encountered in the oral cavity that should be diagnosed in the early stages. Some of these lesions have a very high malignant transformation rate making their early diagnosis and management is of utmost importance.

12.1 Definitions

Premalignant Lesions

A premalignant lesion (or potentially malignant lesion) is an altered tissue in which cancer is more likely to occur and is characterized by presence of epithelial dysplasia. They should be differentiated from precancerous conditions.

Precancerous Conditions

Are conditions associated with increased risk of cancer but without the evidence of epithelial dysplasia. Epithelial dysplasia may develop later on as a step by which the lesion progresses into cancer. Some examples are:

- Syphilis of tongue.
- Most benign tumors.

- Xerodermia pigmentosa.
- Plumer-Vinson syndrome.
- Gardener syndrome.

Relevant Definitions

1. Acanthosis

   Is the increase in the size of prickle cell layer due to increase in the number of its cells.

2. Hyperkeratosis

   Is the increased thickness of keratin layer. Keratin may be parakeratin, which retain nuclear remnants or orthokeratin, which is devoid of such remnants.

3. Hyperplasia

   Is the increase in the size of an organ due to increase in the number of its cells.

4. Hypertrophy

   Is the increase in the size of an organ due to increase in the size of its cells.

5. Anaplasia

   Is the reversion of cells into a more undifferentiated form.

6. Metaplasia

   Is the change of one type of cell into another type within the same category.

7. Atypia

   A Condition in which cells do not conform to a type.

12.2 Epithelial Dysplasia

12.2.1 Overview

Epithelial dysplasia is a microscopic term denoting malignancy or premalignancy. The old term for epithelial dysplasia was malignant dyskeratosis, which is abandoned now. Epithelial dysplasia should be differentiated from benign dyskeratosis, which is the premature keratinization of epithelial cells that have not reached the keratinizing surface layer. Benign dyskeratosis is usually found in the following lesions:

- Hereditary benign intraepithelial dyskeratosis.
- Keratoacanthoma.
- Dyskeratosis congenita.
- Pachonychia congenita.
- Darier's disease.
- Molluscum contagiosum.

12.2.2 Criteria of epithelial dysplasia

1. Loss of polarity

Basal cells are considered to be polar cells that is to say they grow in only one direction namely from the basement membrane to the keratin layer and in order to achieve this target, basal cells should be positioned perpendicular to the basement membrane. Failure of basal cells to be perpendicular to the basement membrane will result in cells grown in different planes with the consequent formation of cell aggregates within the epithelium usually known as cell nests.

2. Basilar hyperplasia

Hyperplasia of basal cell layer and presence of more than one layer of basal cells is termed basilar hyperplasia.

3. Individual cell keratinization

A condition resulting from premature keratin formation inside prickle cells

4. Formation of cell nests and keratin pearls

Cell nests are aggregates of epithelial cells and when such cells undergo keratinization the term keratin pearl is given.

Cell nests result as a direct consequence to loss of polarity of basal cells

5. Increased nuclear cytoplasmic ratio

The normal nuclear cytoplasmic ratio is usually 1:4 and when this ratio in increased it denotes hyperactive nuclei.

6. Large prominent nucleoli

Nucleoli are essential for the process of mitosis as they contain the nucleolar oraganizer region.

7. Abnormal mitosis

The abnormality usually involves rate (being increased), Pattern (being abnormal) and site of mitosis (being in the superficial layers of the epithelium). Mitosis is normally confined to the basal and the first two layers of prickle cells.

8. Hyperchromatism of nuclei

Nuclei become deeply stained due to presence of excess quantities of DNA.

9. Dyskaryosis

Dyskaryosis is sometimes refereed to as nuclear pleomorphism, a condition that means bizarre shaped nuclei.

10. Poikilokaryonosis

Is the division of the nucleus without division of the cytoplasm.

12.2.3 Grading of dysplasia

Oral epithelial dysplasia is graded into three prognostically significant categories:

1. Mild (grade I): Presence of dysplastic cells in the basal and parabasal region but not extending beyond the lower third of the epithelium.
2. Moderate (grade II): As grade I with extension not exceeding beyond the middle one third of the epithelium.
3. Severe (grade III): Dysplastic cells occupy the whole thickness of the epithelium (top to bottom changes with lateral spread). Carcinoma in situ is considered by many authors to be grade III.

Certain grading criteria are in general use:

- There is no evidence of invasion into underlying stroma (the diagnosis would then change to carcinoma).
- The final grading or diagnosis should be based on the most severely involved area of change, even if that area includes no more than a few rete

processes. This is because the epithelium with the greatest proportion of atypical cells has the greatest risk of being or becoming a carcinoma.

Correlation of dysplasia with eventual malignant transformation

Investigations have followed lesions with specific dysplastic grades or changes in order to determine their natural history. This is, of course, made quite difficult by the following facts:

- The biopsy procedure itself has removed the cells upon which the diagnosis is based.
- The grading of dysplasias is an extremely subjective issue and there is often poor correlation between pathologists, even between very experienced pathologists.

Investigations have found that 20-35% of severely dysplastic lesions develop carcinoma, which is similar to the figures for carcinoma in situ. At the opposite end of the spectrum, mild epithelial dysplasias as found in leukoplakias show malignant transformation rate ranging from 1 to 10% of cases.

A greater risk of malignant change in an epithelial dysplasia has been associated with the following factors:

1. Erythroplakia within a leukoplakia
2. A proliferative verrucous appearance
3. Location at a high-risk anatomic site such as the tongue or floor of mouth
4. The presence of multiple lesions
5. Paradoxically, a history of not smoking cigarettes.

12.2.4 Microbiology of Oral Dysplasia

Several microorganisms are associated with proliferative epithelial lesions. Human papilloma virus, herpes virus, Epstein-Barr virus and candida albicans fungus show strong association with oral dysplastic lesions.

1- Human papilloma virus (HPV)

- Some strains of HPV show correlation with oral dysplasia and squamous cell carcinoma
- High-risk HPVs are found in 15–42% of leukoplakias, in 50% of erythroplakias, in 50–100% of oral squamous cell carcinomas, and in up to 10% of normal oral mucosa.
- The possible mode of action of HPV is to inactivate p53
- There is lack of a positive correlation between HPV presence and the severity of the histopathologic grade of epithelial dysplasia
- Survival from oral carcinoma does not appear to be associated with the presence or lack of HPV.

2- Herpes simplex virus (HSV)

- Herpes simplex virus (HSV), especially type 2 HSV, was once considered to be the cause of a large proportion of cancers of the uterine cervix, and it has been suggested that it plays a role in oral carcinoma.
- Currently, the evidence to prove a causal relationship between HSV and oral precancers or cancers is insufficient, but continued research may eventually show a relationship.

3- Epstein-Barr virus

- Is thought to play a role in the production of hairy leukoplakia and also in nasopharyngeal carcinomas.
- EBV is acquired by over 90% of the world population during childhood or adolescence and thereafter remains in a carrier state for the lifetime of the infected host.

4- Candida albicans

- Show strong association with oral dysplasia.
- Candida albicans could be culture from about 50% of leukoplakia.
- Some authors prefer to include this group in a separate leukoplakia subtype called candida leukoplakia, chronic hyperplastic candidiasis, or candida hyperplasia.
- The association of candida albicans with oral dysplasia may be a secondary phenomenon by which the dysplastic epithelium acts as a favorable media for fungus growth or that the fungus is producing the keratosis and dysplasia; evidence for the later assumption are:
    1. Laboratory experiments have shown that the yeast is capable of actually producing keratotic plaques on the tongues of rats.
    2. Certain strains of candida have been shown to produce carcinogenic nitrosamines.
    3. It has also been shown that at least some candida leukoplakias diminish in size or become less irregular in appearance when treated with antifungal therapy.
    4. Some oral pathologists are now recommending a course of antifungal therapy prior to biopsy of a suspected candida leukoplakia in order to reduce the abnormal histopathologic appearances of epithelial cells in the biopsied tissue.

12.2.5 Oral premalignant lesions

1. Leukoplakia
2. Carcinoma in situ
3. Erythroplakia
4. Oral submucous fibrosis
5. Actinic keratosis
6. Lichen planus

12.3 Leukoplakia

Definition

- Unfortunately, there is lack of consensus regarding a precise definition of leukoplakia.
- The World Health Organization first defined oral leukoplakia as a white patch or plaque that could not be characterized clinically or pathologically as any other disease; therefore, a process of exclusion establishes the diagnosis of the disease and hence lichen planus, candidiasis, and white sponge nevus were excluded.
- At the 1983 international seminar, the current definition was composed:
- Leukoplakia is a whitish patch or plaque that cannot be characterized clinically or pathologically as any other disease, and is not associated with any physical or chemical causative agent, except the use of tobacco.
- The presence of epithelial dysplasia in all cases of leukoplakia is still a controversial issue and many authors suggest that most leukoplakias show little evidence of dysplastic histologic changes or aneuploidy. The

term non-dysplastic leukoplakia was given for such cases of leukoplakia showing no signs of epithelial dysplasia.

- Because leukoplakia is diagnosed by the process of eliminating other possible etiologies, it is often termed idiopathic leukoplakia.

Etiology

- The etiology of premalignant lesions is very much related to the etiology of malignancy and in fact both conditions should share the same etiologic process.
- Refer to the chapter "Malignant Non-Odontogenic Tumors", page (311) for further details.
- No etiologic factor can be identified for most persistent oral leukoplakias (idiopathic leukoplakia).
- Briefly speaking oral premalignant lesions are usually associated with the following risk factors:

1. Smoking
2. Spirits
3. Spicy food
4. Sepsis
5. Syphilis
6. Galvanism
7. Candida infection
8. Chronic mechanical irritation
9. Actinic rays, especially in the lower lip.

Clinically

- **Age:** Usually after 40 years.
- **Sex:** Males are affected more than females.
- **Site:** Usually buccal mucosa, alveolar mucosa, tongue and palate.
- **Features:** Leukoplakias are white lesions that cannot be wiped off. Most leukoplakias are smooth, white plaques (homogeneous leukoplakias).

Some leukoplakias are white and warty (verrucous leukoplakia). Some leukoplakias are mixed white and red lesions (erythroleukoplakias or speckled leukoplakias). Rare cases of leukoplakia show nodular appearance (nodular leukoplakia). The presence of a nodule indicates malignant potential.

- Generally speaking, 3 stages of leukoplakia can be observed:
    1. First stage:

       White patch, non-palpable, soft can not be wiped off.
    2. Second stage:

       Palpable and rough white patch
    3. Third stage:

       Indurated, fissured and ulcerated patches.

Histologically

- Hyperkeratosis.
- Acanthosis.
- Signs of epithelial dysplasia (is still controversial).
- Intact basement membrane.

12.4   Hairy leukoplakia

Definition

- Oral hairy leukoplakia (OHL) was first observed in 1981 and reported in 1984 as a, benign, asymptomatic, white, non-removable lesion of the lateral borders of the tongue in patients with HIV infection and AIDS.

- In patients with HIV infection, when laboratory estimates are not available, OHL may be a useful clinical marker of the presence, severity and progression of HIV disease.
- The lesion is rare in the healthy population.
- OHL has been also observed in immunodeficient patients with other causes of immunosuppression (chemotherapy, long term steroid use, organ transplantation). Thus, it is regarded as a clinical marker of impaired immune status, in general, and its appearance should prompt the clinician to carry out further investigations in order to establish the underlying cause of immunosuppression.

Etiology

- Thought to be due to Epstein-Barr virus (EBV) infection facilitated by immunodeficiency.
- EBV is acquired by over 90% of the world population during childhood or adolescence and thereafter remains in a carrier state for the lifetime of the infected host.
- The virus is shed in saliva and cellular EBV receptors are found in the upper layers of parakeratinized oral epithelium.
- The close relationship between EBV infection and OHL is evident since EBV antigens have been demonstrated in tissue sections by immunohistochemical analysis and EBV-DNA has been demonstrated in tissue by molecular techniques such as Southern blotting and in situ hybridization (ISH).
- The pathogenesis is thought to be due to action of EBV proteins, which delay apoptosis of oral epithelial cells allowing very intense viral replication.

- It is unclear how OHL is initiated and whether it develops after EBV re-activation from latency state or is a result of re-infection of upper epithelial cells by the virus derived from saliva or other infected cells.
- Intracellular herpes virus particles have also been observed by electron microscopy but its role in the pathogenesis is unclear.
- Also, the mystery of why OHL is localized mainly on the lateral borders of the tongue has not been adequately clarified.

Clinical Picture

- Oral hairy leukoplakia presents as unilateral or more often bilateral, white patches mainly on the lateral borders of the tongue and sometimes the dorsum or ventrum of the tongue. The surface of the patches has usually a corrugated appearance forming prominent folds or projections (sometimes so marked as to resemble "hairs", hence its name).
- The corrugations are usually vertically oriented.
- OHL may occur (rarely) on other mucosal surfaces such as buccal mucosa, floor of the mouth and soft palate.
- OHL has so far not been observed in other areas than the oral cavity.
- Although usually symptomless, it may cause a burning sensation, while patients may complain of its unsightly appearance, especially when it is extended on all lingual surfaces.

Histopathology

- Hyperparakeratosis
- Acanthosis
- Epithelial cells show nuclear beading and ***Cowdry*** inclusion bodies. Nuclear beading refers to scattered cells with peripheral margination of chromatin by EBV replication

Chapter 12. Premalignant Lesions of the Oral Cavity

- Minimal or absent dysplastic changes
- Minimal or absent inflammatory reaction in the connective tissue

Diagnosis

A definitive diagnosis of hairy leukoplakia requires both an appropriate histologic appearance and the demonstration of EBV DNA, RNA using immunohistochemistry or in situ hybridization.

Treatment

- Since OHL is usually symptomless and their premalignant potential is in dispute, treatment is seldom required.
- Several treatment options are available for symptomatic lesions, such as topical retinoids, surgical excision and cryotherapy, but none prevent the recurrence of the lesion after therapy.
- Antifungal therapy may lead to some reduction in the extent of the lesion but does not eradicate the infection.
- Antiviral agents can result in amelioration of OHL, but lesions recur soon after discontinuation of therapy while side effects may occur and resistant viral strains may arise.
- It has been documented that OHL improves spontaneously in about 10% of the cases.

12.5 Carcinoma in Situ

(Intraepithelial Carcinoma)

Definition

A Microscopic terms denoting severe epithelial dysplasia with top to bottom changes and lateral spread. Bowen's disease of skin is a special form of carcinoma in situ resulting from arsenic therapy.

Etiology

The same as that of leukoplakia.

Clinically

- Appears as leukoplakia, or
- Appears as erythroplakia, or
- Appears as speckled leukoplakia or sometimes as speckled erythroplakia

Histologically

- Severe epithelial dysplasia.
- Intact basement membrane.

12.6 Erythroplakia (Erythoplasia of Quirat)

Definition

A red patch characterized by epithelial dysplasia.

Etiology

The same as that of leukoplakia.

Clinically

- A red velvety patch can not be wiped off.
- Sometimes appears as speckled erythroplakia.
- The red appearance of this lesion clinically is due to lack of keratinization and presence of high connective tissue papilla.

Histologically

The microscopic picture of erythroplakia is either:

- Carcinoma in situ i.e. severe epithelial dysplasia.
- Or rarely squamous cell carcinoma.

12.7 Oral Submucous Fibrosis

Definition

A disease characterized by atrophy of the epithelium followed by epithelial dysplasia.

Etiology

- The disease is usually related to tobacco chewing or beetle nut (areca nut) chewing (quid).
- Other postulated etiologic factors are:

- Genetic basis
- Autoimmunity
- Iron and Vitamin B12 deficiency

Clinically

- Red patch, which may be ulcerated. Areas of leukoplakia may be present
- Loss of elasticity of the oral mucosa
- The affected mucosa becomes pale in color and feels firm on palpation
- Associated with burning sensation

Histologically

The disease occurs in the following steps:

- Juxta epithelial inflammatory reaction.
- Juxta epithelial fibrosis with decreased vascularity and cellularity.
- Juxta epithelial hyalinization.
- Followed by atrophy of the epithelium and epithelial dysplasia.
- See figure ((12.1))

12.8 Lichen Planus

The premalignant or malignant potential of lichen planus is in dispute. Some believe that the occasional epithelial dysplasia or carcinoma found in patients with this lesion may be either coincidental or evidence that the initial diagnosis of lichen planus was erroneous. It is frequently difficult to differentiate lichen planus from epithelial dysplasia; one study found that 24% of oral lichen planus cases had 5 of the 12 World Health Organization (WHO) diag-

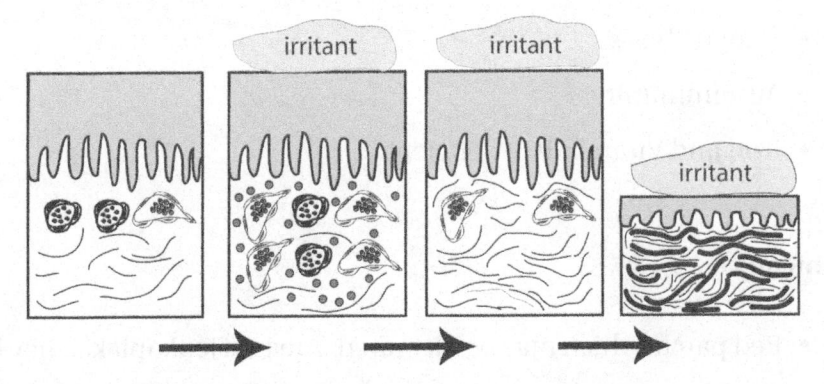

Figure 12.1: Diagrammatic representation of stages of oral submucous fibrosis. From the left to the right, normal mucosa, juxtaepithelial inflammatory reaction, juxtaepithelial fibrosis with diminution of vascularity and finally juxtaepithelial hyalinization with atrophy of the epithelium.

nostic criteria for epithelial dysplasia. Therefore, it is a reasonable practice to biopsy the lesion at the initial visit to confirm the diagnosis and to monitor it thereafter for clinical changes suggesting a premalignant or malignant change.

12.9 Actinic Keratosis

(Solar keratosis, Actinic cheilitis, Senile keratosis)

Definition

Actinic keratosis is a lesion which is directly related to long-term exposure to sun particularly in fair-skinned people. The malignant potentiality of the lesion is well established. There is also a positive relationship between exposure to ultraviolet rays and carcinoma.

Etiology

- Ultraviolet rays of sun are the responsible factor.
- This radiant energy affects not only the epithelium but also the supporting connective tissue.

Clinically

- The lesion usually affects the vermilion border of the lower lip.
- Other exposed areas of the skin may be affected.
- Hence the lesion usually occurs in persons with outdoor occupations such as farmers.
- The lesion appears as a white patch with rough crusted surface.
- Mottled areas of hyperpigmentation are often noted.
- The lesion shows definite malignant potentiality.

Histologically

- Hyperkeratosis.
- Atrophy of the epithelium affecting mainly the prickle cell layer.
- Basophilic changes of collagen.
- Telangiectasias (dilatation of blood vessels).

Treatment

- Lip protection is indicated using lip balm containing the sunscreen agent para-aminobenzoic acid.
- Sun blocking opaque agents also boosts the effectiveness of lip balm.
- Suspicious lesions are removed using laser surgery or cryosurgery.

12.10 Management of Oral Premalignancy

Elimination of the Predisposing Factors

If possible, the local or systemic predisposing factors should be eliminated. After completion of treatment, the patient is followed up for a period of 5 years (periodic recall every 3-4 months).

Surgical Intervention

Surgical excision, with a scalpel or a CO2 laser, is the treatment of choice for epithelial dysplasia of the oral cavity. Once an incisional biopsy has established the diagnosis of epithelial dysplasia, the remainder of the lesion should be removed completely, as the probability of malignant transformation, although unknown exactly, must be considered substantial. Reported recurrence rates for premalignant lesions are as high as 34.4%. One study found an 18% recurrence rate in cases of severe epithelial dysplasia or carcinoma in situ in which the lesion had been excised with a 3–5 mm margin of normal tissue. Whether recurrence relates to continued exposure to risk factors or to an underlying mechanism that initiated the original lesion is not known.

Chemoprevention

If the size of the lesion, its location, or the medical status of the patient would make surgical removal challenging, use of some medications should be considered as "chemoprevention" to try to prevent progression to carcinoma. Beta-carotene, retinoids and metformin are the most commonly used medications for chemoprevention of oral cancer.

Beta-carotene is a carotenoid found primarily in dark green, orange, or yellow vegetables. Several clinical trials have found that treating oral leukoplakia solely with beta-carotene supplements is associated with clinical improvement; rates have ranged from 14.8% to 71%. No side effects have been reported in patients given beta-carotene supplements; but there is little information about recurrence following discontinuation of this substance.

Retinoids are compounds consisting of natural forms or synthetic analogues of retinol. Of the synthetic analogues of vitamin A, 13-cis-retinoic acid (13-cRA), also known as isotretinoin or Accutane®, has generated the most interest. 13-cRA has been shown to cause temporary remission of oral leukoplakia, but it also causes side effects in a high percentage of patients. The recommended dose is 1–2 mg / kg / day of for 3 months. A rise in serum triglycerides has been reported with use of 13-cRA.

To date, no combination of antioxidants has demonstrated its clear superiority. Beta-carotene with ascorbic acid and/or alpha tocopherol is attractive because of a lack of side effects, but clinical improvement typically takes several months.

Topical antifungal drugs should be used for 1–2 months as Candida infection acts as an important predisposing factor for some cases of oral premalingancy.

Metformin which is the drug used in the control of diabetes is showing a promising effect for the treatment of oral premalignant lesions.

Chapter 13
Malignant Non-Odontogenic Tumors

Malignant tumors arising from the odontogenic tissues will be discussed in a separate chapter.

13.1 Classification of Malignancy

Malignant tumors are classified according to:

1. Histogenesis
2. Degree of differentiation (Broder's classification; used mainly for squamous cell carcinoma)
3. Clinical picture (TNM)

Classification According to Histogenesis

I- Malignant tumors of epithelium: (carcinomas)

1. Malignant tumors of surface epithelium:
   (a) Squamous cell carcinoma, some variants exist:
      i. Spindle cell carcinoma
      ii. Adenoid squamous cell carcinoma.
      iii. Verrucous carcinoma.
   (b) Basal cell carcinoma.

(c) Nasopharyngeal Carcinoma

2. Malignant tumors of glandular epithelium (see chapter "16", page (16) for further details):

   (a) Malignant pleomorphic adenoma.

   (b) Mucoepidermoid carcinoma.

   (c) Adenocystic carcinoma

3. Malignant tumors of odontogenic epithelium (see chapter "14", page (14) for further details)::

   (a) Malignant ameloblastoma.

   (b) Ameloblastic carcinoma.

   (c) Primary intraossous carcinoma of jaws.

II- Malignant tumors of connective tissue (sarcomas)[1]

A) Undifferentiated:

1. Spindle cell sarcoma
2. Small rounded cell sarcoma
3. Large rounded cell sarcoma.
4. Mixed cell sarcoma.

B) Differentiated sarcoma:

1. Fibrosarcoma.
2. Osteogenic sarcoma.
3. Chondrosarcoma
4. Ewing's sarcoma.
5. Kaposi sarcoma.

III- Malignant melanoma

IV- Metastatic tumors of the jaw

---

[1] Malignant and benign tumors of the connective tissues are also known as "soft tissue tumors" and also known as mesenchymal tumors as they almost all originate from the mesenchyme (ectomesenchyme).

Classification According to Differentiation

(Broder's classification, Histologic grading of malignancy)

Broder classified tumors according to the degree of differentiation into 4 grades. Grade I and II are the less dangerous and they contain more keratin pearls and show delayed metastasis. Although, the classical Broder's classification was used *mainly* for squamous cell carcinoma, modified forms of this classification were developed for other tumors as well. Broder classified squamous cell carcinomas as follows:

- Grade I: 75 – 100 % of cells are differentiated in the microscopic fields
- Grade II: 50 – 75 % of cells are differentiated.
- Grade III: 25 – 50 % of cells are differentiated.
- Grade VI: 0 – 25 % of cells are differentiated.

Classification According to Clinical Picture (TNM)

T = tumor -**N** = lymph node -**M** = metastasis.

Table (13.1) shows the most simplified TNM staging system. More sophisticated staging systems have been put forward to resolve some of the limitations of the classical staging.

13.2 Malignant Epithelial Tumors (Carcinomas)

13.2.1 Squamous Cell Carcinoma

(*Epidermoid carcinoma, Epithelioma*)

Chapter 13. Malignant Non-Odontogenic Tumors

Table 13.1: TNM of Oral Carcinomas

T0 = carcinoma in situ.
T1 = tumor 2 cm or less in its greatest diameter.
T2 = tumor more than 2 cm but less than 4 cm in its greatest diameter.
T3 = tumor 4 cm or more.
T4 = extending to adjacent structures e.g. bone or sinus

N0 = no palpable lymph node or palpable but not hard enough to suspect malignancy
N1 = palpable but not fixed on the same side (epsilateral)
N2 = palpable but not fixed bilateral or on the controlateral side
N3 = palpable and fixed.

M0 = no evidence of distant metastasis via blood.
M1 = evidence of distant metastasis.

Scores are compiled to designate the stage as follows:
Stage 1: T1N0M0
Stage 2: T2N0M0
Stage 3: T3N0M0, any T (except T4) + N1 + M0
Stage 4: Any T4, any N2, any N3, any M1

Definition

Squamous cell carcinoma is a malignant tumor of surface epithelium. Squamous cell carcinoma is the most common malignant tumor of the oral cavity.

Etiology

Important risk factors for oral squamous cell carcinoma are:

- Carcinogenic agents
- Tobacco
- Alcohol
- Areca nut (betel nut)
- Sunlight (lip only)
- Infections
- Candidosis
- Syphilis
- Viruses (some strains of HPV)
- Mucosal diseases
- Epithelial dysplasia
- Oral submucous fibrosis
- Lichen planus
- Genetic disorders
- Dyskeratosis congenital
- Fanconi's anemia
- Plumer-Venson syndrome

Clinically

- Age: over 50 years.
- Sex: males are affected more than females.
- Site: the lower lip is the most frequent site of oral cancer, while the tongue is the most frequently affected site within the mouth. The majority of intraoral squamous cell carcinomas are concentrated in the lower part of the mouth in a horseshoe or U-shaped area consisting of the lateral borders of the tongue, floor of the mouth and adjacent lingual mucosa, lingual sulcus and retromolar region.
- Incidence of intraoral squamous cell carcinoma is 52% in the tongue, 16% in the floor of mouth, 12% in the alveolar gingiva, 11% in the palate and 9% in the cheek mucosa.
- Features: the lesion appears clinically as either an exophytic or productive growth, which soon ulcerates, or as an ulcer from the start (destructive or endophytic growth). The characteristics of the ulcer are; everted or rolled out waxy edges, indurated base, necrotic floor, foul odor, bloody discharge and irregular outline. In the late stages, tissue

Chapter 13. Malignant Non-Odontogenic Tumors

destruction and necrosis lead to intense discomfort, pain and infection. See figure (13.1)

- Carcinoma of the lip is the most common site of oral cancer. Actinic rays of the sun appear to be a major cause of carcinoma at this site. The usual site is the vermilion border of the lower lip to one side of the midline. The lower lip is far more commonly affected than the upper lip. Metastases to the submental and submandibular lymph nodes is usually a late event.

- Carcinoma of the tongue most frequently affects the anterior two-thirds, particularly the lateral border. The dorsum of the tongue is an exceedingly rare site for the development of carcinoma. Spread to regional lymph nodes depends on the location of the tumor. Tumors at the tip of the tongue tend to spread to the submental lymph nodes whereas more distal tumors spread to the submandibular lymph nodes. Sometimes carcinoma of tongue may be found on the undersurface or in the posterior one third and is termed "hidden carcinoma of tongue". The following are valuable criteria in diagnosing hidden cancer of tongue:

    1. Deviation of the tongue towards the affected side on protrusion.
    2. Defect in patient speech.
    3. Dimpling which is the presence of a minute dimple on the surface of the tongue due to retraction of the mucous membrane by fibrosis.
    4. Discharge of blood.
    5. Defect of the surface i.e. minute ulcer.
    6. Induration.

- Carcinoma of the floor of the mouth tends to invade adjacent structures extensively. The tumor may form an exophytic mass but, more commonly; the presenting lesion is a typical malignant ulcer. The lesion might involve the under side of the tongue, and is then referred to as

"Oyster carcinoma". The submandibular nodes are the most frequent sites of secondary spread.

- Carcinoma of the buccal mucosa is probably related to the habit of betel nut and tobacco-chewing. It usually involves the mucosa opposite the third molar tooth and retromolar pad. Metastasis is usually to the submandibular lymph nodes.

- Other less common sites for intraoral carcinoma are the gingiva, the alveolar mucosa and the palate. These sites show similar features to those already described, but tend to involve the bone at a relatively early stage.

Complications

The major complications and causes of death of malignancy are loss of function of an organ, hyperfunction of an organ (as in endocrine glands), sever hemorrhage due to erosion of major blood vessels, toxemia, cachexia and severe pain (particularly in the later stages).

Methods of Spread

Squamous cell carcinoma usually spread in the following order.

1. Local spread.
2. Lymphatic spread.
3. Later on blood spread. However some carcinomas show early spread by blood e.g. carcinoma of breast, thyroid, prostate, suprarenal and lung.

Histopathology

- Invasion of the connective tissue by masses of malignant epithelial cells forming cell nests and keratin pearls, these cells show signs of epithelial dysplasia.
- In well-differentiated carcinomas the invading tumor cells retain, to some extent, the function of normal prickle cells. Nests of epithelial cells surrounded by basement membrane and showing keratin formation is a prominent feature of such lesions. In less well-differentiated tumors (moderately-differentiated) keratin pearl formation is absent and the masses of invading tumor cells are surrounded by a discontinuous basement membrane. In poorly-differentiated (anaplastic) lesions the cells tend to be more irregular and show extreme degrees of pleomorphism and hyperchromatism with frequent abnormal mitoses. Basement membrane formation is lost and the resemblance to the mother tissue is minimal.
- Sometimes, there is infiltration of the surrounding connective tissue with chronic inflammatory cells around the invading tumor masses. The presence of such inflammatory reaction is of good prognosis.

13.2.2 Variants of Squamous Cell Carcinoma

1- Spindle Cell Carcinoma

Definition

Rare undifferentiated variant of squamous cell carcinoma.

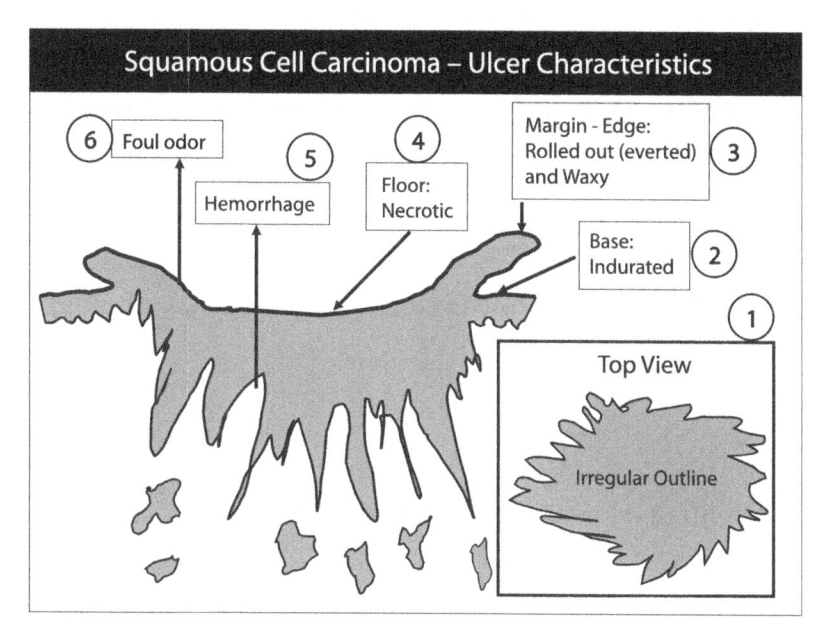

Figure 13.1: Clinical characteristic features of squamous cell carcinoma ulcer

Etiology

Usually there is a previous history of traumatic injury such as thermal burn, irradiation or physical trauma.

Clinically

The lesion usually affects the lower lip and appears clinically similar to squamous cell carcinoma.

Histopathology

The microscopic appearance of these lesions might resemble sarcomas, particularly fibrosarcoma and it might be necessary to use immunohistochemical markers to confirm the epithelial nature of the tumor. The lesion consists of:

1. Masses of spindle shaped cells with no keratinization
2. Hyperchromatic nuclei and frequent abnormal mitoses are prominent.

2- Adenoid Squamous Cell Carcinoma

(psuedoglandular squamous cell carcinoma, adenoacanthoma)

Definition

Rare differentiated form of squamous cell carcinoma

Etiology

Usually follows senile keratosis of the lip

Clinically

The most common site of this lesion is the lip. Crust formation and ulceration are common clinical features. Prognosis is better than squamous cell carcinoma.

Histopathology

Microscopically the lesion resembles squamous cell carcinoma but the deeper epithelial extensions show duct like structures lined by a layer of cuboidal cells.

3- Verrucous Carcinoma

(Snuff Dippers's Carcinoma, Ackerman's Carcinoma)

Definition

This is a variant of squamous cell carcinoma and is of low malignancy. It is a differentiated form of squamous cell carcinoma.

Etiology

Tobacco-chewing and snuff-dipping are common etiologic factors.

Clinically

- Age: It is usually seen in elderly patients.
- Sex: males affected more than females.
- Site: The most frequent oral site is the lower buccal sulcus and adjacent alveolar mucosa.
- Features: the lesion forms a slowly growing, warty, exophytic white mass that is papular rather than ulcerative. Invasion of the underlying soft tissue and bone could be a late complication. Metastasis is rare.

Histopathology

Verrucous carcinoma consists of closely packed papillary masses of well differentiated squamous epithelium showing:

1. Heavy keratinization
2. Blunt rete pegs tending to be all on the same level, giving the characteristic pushing margin of the tumor.
3. Intact basement membrane.
4. Dense chronic inflammatory infiltrate in the stroma.

13.2.3 Nasopharyngeal Carcinoma

(Lymphoepithelioma, Rounded cell carcinoma)

Definition

This is a rare highly malignant undifferentiated tumor. In old medical literature, the obsolete term transitional cell carcinoma was used to refer to this tumor. Epstein-Barr virus genome is identified in most nasopharyngeal carcinomas and is thought to play an important role in its pathogenesis.

Clinically

The most common site of this tumor is the posterior part of the tongue, tonsils and nasopharynx and rarely occurs on the palate. Thus the tumor is often hidden. This tumor is highly malignant and has a rapid clinical course causing early wide spread metastasis.

Histopathology

The lesion consists of two elements:

- The epithelial element which consists of masses of large epithelial cells with vesicular nuclei and prominent nucleoli showing ill-defined cell borders
- Dense lymphocytic infiltrate between epithelial cell masses with occasional presence of plasma cells
- The tumor cells are immunoreactive for pan-cytokeratin and epithelial membrane antigen. EBV encoded RNA (EBER) has been demonstrated by in-situ hybridization in some patients particularly Chinese

13.2.4 Basal Cell Carcinoma (Rodent Ulcer)

Definition

Basal cell carcinoma is a locally invasive tumor of surface epithelium.

Etiology

Prolonged exposure to sun light is the most common etiologic factor.

Clinically

- **Age:** old age. An exception is seen in patients with the neviod basal cell carcinoma syndrome (Gorlin - Goltz syndrome), in which tumors develop in young aged patients.
- **Sex:** Males are affected more common than females.
- **Race:** More common in white races. The protective role of skin pigmentation has been shown to form the relative rarity of skin cancer in Negroes.
- **Site:** Most frequently in the middle third of the face but may occur anywhere in the skin. There is no convincing evidence that basal cell carcinoma arise from oral mucosa, yet the mucosa of the upper lip might be involved as an extension from the skin surface.
- **Features:** Basal cell carcinoma forms a slightly elevated, slowly growing, nodule which eventually undergoes central ulceration. The ulcer is irregular, with inverted edges, indurated base, covered by a scab or crust and bloody discharge. Basal cell carcinoma rarely metastasizes. Although most basal cell carcinomas are solitary tumors, those occurring in the Gorlin - Goltz syndrome are multiple. See figure (13.2)

Histopathology

- Invasion of the connective tissue by epithelial cells that form nests or islands. The periphery of these nests is composed of an outer layer of columnar cells with palisading nuclei resembling the basal cells of the epithelium. The central cells are polyhydral. These cells show signs of epithelial dysplasia.

- As the basal cells are pleuripotent, it is expected to find hair follicles, sebaceous glands, sweat glands or squamous epithelium and keratin in basal cell carcinoma.

Variants of basal cell carcinoma

1. Trichoepithelioma: if the tumor arises from hair follicles.
2. Adenoid basal cell carcinoma: if the tumor forms or arises from sebaceous glands.
3. Basosquamous cell carcinoma: if the central cells form keratin. Recently, it is considered as an aggressive variant of squamous cell carcinoma.
4. Krompeckers carcinoma: if the tumor occurs in the oral cavity.
5. Cystic basal cell carcinoma: If the central cells undergo cystic degeneration.

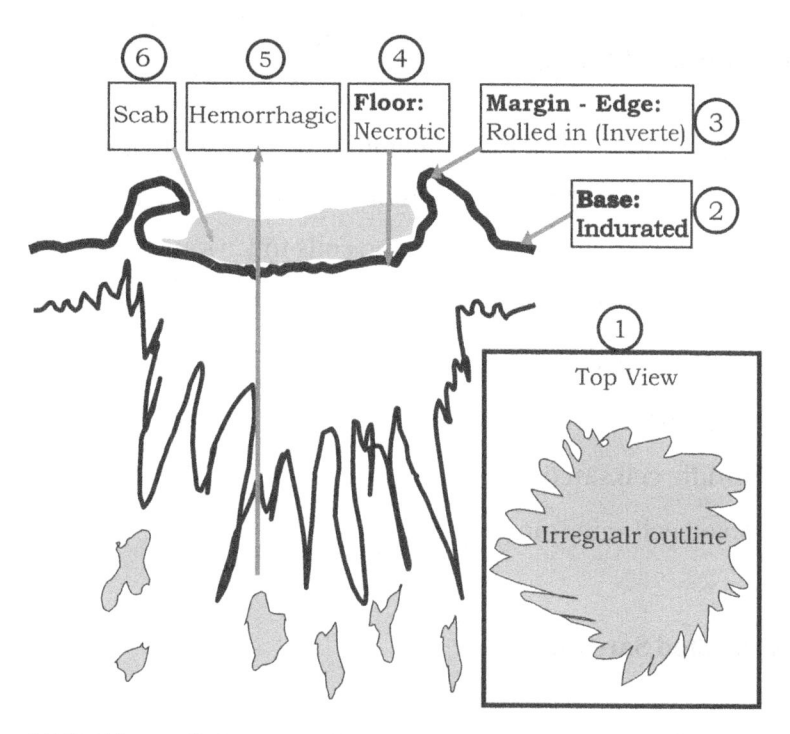

Figure 13.2: Clinical characteristic features of basal cell carcinoma ulcer

13.3 Malignant Mesenchymal Tumors (Sarcomas)

13.3.1 Introduction

Sarcomas of any type can affect the oral tissues. They are less frequent than carcinomas. These neoplasms tend to affect considerably younger age groups than carcinomas. Sarcomas grow rapidly, are invasive and destructive to the surrounding tissues. Metastasis of sarcomas is mainly through the bloodstream thereby producing more widespread foci of secondary tumor growth.

Sarcomas occur either in differentiated or undifferentiated forms

Undifferentiated Sarcomas

The cells are scattered all over the field. They have a hyperchromatic nucleus and present unequal mitosis. Sarcoma presents very thin walled-blood vessels; blood is seen to run between the cells in various parts. Undifferentiated sarcomas are subdivided according to the type of cells present into:

1. Small round cell sarcoma.
2. Large round cell sarcoma.
3. Spindle cell sarcoma.
4. Mixed cell sarcoma.

Differentiated Sarcomas

These tumors present histologically varying amount of matrix between the cells. The names given to these tumors are those of the matrix found, so there are fibrosarcoma, myxosarcoma, chondrosarcoma and osteosarcoma etc.

13.3.2 Fibrosarcoma

Definition

This is a malignant neoplasm of fibrous tissue.

Clinically

- **Age:** Young age
- **Sex:** Males and females are equally affected.
- **Site:** In the fibrous tissue of the cheek, maxillary sinus, lip, palate, gingiva and tongue.

- **Features:** Bulky, fleshy mass or swelling producing early facial asymmetry. Ulceration, hemorrhage and secondary infection are seen in some cases. Fibrosarcoma does not exhibit early metastasis.

Histopathology

- Some fibrosarcomas appear highly differentiated and closely resemble the normal parent tissue, while others are poorly differentiated.
- The lesion consists of:
    1. Proliferating spindle shaped fibroblasts with elongated and deeply stained nuclei.
    2. Interlacing bands of collagen fibrils.
    3. Thin walled blood vessels.

13.3.3 Osteosarcoma (Osteogenic Sarcoma)

Definition

Osteosarcoma is a malignant neoplasm of bone that have the ability to form osteoid or disorganized bone. It is the most common primary neoplasm of bone, but overall is rare, especially in the jaws. Some authors consider osteosarcoma of jaw as a separate entity due to its distinctive clinical and biologic features.

Etiology

- The exact etiologic factors for the development of osteosarcoma are unknown.

- Irradiation, trauma or pre-existing bone disorder such as Paget's disease or fibrous dysplasia might be predisposing conditions for the development of osteosarcoma.

Classification

1. According to clinical appearance:
   (a) Conventional (endosteal, central) osteosarcoma: here the tumor arises from the osteoblasts in the endosteum and grows within the marrow spaces. It penetrates or partially destroys the overlying cortex to extend beneath the periosteum.
   (b) Parosteal osteosarcoma (surface): this uncommon variant of osteosarcoma has a somewhat better prognosis. The tumor grows from the external surface of the bone. These tumors tend to grow slowly and metastasize late.
   (c) Extraskeletal (arising within soft tissue): Occurs in the soft tissue and is very rare.
2. According to radiographic picture:
   (a) Osteoblastic (sclerosing) type
   (b) Osteolytic type
3. According to histologic features:
   (a) Osteoblastic osteosarcoma.
   (b) Fibroblastic osteosarcoma.
   (c) Chondroblastic osteosarcoma.
   (d) Telangiectatic osteosarcoma.

Pathogenesis

Mutations in the TP53 tumor suppressor gene or overexpression of the MDM2 oncogene . MDM2 protein binds to and inactivates the TP53 gene product. Also, hereditary retinoblastoma (RB1) predispose to osteosarcoma.

Risk Factors:

- Radiation exposure
- Alkylating agents
- Paget's disease of bone
- Li-Fraumeni syndrome
- Hereditary retinoblastoma
- Rothmund-Thomson syndrome[2]

Clinically

- **Age:** Young age.
- **Sex:** Males more than females.
- **Site:** This lesion mainly affects the long bones and is rare intraorally. Orally, the mandible is more affected than the maxilla.
- **Features:**
    - Pain and swelling of the affected bone.
    - History of trauma.
    - Osteosarcoma of the jaw is a rapidly invasive lesion, there is facial asymmetry, pain, loosens of the teeth and bleeding.

---

[2] A rare autosomal recessive skin disease characterized by sun-sensitive rash.

Radiographic Features

- The radiographic features of osteosarcoma are variable depending on the degree of bone formation in the tumor. In the osteoblastic or sclerosing type irregular foci of radiopacity intermingled with areas of radiolucency is noted. In the osteolytic type irregular radiolucent area with no radiopacities can be seen.

- In rapidly growing tumors when the periosteum is raised, specules of new bone are laid down perpendicular to the cortex giving the **"sun ray appearance"**, while at the junction between raised and normal periosteum a wedge of reactive bone referred to as **"Codman's triangle"** may develop. See diagrammatic representation in figure (13.3).

- Symmetrical widening of the periodontal ligament space of one or more teeth is considered an early and diagnostic feature of osteosarcoma in dental periapical radiographs.

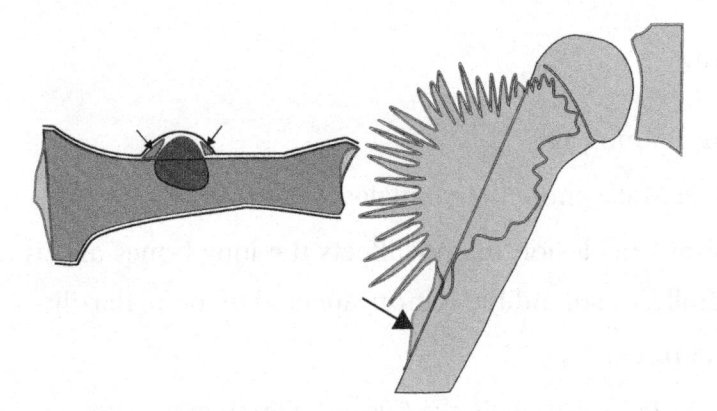

Figure 13.3: Diagrammatic representation of the radiographical features of osteosarcoma. Left panel, the arrows indicate the Codman's triangle formed under the elevated periosteum. The Codman's triangle is normal bone unlike the sarcomatous bone formed by the lesion. Right panel shows the characteristic sun-ray appearance and the red arrow points also to Codman's triangle.

Histopathology

- Osteosarcomas originate from bone cells (osteoblasts) that are variable in appearance and have wide potentialities. The microscopic appearance of the tumor is therefore widely variable, even within an individual lesion. The lesion consists of:
- Collections of atypical neoplastic osteoblasts showing considerable variation in size and shape, they may be small and angular or large and hyperchromatic. Mitoses may be prominent, particularly in the most cellular areas of the tumor.
- The formation of tumor osteoid or bone is a diagnostic histologic criterion of the lesion. The neoplastic cells do not rim the tumor bone in the manner seen in normal or reactive bone. The trabeculae of tumor bone tend to be delicate and irregularly arranged.
- **Osteoblastic osteosarcoma** – is a variant of osteosarcoma showing extensive formation of tumor osteoid and bone.
- **Fibroblastic osteosarcoma** – shows the tendency of the tumor cells to form varying amounts of collagen. Tumor osteoid and bone are sparse or absent.
- **Chondroblastic osteosarcoma** – is an aggressive variant of osteosarcoma in which the tumor cells form malignant chondroid tissue.
- **Telangiectatic osteosarcoma** – is a tumor characterized by the presence of large blood filled cystic spaces.

Treatment

- Wide surgical resection.
- The additional use of chemotherapy and/ or radiotherapy is controversial but may be considered in some cases.

13.3.4 Chondrosarcoma

Definition

This is the malignant counterpart of chondroma. It is less common than osteosarcoma.

Classification

Chondrosarcoma is classified into primary and secondary types. The secondary type is that chondrosarcoma arising in a pre-existing benign cartilaginous tumor, whereas the primary type develops in the absence of a pre-existing benign cartilaginous tumor.

Clinically

- **Age:** Most patients are between the age of 40–60 years.
- **Sex:** Males are affected more than females (2:1).
- **Site:** In the mandible chondrosarcoma occurs in the premolar and molar regions, in the symphysis or in the coronoid and condylar process. In the maxilla, the anterior alveolar ridge is the most common site (anterior part of maxilla and posterior part of mandible).
- **Features:** Pain, swelling and loosening of the teeth are clinical signs of chondrosarcoma and, although metastases tend to be late, many patients die from extensive local tissue invasion. Radical surgical excision offers the only hope of cure; but this is difficult, as it is frequently impossible to define the extent of the tumor, clinically or radiographically. Local recurrences are common and the overall prognosis for chondrosarcoma of the jaws is worse than that for osteosarcoma.

Radiographically

Chondrosarcomas appears as a unilocular or multilocular radiolucency with some spotty radiopacities.

Histopathology

The microscopic picture of chondrosarcoma is variable. The tumor is richly cellular with pleomorphic and hyperchromatic chondrocytes, many of which have several nuclei. Mitoses, however, are rare.

13.3.5 Ewing's Sarcoma

Definition

This is a rare highly malignant tumor of bone.

Histogenesis

- The histogenesis of Ewing's sarcoma remains uncertain.
- An endothelial, neural or nuroectodermal origins were suggested.

Clinically

- Age: children and young adults is the common age (5–20 years).
- Sex: males are affected more than females (2:1).
- Site: This lesion mainly affects the long bones and is rare intraorally. Orally the mandible is more affected than the maxilla.
- Features: bone swelling and often pain, progressing over a period of months are typical symptoms. Teeth may be come loosened by bone

destruction. The overlying mucous may ulcerate. Fever, leukocytosis, a raised ESR and anemia may be associated and indicate a poor prognosis.
- Distant spread is usually to the lungs and other bones, and Ewing's sarcoma in the jaws may therefore be a metastasis from another bone. Lymph nodes are rarely involved.

Radiographically

Ewing's sarcoma forms an irregular diffuse radiolucent area with or without cortical expansion. Reactive subperiosteal new bone formation giving the *"onion skin"* appearance could be seen in jaw lesions.

Histopathology

Ewing's sarcoma cells have a darkly staining nuclei surrounded by a rim of cytoplasm, which is typically vacuolated. They resemble mature lymphocytes but are about twice their size. Intracellular glycogen is detected in approximately 75% of cases. The tumor cells are in diffuse sheets or in loose lobules, separated by septa.

13.3.6 Kaposi's Sarcoma

(Multiple Idiopathic Hemorrhagic Sarcoma of Kaposi)
- Kaposi (1872) originally described this vascular tumor as a rare entity among elderly persons of central European or Mediterranean origin. However, the disease is common in central Africa, particularly Zaire, where it formed up to 12% of all malignant tumors. "Classical Kaposi's" sarcoma is predominantly cutaneous, mainly affects the lower extremities and has an indolent course with late visceral involvement.

- Since 1981, however, Kaposi's sarcoma has become common, as a feature of the acquired immune deficiency syndrome (AIDS), but had also been noted as an occasional complication of deep immunosuppression.

Clinically

- The clinical features of classical Kaposi's sarcoma and AIDS-associated Kaposi's sarcoma are generally the same.
- However, the AIDS-associated type predominantly affects younger males and involves the head and neck region in about 50% of patients.
- In AIDS patients, Kaposi's sarcoma frequently involves the oral cavity, where it often appears as a flat or nodular purplish, easily bleeding lesion on the palate, but can affect any site.

Histopathology

- Kaposi's sarcoma appears to originate from endothelial cells as indicated by immunohistochemical investigations. The appearance varies with the stage of development of the neoplasm.
- Initially, the lesion consists of a mass of irregular vascular capillaries with perivascular cuffing by plasma cells and lymphocytes. This appearance may be very similar to granulation tissues. Histological recognition at this stage may, therefore, be very difficult.
- In intermediate stage, angiomatous proliferation becomes widespread and the vascular spaces appear in longitudinal sections as slit-like. There is also perivascular proliferation of spindle-shaped and angular cells.
- In the late stages of the lesion, proliferation of the interstitial spindle-shaped and angular cells tend to dominate, mitotic activity may be come conspicuous, and there is extravasation of erythrocytes.

13.3.7 Lymphomas

- Lymphomas are primary tumors of the lymphoreticular system, almost all of which arise from lymphocytes. Most lymphomas arise in lymph nodes, but 30–40% develop in extranodal sites such as the stomach, though almost any organ may be primarily involved.
- They usually produce lymph node enlargement which may be localized or generalized, with widespread involvement of the lymphoreticular system at presentation.
- Typically, lymphoma presents as a solid tumor of lymphoid cells.
- Lymphomas are closely related to *lymphoid leukemias*, which also originate in lymphocytes but typically involve only circulating blood and the bone marrow and do not usually form solid tumors.

13.3.8 Burkitt's Lymphoma

(African Jaw Lymphoma)

Definition

- Burkitt's lymphoma is a high-grade B-cell neoplasm that has 2 major forms, the endemic (African) form and the non-endemic (sporadic) form.
- Burkitt's lymphoma is named after Burkitt, who mapped its peculiar geographic distribution across Africa.
- Burkitt's lymphoma is a childhood tumor but it is observed in adult patients. Burkitt's lymphoma is one of the fastest growing malignancies in humans, with a very high growth fraction.

Pathogenesis

- The Epstein-Barr virus (EBV) has been implicated strongly in the African form, while the relationship is less clear in the sporadic form.
- EBV is associated with about 20% of sporadic cases.
- The lymphocytes have receptors for EBV and are its specific target.
- In the African form, the hosts are believed to be unable to mount an appropriate immune response to primary EBV infection, possibly because of coexistent malaria or another infection that is immunosuppressive. Months to years later, excessive B cell proliferation occurs.
- Rare adult cases are associated with immunodeficiency, particularly AIDS.

Clinically

- About 50 – 70 of African cases occurs in the jaws
- Young age (peak at about 7 years of age)
- Males more than females
- The posterior part of the jaws are more commonly affected
- Maxilla is involved more commonly than the mandible (a 2:1 ratio)
- Produce facial swelling and proptosis
- Pain, tenderness, and paresthesia
- Tooth mobility may be present because of the aggressive destruction of the alveolar bone
- Premature exfoliation of deciduous teeth

Radiographically

Aggressive radiolucent destruction of the bone with ragged, ill-defined margins

Chapter 13. Malignant Non-Odontogenic Tumors

Histologically

- Consists of undifferentiated, small, noncleaved[3] cells in broad sheets of tumor cells
- Numerous mitoses are seen
- Burkitt's lymphoma demonstrates starry sky appearance, the stars are represented by the macrophage ingesting degenerating tumor cells. The sky is represented by the numerous dark lymphocytes

13.3.9 Plasma Cell Myeloma (Plasmacytoma)

Definition

- Is the malignant neoplasm of a single clone of plasma cells.
- Plasma cells are characterized by the production of immunoglobulin and therefore, there are large amounts of a single type of immunoglobulin, most commonly IgG.
- High levels of the homogeneous immunoglobulin and/or its constituent polypeptide chains appear in serum, and are termed paraproteins or "M" components (in reference to myeloma).
- Although a high level of M protein in the blood is a hallmark of myeloma disease, about 15% to 20% of patients with myeloma produce incomplete immunoglobulins, containing only the light chain portion of the immunoglobulin (also known as **Bence Jones proteins**, after the chemist who discovered them).
- These patients are said to have light chain myeloma, or Bence Jones myeloma. In these patients, M protein is found primarily in the urine, rather than in the blood. These Bence Jones proteins may deposit in the kidney and clog the tiny tubules that make up the kidney's filtering

---
[3]Cleaved cell: Is the cell with cleft in the cell membrane

system, which can eventually cause kidney damage and result in kidney failure.

- Bence Jones proteins will not be detected by routine urinalysis.
- A more complex test called immunoelectrophoresis can measure the exact amount of Bence Jones proteins in the urine.
- Because many organs can be affected by myeloma, the symptoms and signs vary greatly. A mnemonic sometimes used to remember the common tetrad of multiple myeloma is CRAB - C = Calcium (elevated), R =Renal failure, A = Anemia, B = Bone lesions.
- Myeloma has many possible symptoms, and all symptoms may be due to other causes.

Types

1. Multiple plasma cell Myeloma (multiple myeloma) Which is the most common form
2. Solitary plasma cell myeloma (solitary plasmacytoma) Which is the less common form. Some, but not all, patients with solitary lesions eventually develop multiple myeloma
3. Soft Tissue Plasmacytoma (Single plasma cell tumor in soft tissue), usually in nasopharynx or oropharynx, minimal M-component (immunoglobulin) in serum. Low risk of progression into multiple myeloma.

Clinically

- Occurs most frequently in patients between 50 and 70 years of age.
- Jaw lesions may occur as part of multiple myeloma or as a solitary lesion.
- Extramedullary plasmacytoma may also occur rarely in the oral soft tissues, presenting as diffuse swellings.

- Although any bone may be involved, the skull, vertebrae, sternum, ribs, and pelvic bones are most commonly affected.
- These are sites where red marrow is normally present.
- Jaw lesions may be the initial manifestation of disease, but more commonly they are purely secondary to other remote lesions.
- The proliferation of plasma cells may interfere with the normal production of blood cells, resulting in leucopenia, anemia, and thrombocytopenia. The cells may cause soft tissue masses (plasmacytomas) or lytic lesions in the skeleton.
- Possible complications of this malignancy are bone pain, hypercalcemia, and spinal cord compression.
- The aberrant antibodies that are produced lead to impaired humoral immunity, and patients have a high prevalence of infection.
- The overproduction of these antibodies may lead to hyperviscosity of the blood, amyloidosis, and renal failure. About 8% of myeloma patients develop amyloidosis.

X-Ray

The classical radiographic feature is of sharply demarcated, round or oval osteolytic lesions with a characteristic *punched-out appearance*.

Histologically

- The lesions are densely cellular and consist of sheets of myeloma cells which bear a striking resemblance to mature plasma cells or their immediate precursors.
- Russell bodies may be present, they represent aging plasma cells.

Treatment

Partial remission may be achieved with systemic chemotherapy using prednisone, cyclophosphamide and melphalan.

Prognosis

Despite therapy, is generally poor.

Solitary Plasma Cell Myeloma

(Solitary plasmacytoma)

- Absence of a plasma cell infiltrate in random marrow biopsies
- No evidence of other bone lesions by radiographic examination
- Absence of renal failure, hypercalcemia or anemia

Extramedullary Plasmacytoma

- Plasma cell tumors that arise outside the bone marrow and no features of Multiple Myeloma
- Most Common Primary Sites - Head and Neck region: Upper air passages and oropharynx (May involve draining lymph nodes).
- Less Common Sites – Lymph nodes (primary), salivary glands, spleen, liver, etc.
- 25% have small monoclonal spike
- Rare dissemination, rarer evolution to myeloma
- Management:
    - ★ If completely resected during biopsy, no further therapy
    - ★ If incompletely resected, radiation therapy locally

13.3.10 Vascular Tumors

Angiosarcoma

Definition

- Angiosarcomas are malignant tumors that arise from either vascular or lymphatic endothelium.
- One of their common sites is the skin of the maxillofacial area and the scalp (52%).

Clinically

- They may occur at any age but are more common in old age.
- More common in males than females.
- The tumor usually begins as a flat, red area with a firm, indurated edge.
- As the lesions mature, they become nodular and fleshy and will ulcerate.
- Most are painless.

Differential Diagnosis

- Induration and ulceration lead to a suspicion of malignancy.
- Basal cell carcinoma, melanoma, skin squamous cell carcinoma, and eccrine tumors of sweat gland origin.

Histopathology

- Usually form irregular vascular channels that often intercommunicate to form a network.

- The endothelial cells lining the channels are plump and hyperchromatic and may proliferate to form papillary projections.
- Nuclear pleomorphism and atypical mitoses.
- Immunohistochemical staining for factor VIII antigen, which is a marker of vascular differentiation, is present in almost all tissues and is therefore not reliable.

Treatment

- Radical excision with 5 cm margins and/or radical electron-beam radiotherapy.
- lymph node metastasis is common, necessitating surgical lymphadenectomy or radiotherapy.

Hemangioendothelioma

- Are variants of angiosarcomas that are characterized by either a benign or usually of intermediate behavior.
- Thus, most lesions are considered as low grade malignancy.
- Their clinical and histological appearances are very similar to angiosarcoma but run an indolent course.

Hemangiopericytoma

Definition

- Benign hemangiopericytomas arise from a vascular supporting cell, the pericyte.
- Its behavior rangs from benign, intermediate and malignant.

Clinically

- A mass within muscle or within deeper fascial spaces, rarely superficial.
- Men and women are affected equally.
- The peak incidence is between the ages of 30 and 50 years.
- Slowly growing.
- Most are of significant size at the time of diagnosis.
- The tumor mass is painless but often contains pulsations.

Differential Diagnosis

If pulsations are noted, it may suggest an arteriovenous hemangioma or, if the nasal cavity or medial orbit is involved, a nasopharyngeal angiofibroma.

Histopathology

- Thin, vascular pseudocapsule.
- Ovoid to spindle cells, surrounding endothelially lined vascular spaces.
- The vessels may be distended and often have a staghorn[4] appearance.
- A *silver stain* will stain the basement membrane of the endothelial cells so that the proliferating cells are seen outside the vessel, thus clearly distinguishing these tumors from those of endothelial origin.

Treatment

- Local excision with margins of 0.5 to 1.0 cm.
- Because many have feeder vessels and the lesion itself is vascular, ligation of all feeding vessels in the immediate area is advised.

---
[4] Like a horn with many branches

Prognosis

The prognosis of this tumor is excellent; no recurrences are expected when it is excised with clear margins.

13.4 Malignant Melanoma

13.4.1 Cutaneous Melanomas

Definition

Melanomas are malignant tumors of melanocytes. Melanomas can arise de novo or from a preexisting lesion (congenital nevus). The precise fraction that arises in nevi or de novo is difficult to determine.

Etiology and pathogenesis

- The most important etiologic factor is UV light.
- Molecular analysis revealed mutation of the CDKI2A (CDKN2A, p16) in about 50% of melanoma patients. CDKI acts as a tumor suppressor gene.
- Surprisingly, unlike in most malignancies, deletion or mutation of p53 is uncommon in melanomas.
- Risk factors for developing malignant melanomas are:
- Exposure to excessive sunlight is the most important risk factor
- A history of severe sunburn
- Fair skin, blue eyes, blond or red hair

- Dysplastic nevus syndrome (Dysplastic nevi are multiple scattered nevi over the entire body with individual lesions that have a diameter greater than 1 cm).
- Freckling on exposure to sun (melanoma syndrome)
- Melanoma in a first/second degree relative
- Xeroderma pigmentosa (autosomal recessive disease with a lack of DNA repair enzymes)

Clinicopathologic Features

An important feature of malignant melanoma is the concept of radial and vertical growth phases.

Radial growth phase:

Radial growth is the initial tendency of melanoma to grow horizontally within the epidermal and superficial dermal layers, often for a prolonged period of time. During this phase melanoma cells do not have the capacity to metastasize and there is no evidence of angiogenesis.

Vertical growth phase:

With time, the melanoma cells grow downward into the deeper dermal layers as an expansile mass lacking cellular maturation. Cells acquire the metastatic potentiality and can exert angiogenesis. This phase is represented clinically as a nodular mass instead of the relatively flat lesion of the radial growth phase.

See figure ((13.4))

Radial Growth Phase	Vertical Growth Phase
1- No metastasis	1- Can metastasis
2- Little angiogenesis	2- Increased angiogenesis
3- Usually flat	3- Usually nodular

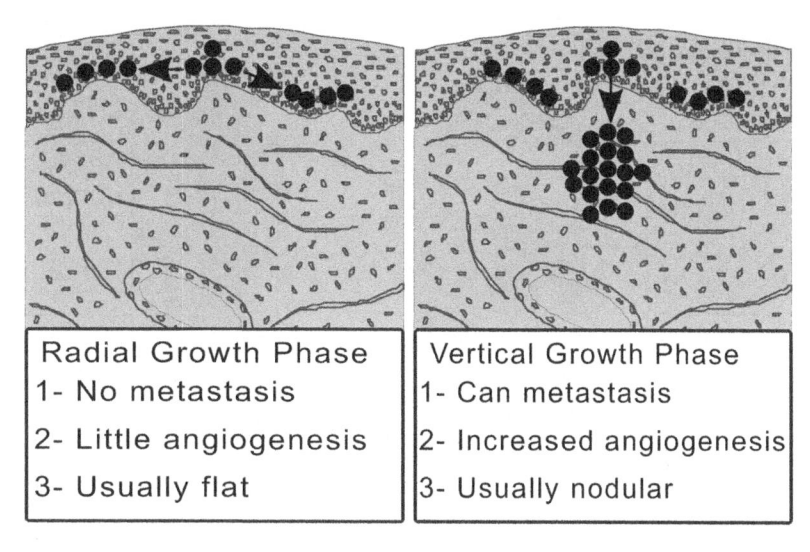

Figure 13.4: Melanoma in radial and vertical growth phases.

Clinically

- Melanoma of the skin is usually asymptomatic, although itching may be an early sign
- Lesions may be pigmented or non-pigmented, non-pigmented lesions are known as amelanotic melanomas.
- Unlike nevi, pigmented melanomas show striking variations in pigmentation, appearing in shades of black, brown, red, dark blue and gray.
- The borders of melanomas are irregular and often notched.
- The warning signs of melanoma are (see figure ((13.5)):
    1. Enlargement of a pre-existing nevus.
    2. Itching or pain in a pre-existing nevus.
    3. Variation of color within a pigmented lesion.
    4. Development of a new pigmented lesion.
    5. Irregularity of the borders of a pigmented lesion.

Chapter 13. Malignant Non-Odontogenic Tumors

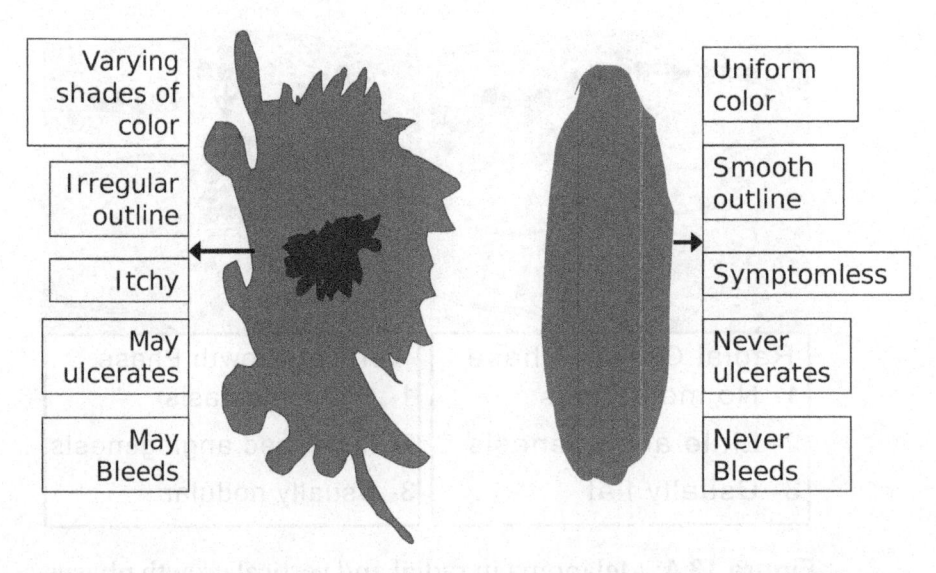

Figure 13.5: Melanoma vs pigmented nevus and the warning signs of melanoma, left panel shows melanoma and the right one shows pigmented nevus

ABCDE Clinical Evaluation System

ABCDE clinical evalution system was developed to differentiate melanoma from its bengin counparts, see table ((13.2)).

Clinical Variants

1. Acral lentiginous melanoma
    - Occurs in the palms and soles.
    - Rare in white race, the commonest form is in blacks and Japanese.
2. Lentigo maligna melanoma
    - Also known as malignant melanoma in situ (In situ melanoma).
    - Occurs on the sun-damaged areas of the face in elderly people.
    - More indolent course.
    - Occurs on top of lentigo maligna (Hutchinson's melanotic freckles). Lentigo maligna is a skin lesion in which there is prolifera-

Table 13.2: The ABCDE system of melanoma

> **Always Remember**
>
> - **A**symmetry (because of its uncontrolled growth pattern)
> - **B**order irregularity (often with notching)
> - **C**olor variegation (which varies from shades of brown to black, white, red, and blue, depending on the amount and depth of melanin pigmentation)
> - **D**iameter greater than 6 mm (which is the diameter of a pencil eraser)
> - **E**volving (lesions that have changed with respect to size, shape, color, surface, or symptoms over time)

tion of atypical melanocytes in the basal epidermis. Lentigo maligna differs from junctional nevus in two aspects, the first is that melanocytes in lentigo maligna are restricted to the basal cell layer not extending into the dermo-epidermal junction, and the second is that melanocytes are atypical in lentigo maligna.

- When nodularity appears within the lentigo maligna, invasive or vertical growth phase has started, then the condition is now termed lentigo maligna melanoma.

3. Superficial spreading melanoma
   - Superficial spreading melanoma is the most common form.
   - Usually is smaller than 3 cm in greatest diameter but may be much larger.
   - Most lesions are slightly elevated and invasion is indicated by the appearance of surface nodules or induration.

4. Nodular melanoma

- Does not have a preliminary radial or horizontal phase but begins its vertical growth phase immediately.
- Presents as a nodular elevation as it simultaneously invades the connective tissue.
- Usually is deeply pigmented and exophytic.

Histologically

- Rounded or spindle-shaped large melanocytes with atypical hyperchromatic nuclei. They are often arranged in nests.
- The nests are scattered in pagetoid pattern (resembles an intraepithelial adenocarcinoma known as Paget's disease of the skin).
- The atypical melanocytes are larger than the normal melanocytes and markedly larger and more pleomorphic than any adjacent nevus cells. The large nuclei have irregular contours with chromatin clumps characteristically at the periphery of the nuclear membrane and there are prominent nucleoli.
- Usually, melanoma cells contain melanin granules but sometimes there are none (amelanotic melanoma).
- Cellular pleomorphism and nuclear hyperchromatism are very common in all types of melanoma.

13.4.2 Mucosal Melanomas

- Melanomas are malignant tumor of melanocytes, in the oral cavity and eye, they are known as mucosal melanomas.
- Within the oral cavity, mucosal melanoma is most frequently found involving the upper alveolus and the hard palate. It is most common in males, between 40 and 60 years of age.
- No specific risk factors or premalignant lesions have been identified.

- Oral mucosal melanoma typically appears as a flat or nodular pigmented lesion, frequently associated with ulceration. Amelanotic melanoma is, fortunately, rare (15% of cases, and appears pink). Patients usually seek medical attention at an advanced stage of the disease, when pain develops or when they notice a change in the fit of their dentures. Approximately 25% of patients have nodal metastases at presentation. Tumors thicker than 5 mm are associated with an increased likelihood of nodal metastases at presentation.
- No formal staging system has been developed for mucosal melanoma.
- The diagnosis is made by means of biopsy and immunohistochemical staining. Any suspicious pigmented lesion in the oral cavity should undergo biopsy to rule out melanoma. Amalgam tattoos are common in the oral cavity and can often be diagnosed on the basis of the presence of metallic fragments on dental radiographs.
- Histologically, consists of neoplastic melanocytes, both within the epithelium and invading deeper tissues. These cells are round to spindle shaped and typically heavily pigmented with melanin. In amelanotic melanomas, the absence of pigment makes these cells more difficult to recognize. Histopathological diagnosis is greatly helped by immunohistochemistry. Melanomas are typically S-100, and MMA (melanoma-associated antigen) positive.
- Mucosal melanoma is managed primarily with surgical resection.
- The role of radiation therapy in this setting remains controversial. Some clinicians recommend postoperative radiotherapy for all cases of mucosal melanoma; others recommend it only for patients with positive margins. Because of the high incidence of nodes at presentation and the high regional recurrence rates reported in some studies, consideration should be given to treating the neck prophylactically by extending the postoperative radiation fields to cover this region.

- Prognosis of melanomas is bad. The survival rate for oral melanomas at 5 years ranges from 15% to 45%, with most patients dying of distant disease. Nodal involvement further reduces survival. Melanoma of the gingiva has a slightly better prognosis than melanoma of the palate.

13.5 Metastatic tumors of the jaws

- Sometimes termed secondary tumors of the jaws.
- Metastatic carcinoma is the most common form of cancer involving bone.
- The most common primary sites for carcinomas that metastasize to bone are the breast, lung, thyroid, prostate, and kidney.
- Metastatic spread of a carcinoma to the jaws usually occurs by blood route.
- In autopsy microscopic studies, it was found that around 16% of extra-oral carcinomas do metastasize to jaws but they remain clinically, radiographically and grossly undetectable.
- Sarcomas arising in soft tissues or other bones metastasize to the jaws very rarely.
- Clinical features of jaw metastasis may include pain, swelling, tooth mobility, trismus, and paresthesia.
- Sometimes, diagnosis of a jaw metastasis is the first indication that the patient has a primary tumor at some other anatomic site. Location of the hidden primary tumor may be difficult and may require extensive investigations.
- Radiographically evident jaw metastases appear as ill-defined or "moth-eaten" radiolucencies. However, some examples particularly *metastatic*

prostate[5] and *breast carcinomas* may appear radiopaque or sometimes as mixed radiocent-radiopaque.

- Histologically, appearance of metastatic carcinoma in bone varies. In some cases, the metastasis exhibits well-differentiated features that suggest an origin from a specific site, such as the kidney, colon, or thyroid. In other cases, metastatic carcinomas are poorly differentiated, and the tumor origin cannot be determined accurately. In such cases, immunohistochemistry may aid in diagnosis.

---

[5] Prostate, in particular is rich in alkaline phosphatase which is an osteoblastic agent i.e. increasing the possibility of calcific tissue formation.

CHAPTER 14

BENIGN ODONTOGENIC TUMORS AND TUMOR-LIKE LESIONS

Odontogenic tumors are tumors arising from odontogenic tissues. Although most of these tumors are true neoplasms, many of them are developmental disturbances (hamartomas).

Odontogenic tissues which may act as a source for these tumors are:

1. Ectodermal tissues

    (a) Dental lamina and its remnants (Serries pearl).

    (b) Enamel organ and its remnants (reduced dental epithelium).

    (c) Epithelial root sheath of Hertwig and its remnants (epithelial rests of Malassez).

2. Ectomesenchyme tissues[1] (in old literature was termed mesenchymal tissues)

    (a) Dental papilla and its remnants is represented by the dental pulp.

    (b) Tooth sac and its remnants is represented by the periodontal ligament.

It is worthy to note that the incidence rates of odontogenic tumors mentioned in this chapter are subject to variations depending upon geographic, racial and ethnic factors.

---

[1] Ectomesenchyme is a form of mesenchyme which originates from neural crest cells and forms the tissues of the head and neck; while mesenchyme is that part of the mesoderm of an embryo that develops into connective tissue, bone, cartilage, etc. other than that of the head and neck.

Classification of Odontogenic Tumors

There are 3 ways to classify odontogenic tumors, the first one is according to the histogenesis (tissue of origin) into ectodermal, ectomesenchymal and mixed, the second one according to the behavior into benign and malignant and the third one is according to the presence of hard tissues into hard, soft and mixed. The presence of hard tissues depends on the inductive process between the ectodermal and ectomesenchymal tissues. Almost all odontogenic tumors can exhibit variable degrees of hard tissue formation *except* ameloblastoma and to a lesser extent ameloblastic fibroma.

1. Benign odontogenic tumors
    (a) Epithelial odontogenic tumors
        i. Ameloblastoma
        ii. Calcifying epithelial odontogenic tumor (Pindborg tumor)
        iii. Adenomatoid odontogenic tumor
        iv. Calcifying epithelial odontogenic cyst (Gorlin Cyst)
        v. Squamous odontogenic tumor
        vi. Enameloma
    (b) Ectomesenchymal Odontogenic Tumors
        i. Odontogenic fibroma
        ii. Odontogenic myxoma
        iii. Dentinoma
        iv. Cementomas and cemental dysplasias
            A. Benign cementoblastoma
            B. Cementifying fibroma
            C. Juvenile ossifying fibroma
            D. Focal cemento-osseous dysplasia
            E. Periapical cemental dysplasia

        F. Florid cemento-osseous dysplasia

        G. Familial gigantiform cementoma

   (c) Mixed Odontogenic Tumors

        i. Ameloblastic fibroma

        ii. Compound composite odontome

        iii. Complex composite odontome

        iv. Ameloblastic fibro-odontome

        v. Ameloblastic odontome (Odonto-ameloblastoma)

2. Malignant odontogenic tumors

   (a) Malignant Ameloblastoma

   (b) Ameloblastic Carcinoma

   (c) Odontogenic Carcinoma

   (d) Primary Intraosseous Carcinoma of Jaw

        i. Solid primary intraosseous carcinoma

        ii. Cystic primary intraosseous carcinoma

   (e) Ghost cell odontogenic carcinoma

   (f) Clear cell odontogenic carcinoma

   (g) Ameloblastic fibrosarcoma

14.1 Benign Epithelial Odontogenic Tumors

14.1.1 Ameloblastoma

Definition

A locally invasive tumor consists of cells similar to ameloblasts

Clinical Classification

1. Conventional ameloblastoma (also called multicystic, polycystic, common ameloblastoma)
2. Unicystic ameloblastoma
3. Peripheral ameloblastoma

Multicystic Ameloblastoma

Definition

A locally invasive tumor consists of cells similar to ameloblasts and characterized by multiple cystic cavities.

Clinically

Age Usually 20–40 years age.

Sex No sex predilection

Race Usually Africans.

Site Mandible more than maxilla, in the mandible usually affects the molar-ramus area. In the maxilla usually affects the tuberosity area.

Features Swelling slowly growing, rarely painful and usually associated with an impacted tooth.

X - Ray

- Usually appear as a multilocular radiolucent area, honey comb appearance or soap bubble appearance. One of the loculi may enlarge on the expense of others (mother cyst). This picture is due to the tendency of the tumor to spread into marrow spaces and the focal destruction of the cortical plate. This picture is not pathognomonic as many lesions produce the same picture.

- Rarely appears as a monolocular radiolucent area.
- Root resorption could be detected in some cases.

Macroscopically

The lesion appears as a multicystic mass containing a fluid rich in albumin and rarely containing cholesterol.

Microscopically

Two histologic patterns have been recognized:

1- Follicular Pattern

Consists of follicles in a connective tissue stroma. Each follicle consists of an outer layer of columnar cells similar to ameloblasts and an inner mass of cells similar to stellate reticulum. The nuclei of the ameloblast like cells are situated at the apex of the cell (reverse polarization). Some times a mass of cells similar to stratum intermedium may be found. In some tumors, a zone 30u thick, of the stroma around the epithelium shows hyalinization which is mainly collagenous. The ameloblast-like cells which characterizes the tumor express amelogenin, a protein that is unique to enamel matrix. However, enamel and dentin are not formed in ameloblastomas. This classical form of ameloblastoma is often termed in some texts as simple ameloblastoma.[2]

---

[2] Regarding the term simple ameloblastoma, unfortunately, there is lack of consensus regarding what is meant by simple ameloblastoma. Many text books refer to simple ameloblastoma as the solid follicular or solid plexiform without any variations such as cystic, granular, acanthomatous, or hemorrhagic. Other texts refer to simple ameloblastoma as the benign form of ameloblastoma with all possible variations except malignancy.

Histological Variants of Follicular Pattern

Three main histologic variants have been recognized. Mixtures of different patterns are commonly observed and the lesions are usually classified based on the predominant pattern present.

(a) Cystic Ameloblastoma

Is due to cystic degeneration affecting stellate reticulum-like cells. Cystic fluid is rich in albumin and rarely contains cholesterol.

(b) Acanthomatous Ameloblastoma

Squamous metaplasia may affect stellate reticulum like cells with formation of keratin. This condition appears to increase by previous surgery or irradiation.

(c) Granular Cell Ameloblastoma

The stellate reticulum like cells may change into eosinophilic granular cells which are rounded cells with eccentric nucleus and finely granular cytoplasm. The granules are PAS positive and represents excessive formation of lysosomes.

2- Plexiform Pattern

Consists of a plexus or anastomosing strands of odontogenic epithelium in a connective tissue stroma. Each strand consists of an outer layer of columnar cells with apical nucleus and an inner mass of cells similar to stellate reticulum.

2 variations do exist:

(a) Cystic Degeneration

This may affect the epithelium (intraepithelial cysts) or more often affects the connective tissue stroma (stromal cysts).

(b) Hemangio-Ameloblastoma

This is an obsolete term in which excessive dilation of the blood vessels of the stroma occurs due to lack of support resulting from degeneration of the connective tissue cells and fibers. It was thought in the past that this tumor is a mixed tumor but this view is not valid as the excessive vascularity is due to degeneration rather than neoplasia. Another term "hemorrhagic ameloblastoma" was given for this tumor.

3- Other rare histologic variants have been recognized:

(a) Basal cell variant

- Masses or strands of basoloid cuboidal cells with little palisading at the periphery.
- Surrounding small darkly stained cells without stellate reticulum like cells.

(b) Desmoplastic ameloblastoma

- Excessive formation of fibrous stroma which is dense and scar like.
- Difficult to excise completely.
-

Figure (14.1) summarizes some of the most common variants of multicystic ameloblastoma.

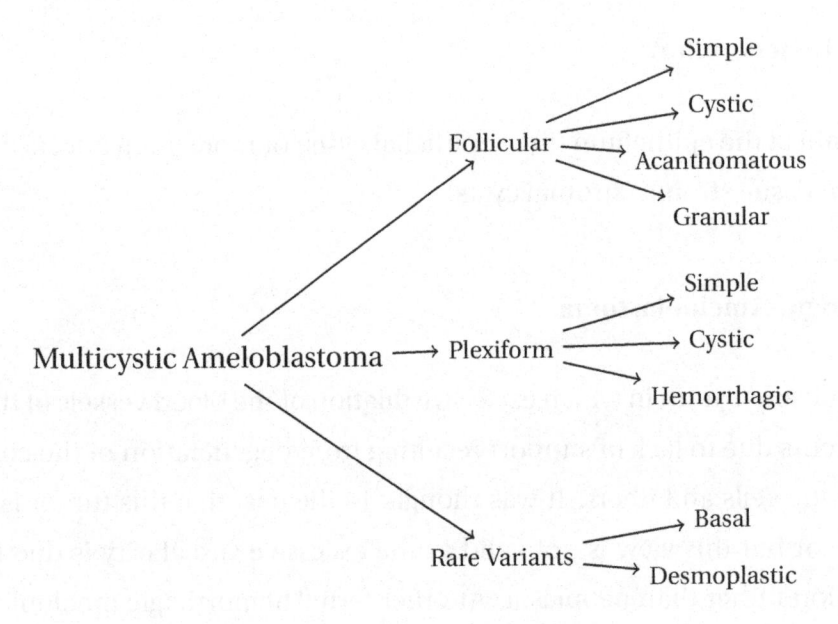

```
                              ┌─→ Simple
                              │─→ Cystic
                   Follicular ─┤
                   ↗          │─→ Acanthomatous
                              └─→ Granular

                                  ┌─→ Simple
Multicystic Ameloblastoma →  Plexiform ─┼─→ Cystic
                   ↘              └─→ Hemorrhagic

                                  ┌─→ Basal
                   Rare Variants ─┤
                                  └─→ Desmoplastic
```

Figure 14.1: Schema Showing Various Subtypes of Multicystic Ameloblastoma

Histogenesis of Ameloblastomas

4 possibilities have been proposed:

- Dental lamina or its remnants. This origin was postulated to explain the origin of some cases of peripheral ameloblastoma
- Enamel organ or its remnants, this is because of the histologic similarity between the structure of enamel organ and follicles of ameloblastoma
- Wall of dentigerous cysts, in this case the tumor is known as (Mural Ameloblastoma)
- Oral mucosa, because of the histologic similarity with basal cell carcinoma and to explain the origin of some cases of peripheral ameloblastoma. However basal cell carcinoma differs from ameloblastoma in being radiosensitive

Treatment

Radical removal with adequate safety margin. Ameloblastoma is not radiosensitive, and chemotherapy is not successful in its treatment.

Prognosis

If adequately treated, prognosis is good. If not, recurrence will occur.

Unicystic Ameloblastoma

Definition

A locally invasive tumor usually consists of a central large cystic cavity and is less aggressive than conventional ameloblastoma

Clinically

Age Usually below 20 years age
Sex No sex predilection
Site Mandible more than maxilla, usually affects the molar region
Features Swelling slowly growing, rarely painful and usually associated with dentigerous cysts and severely displaced third molar

Histologically

- A large cystic cavity lined with odontogenic epithelium showing hyperchromatic and palisaded basal cells with reversed polarization of the nucleus
- Papillary projections arise from the epithelium towards the cystic cavity (intraluminal ameloblastoma). These projections consist of epithelium

with a plexiform pattern that closely resembles that seen in the plexiform ameloblastoma

- Projections arise from the epithelium towards the connective tissue capsule (mural ameloblastoma). These projections consist of epithelium with a follicular pattern that closely resembles that seen in the follicular ameloblastoma

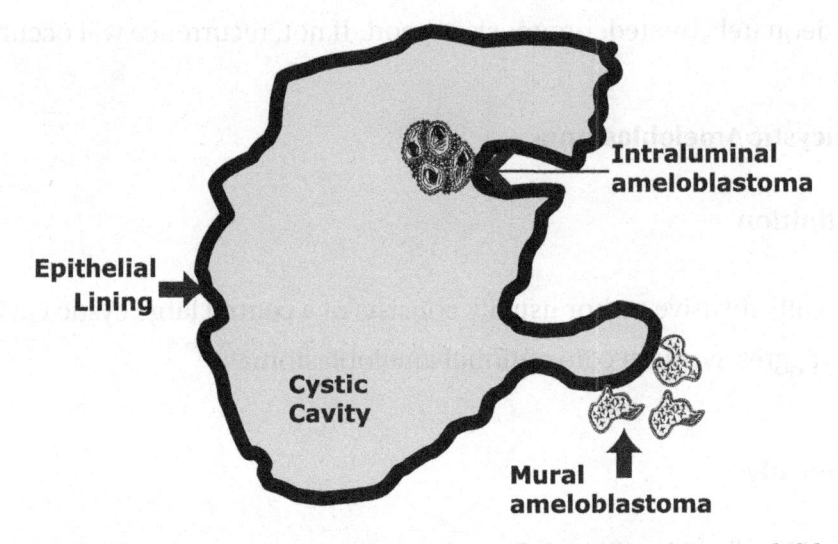

Figure 14.2: Diagrammatic representation of the unicystic ameloblastoma with its possible variations.

X-Ray

Unilocular radiolucent area, usually encroaching on the crown of a tooth

Treatment

Depends on the histologic pattern:

- Intraluminal ameloblastoma is treated by enucleation

- Mural ameloblastoma is treated by marginal resection (block resection) with safety margin

Peripheral Ameloblastoma

Definition

- Peripheral (extraosseous) ameloblastoma is a rare odontogenic tumor which is limited to the soft tissue of the gingiva
- It is less aggressive than conventional ameloblastoma

Histogenesis

- Thought to arise form remnants of the dental lamina
- Origin from oral mucosa was also postulated

Clinically

Age Usually between 23 and 82 years age

Site Mandible more than maxilla

Features firm sessile nodules of the gingiva that range in size from 0.5 to 2.0 cm

X-Ray

- Usually negative in x-ray
- Sometimes causes sauceriazation of bone

Histologically

- Strands of odontogenic epithelium, usually resembling the follicular pattern of intraosseous common ameloblastoma
- Acanthomatous and cystic patterns do exist

Treatment

As the tumor is not aggressive, local excision that includes a small margin of normal tissue is adequate.

14.1.2 Calcifying Epithelial Odontogenic Tumor

(Pindborg Tumor)

Definition

A locally invasive tumor characterized by calcification and keratinization

Clinically

- Occurs as either a central (intraosseous) or peripheral (extraosseous) lesion
- Central lesions occur at a mean age of 40 years; mandible is affected more than maxilla and usually affects the molar region. Appears as a painless slowly growing tumor usually associated with impacted teeth
- Peripheral CEOT is rare and occurs in the anterior part of the mouth. It presents as a superficial soft tissue swelling of the gingiva

X-Ray

Unilocular or multilocular radiolucent area containing radiopacities

Histologically

- Connective tissue stroma
- Sheets of polyhedral epithelial cells showing
- Giant, hyperchromatic and pleomorphic nuclei
- Intercellular bridges (hemidesmosomes)
- Amyloid degeneration occurs in some of these polyhedral cells appearing as eosinophilic masses
- The nature of the eosinophilic deposits has been controversial, amyloid, enamel matrix, keratin or basal lamina were all proposed
- This substance takes the stains of amyloid such as Congo red or thioflavin T
- Calcification occurs in a form of concentric rings called Liesegang rings
- Clear cell variant exists

Histogenesis

Thought to arise from remnants of dental lamina or from the reduced enamel epithelium

Treatment

Block resection

Prognosis

Recurrence rate is common unless the tumor is adequately removed

14.1.3 Adenomatoid Odontogenic Tumor

(Adenoameloblastoma)

Definition

A benign odontogenic tumor characterized by presence of duct like structure

Clinically

Age common in young age

Sex common in females more than males

Site maxilla more than mandible, anterior more than posterior usually between lateral incisor and canine.

Features swelling, painless, slowly growing, usually associated with an impacted tooth, rare cases are peripheral.

X-Ray

Well defined radiolucent area with some radiopacities

Histologically

- Connective tissue capsule
- Connective tissue stroma which may show cystic degeneration
- Duct like structure consists of a central space bounded by tall columnar cells similar to ameloblasts with a basal nucleus, a thin layer of an eosinophilic material is found in the central space contacting the free end of the cells. The nature of this eosinophilic material is controversial. Enameloid matrix, or keratin were proposed.

- Convoluted band which is similar to the duct like structure but without a central space
- Masses of small rounded epithelial cells showing clear cytoplasm and oval nucleus
- Foci of calcification which is thought to be a dysplastic dentin or enamel.

Histogenesis

The tumor is thought to arise from the outer layer of the enamel organ or its remnants, the reduced enamel epithelium.

Treatment

Simple enucleation because the tumor is capsulated.

Prognosis

Good, as the tumor is benign and rarely recurs.

14.1.4 Calcifying Odontogenic Cyst

(Calcifying Cystic Odontogenic Tumor, Gorlin Cyst)

Definition

A benign odontogenic tumor showing some features of cysts

Histogenesis

May originate from the remnants of the dental lamina or rests of Malassez

Clinically

- Occurs as either a central (intraosseous) or rare peripheral (extraosseous) lesion
- Central lesions occur at a mean age of 30 years, mandible is affected more than maxilla and usually anterior to the molar region. Appears as a painless slowly growing tumor usually associated with impacted tooth
- Peripheral lesions are rare and occur in the anterior part of the mouth. It presents as a superficial soft tissue swelling of the gingiva

X-Ray

Unilocular radiolucent area with multiple radiopacities

Histologically

- Some lesions have a single or multiple cystic cavities, while others are solid
- The epithelium consists of a layer of palisaded columnar basal cells with reverse polarization of nuclei and an outer mass similar to stellate reticulum
- Greatly enlarged eosinophilic epithelial cells without visible nuclei, referred to as **"ghost cells"** are present within the stellate reticulum-like cells (nature uncertain, may represent keratin). Recently, ghost cells were found to be amelogenin positive suggesting the ameloblastic differentiation of ghost cells.
- The ghost cells may extend deep into the connective tissue provoking a foreign body reaction

- Multiple spherical and diffuse calcifications within the epithelium and the connective tissue are also seen
- dentin-like material may sometimes also form
- The solid variant of this lesion was termed **"Ghost cell tumor"**.

Treatment

Enucleation, recurrence is rare

14.1.5 Squamous Odontogenic Tumor

Definition

Aggressive odontogenic tumor, consisting of islands of stratified squamous epithelium

Histogenesis

May originate from the remnants of the dental lamina or rests of Malassez

Clinically

Age Usually third decade
Sex No sex predilection
Site Equal distribution between mandible and maxilla, anterior to the molars, may be multifocal
Features swelling, painless, slowly growing, usually associated with an impacted tooth

X-Ray

- Small lesions appear as unilocular radiolucencies
- Large lesions are multilocular

Histologically

- Islands of stratified squamous epithelium
- Bounded by inactive appearing cuboidal cells
- Central cells with prominent intercellular bridges (hemidesmosomes)
- Many of the islands have central areas of microcyst formation
- Calcific bodies are found in the islands and in the connective tissue stroma

Treatment

Small lesions can be controlled with local curettage; large lesions require block resection

14.1.6 Enameloma

- A developmental malformation and not a true neoplasm.
- Sometimes termed enamel pearl.
- Enameloma is a piece of normal enamel usually found in the bifurcation area of upper molars. It may contain a core of dentin and an associated pulp horn.
- Histogenesis differentiation of an area of the epithelial root sheath of Hertwig into ameloblasts.

14.2 Benign Ectomesenchymal Odontogenic Tumors

14.2.1 Peripheral Odontogenic Fibroma

Definition

Benign odontogenic tumor consists of cellular fibrous tissue with islands of embryonic odontogenic epithelium.

Histogenesis

Arises from the tooth sac or its remnants, the periodontal ligament. This is supported by the presence of epithelial rests and cementum masses.

Clinically

Painless slowly growing sessile or pedunculated mass usually affecting the gingiva or interdental papilla.

X - Ray

- Negative in X-ray, however small radiopaque flecks may be observed in some lesions.
- Bone saucerization may also occur.

Histologically

- Primitive fibrous tissue similar to that of the dental papilla.
- Islands or masses of quiescent odontogenic epithelium
- Areas of bone or cementum.

Treatment

Local excision.

14.2.2 Central Odontogenic Fibroma

Definition

Benign odontogenic tumor consists of cellular fibrous tissue with islands of embryonic odontogenic epithelium.

Histogenesis

Arises from the tooth sac or its remnants, the periodontal ligament. This is supported by the presence of epithelial rests and cementum masses.

Clinically

Painless slowly growing swelling usually associated with an impacted tooth.

X - Ray

Will defined unilocular radiolucent area. Sometimes faint radiopaque flecks can be observed.

Histologically

- Primitive fibrous tissue similar to that of the dental papilla.
- Islands or masses of quiescent odontogenic epithelium
- Areas of bone or cementum.

Treatment

Conservative surgical enucleation.

14.2.3 Odontogenic Myxoma

Definition

A locally aggressive tumor consists of myxomatous tissue.

Histogenesis

Is thought to arise from odontogenic mesenchyme, because:

- Presence of odontogenic epithelial remnants.
- Association of the tumor with missed teeth.
- Resemblance of the tumor to the embryonic odontogenic mesenchyme
- Almost complete absence of similar tumors in other bones

Clinically

- Young age
- usually associated with an impacted tooth.

X - Ray

Aggressive multilocular radiolucent area, honey comb or soap bubble appearance.

Macroscopically

None capsulated slimy mass.

Microscopically

- Star shaped or stellate shaped cells with many processes.
- Basophilic mucoid matrix.
- Delicate reticulin or collagen fibers.
- Sometimes the tumor contains excess amounts of collagen fibers deserving the term of fibromyxoma (myxofibroma).
- Masses of quiescent odontogenic epithelium.

Treatment

Removal with safety margin (block resection).

14.2.4 Cementomas and Cemental dysplasias

Cementomas and cemental (cemento-osseous) dysplasias are diverse group of lesions that their nomenclature and classification remain an area of debate. An appropriate classification is shown in table (14.1). Cementomas and cemento-osseous dysplasias could be classified into 3 main categories; benign cementoblastoma, ossifying fibroma and its related disorders such as cemento-osseous dysplasias. These lesions share many similarities and the correct diagnosis can be problematic but is critical for correct treatment. Cemento-osseous dysplasias belong to the group of lesion known as fibro-osseous lesions, to which fibrous dysplasia also belongs. For further details see Chapter "Bone Diseases", page (446). The differential diagnosis of cmento-osseous dysplasias is summarized in table (14.2).

Table 14.1: Classification of Cementomas and Cemento-Osseous Dysplasias

> **Always Remember**
>
> 1. Benign cementoblastoma (true cementoma)
> 2. Ossifying fibroma (cementifying fibroma, cemento-ossifying fibroma)
> 3. Juvenile ossifying fibroma
> 4. Cemento-osseous dysplasia (osseous dysplasia, cemental dysplasia)
>   (a) Focal cemento-osseous dysplasia
>   (b) Periapical cemento-osseous dysplasia (periapical cemental dysplasia)
>   (c) Florid cemento-osseous dysplasia (florid cemental dysplasia)
>   (d) Familial gigantiform cementoma

Benign Cementoblastoma (True Cementoma)

Definition

This is a true neoplasm which contains masses of cementum or cementum-like tissue. Many authorities believe that this tumor represents the only true neoplasm of cementum.

Histogenesis

- Arises from odontogenic mesenchyme

Clinically

Age Children and young adults, 50% of cases under the age of 20 and 75% of cases under the age of 30

Sex No sex predilection

Chapter 14. Benign Odontogenic Tumors

Race No racial predilection

Site Mandible more than maxilla, Usually posterior (premolar-molar region).

Features

- The tumor is usually solitary
- In the majority of cases, the tumor appears as a swelling which is usually tender and painful.
- Deciduous teeth are rarely affected.
- During the operation the tumor is found fused to the root of the involved tooth.
- The involved tooth is typically vital.

X - Ray

- A dense or mottled radiopacity attached to the root and surrounded by a radiolucent rim. This radiolucent rim represents the formative tissue of the tumor.
- It remains separated from bone by a continuation of the periodontal membrane.
- Root resorption may be seen.

Histologically

- Loose vascular connective tissue rich in plump mononuclear cells (cementoblasts).
- Multinucleated giant cells.
- Masses of cementum like tissue with many reversal lines and entrapped cells (cellular cementum). This gives these masses a mosaic appearance.

- Sheet of unmineralized tissue at the periphery.
- The periodontal ligament of the involved tooth is continuous with the unmineralized tissue at the periphery of the lesion.

Differential Diagnosis

From other radiopaque lesions that share some features:

- Complex odontome (not attached to the root).
- Osteoblastoma (not attached to the root).
- Focal sclerosing osteomyelitis (source of inflammation, tenderness and presence of inflammatory cells).
- Hypercementosis (no root resorption)

Treatment

- Surgical extraction of the involved tooth with removal of the fused mass.
- Surgical removal of the mass with resection of the fused root and endodontic treatment may be considered.
- Prognosis is good and recurrence is rare.

Cementifying Fibroma

(Ossifying Fibroma, Cemento-Ossifying Fibroma)

Definition

- This is a true neoplasm which consists of fibrous tissue with bone trabeculae, cementum-like tissue or both.
- The classification of ossifying fibroma with many synonymous nomenclatures has been a matter of controversy. While majority of authors

believe that all these names refer to the same tumor or its variants, others believe that they are separate entities.
- Because of the presence of cementum-like tissue, the odontogenic origin of this tumor was postulated.
- However, on the basis of presence of similar tumors in extra-gnathic bones, the cementum-like masses were considered to be variants of bone and the tumor is now thought to be of osteogenic origin and is best classified as an osteogenic rather than an odontogenic neoplasm.

Histogenesis

- Arises from odontogenic mesenchyme

Clinically

Age 20–40 years is the commonest age
Sex Females are affected more than males
Race No racial predilection
Site Mandible more than maxilla, usually posterior (premolar-molar region).

Features

- The tumor is usually solitary
- The tumor appears as a swelling which is slowly growing.
- Can cause facial asymmetry.

X - Ray

- Well-defined unilocular radiolucency with varying degrees of radiopaque masses.

- Rare cases appears as a completely radiolucent area.
- Cases appearing as a radiopaque mass surrounded with a radiolucent rim are uncommon.

Histologically

- Fibrous tissue with varying degrees of cellularity.
- Trabeculae of osteoid, woven bone, and lamellar bone with peripheral osteoblastic rimming.
- Masses of poorly cellular basophilic cementum-like tissue with brush-like borders that blend with the adjacent stroma.

Differential Diagnosis

From facial fibrous dysplasia, in which bone trabeculae are:

- Mainly of woven bone
- Show no osteoblastic rimming
- Radiographically, ossifying fibroma is more well-defined.
- However, these criteria are unreliable and distinguishing between ossifying fibroma and fibrous dysplasia is a diagnostic challenge. For further diagnostic criteria see table (14.3).

Other differential considerations are osteoblastoma, focal cemento-osseous dysplasia and focal sclerosing osteomyelitis.

Treatment

Enucleation, recurrence is rare.

Focal Cemento-Osseous Dysplasia

Definition

- This is a focal lesion which consists of bone and cementum-like substance.
- Most cases were erroneously diagnosed as a variant of ossifying fibroma

Etiology and Pathogenesis

- The exact etiology is unknown.
- It is postulated that these lesions are reactive or dysplastic rather than neoplastic. The reactive process might be against an unknown local factor.
- Because of the proximity of these lesions to the periodontal ligament, it is postulated that these lesions are of periodontal ligament origin.
- Other investigators postulate that these lesions represent defects in extraligamentary bone remodeling triggered by unknown local factors and modified by hormonal imbalance.

Clinically

Age 30–50 years is the commonest age

Sex 90% of cases occur in females

Race More common in white population

Site Mandible more than maxilla, Usually posterior (premolar-molar region).

Features

- The tumor is usually solitary

- Asymptomatic and discovered accidentally by routine X-ray.
- Usually less than 1.5 cm in diameter.
- Rarely causing bone expansion.
- The related teeth are vital.
- Not fused to roots and there is a healthy periodontal ligament separating the lesions form the root.

X - Ray

3 stages have been recognized:

1. Osteolytic stage: appears as a radiolucent area.
2. Cementoblastic stage: a radiolucent area with radiopacities. Most lesions are discovered in this stage.
3. Mature stage: a radiopaque mass with a radiolucent rim.

Histologically

- Loose vascular connective tissue rich in spindle-shaped fibroblasts or cementoblasts with collagen fibers.
- Areas of hemorrhage.
- A mixture of woven bone, lamellar bone and cementum-like tissues.
- With maturation, the bone trabeculae become thick curvilinear structures resembling the shape of ginger roots.
- Further maturation results in fusion of these masses to form large sheets of relatively acellular and disorganized cemento-osseous material.

Differential Diagnosis

From ossifying fibroma, in which bone trabeculae are:

- More delicate
- Showing osteoblastic rimming
- Showing brush-like borders in intimate contact with the stroma, while in cemento-osseous dysplasia, the cementum-like masses often exhibit retraction from the adjacent stroma.

Treatment

- As the lesion is non-neoplastic, surgical treatment is not required.
- As the lesion is relatively avascular and more prone to infection, good oral hygiene is necessary to avoid dental infections and osteomyelitis.
- Extraction of teeth is best avoided and conservative treatment is preferred because of the risk of osteomyelitis.
- Sequestration of the sclerotic cementum-like masses may occur and needs sequesterectomy, debridement and antibiotics.

Periapical Cemento-Osseous Dysplasia

(Periapical Cemental Dysplasia)

Definition

- A multifocal lesion which consists of bone and cementum-like substance usually affecting the lower anterior teeth.

Etiology and Pathogenesis

The same as focal cemento-osseous dysplasia.

Clinically

Age: 30–50 years is the commonest age

Sex: 90% of cases occur in females

Race: More common in black population

Site: Mandible more than maxilla, usually anterior (incisor region).

Features

- The tumor is usually multiple
- Asymptomatic and discovered accidentally by routine X-ray.
- Individual lesions are usually less than 1 cm in diameter.
- Rarely causing bone expansion.
- The involved teeth are vital.
- Lesions are not fused to roots and there is a healthy periodontal ligament separating the lesions form the root.

X - Ray

3 stages have been recognized:

1. Osteolytic stage: appears as a radiolucent area. In this stage, the lesion could be misdiagnosed as a periapical granuloma or cyst.
2. Cementoblastic stage: a radiolucent area with radiopacities.
3. Mature stage: a radiopaque mass with a radiolucent rim. There is a healthy periodontal ligament separating the lesions from the roots.

Histologically

The same as focal cemento-osseous dysplasia and the two lesions can not be distinguished histologically.

Treatment

- Once diagnosed, no treatment is required.

Florid Cemento-Osseous Dysplasia

(Florid Cemental Dysplasia)

Definition

- Lobulated masses of highly dense, highly mineralized, almost acellular cemento-osseous tissue typically occurring in several parts of the jaws.
- The term florid cemento-osseous dysplasia (FCOD) has been proposed in the 2nd edition of the World Health Organization's (WHO).

Etiology and Pathogenesis

The same as focal cemento-osseous dysplasia.

Clinically

Age 30–50 years is the commonest age
Sex 90% of cases occur in females
Race More common in black population
Site Mandible more than maxilla, affection of the maxilla is rare, usually posterior (premolar-molar region).

Features

- The tumor is usually multiple, often bilateral and symmetrical.
- Asymptomatic and discovered accidentally by routine X-ray.
- Some cases complain of dull pain.
- In some cases, a sinus may be present exposing yellowish avascular bone to the oral cavity.
- Rarely causing bone expansion.
- In some cases, simple bone cyst was reported to co-exist with florid cemento-osseous dysplasia. The relationship between simple bone cyst and florid cemento-osseous dysplasia is not yet known.

X - Ray

3 stages have been recognized:

1. Osteolytic stage: appears as a radiolucent area.
2. Cementoblastic stage: a radiolucent area with radiopacities. Most lesions are discovered in this stage.
3. Mature stage: a radiopaque mass with a radiolucent rim. In some cases, the lesion may blend with the adjacent normal bone (no radiolucent rim).

Histologically

The same as focal cemento-osseous dysplasia and the two lesions can not be distinguished histologically.

Differential Diagnosis

1. From focal sclerosing osteomyelitis, in which:

- Source of inflammation is usually evident.
- Presence of inflammatory cells histologically.
2. From Paget's disease of bone:
    - Elevated serum alkaline phosphatase.
    - Possible involvement of other bones.
3. From familial gigantiform cementoma:
    - Presence of family history.
    - Starts in the first decade of life.
    - Bone expansion is more evident.
    - No sex or racial predilection.

Treatment

- As the lesion is non-neoplastic, surgical treatment is not required.
- As the lesion is relatively avascular and more prone to infection, good oral hygiene is necessary to avoid dental infections and osteomyelitis.
- Extraction of teeth is best avoided and conervative treatment is preferred because of the risk of osteomyelitis.
- Sequestration of the sclerotic cementum-like masses may occur and needs sequesterectomy, debridement and antibiotics.

Familial Gigantiform Cementoma

Definition

- A hereditary condition characterized by the formation of massive masses of mineralized tissues.
- Although the term gigantiform cementoma was used in the past as a synonym for florid cemento-osseous dysplasia, most authorities now

restrict use of this term to the hereditary disorder that is different than the conventional florid cemento-osseous dysplasia.

Etiology and Pathogenesis

- Hereditary, autosomal dominant.
- High penetrance and variable expressivity.

Clinically

Age Starts in the first decade of life

Sex No sex predilection

Race More common in Caucasians and black population

Site Mandible and maxilla are affected equally, usually posterior (premolar-molar region).

Features

- Usually multiple, often bilateral and symmetrical.
- Starts as a rapid and expansive swelling that causes facial deformity.
- Failure of eruption of many teeth with malocclusion.
- The lesion ceases during the fifth decade of life.

X - Ray

Similar to other types of cemento-osseous dysplasias and consists of 3 stages:

1. Osteolytic stage: appears as a radiolucent area.
2. Cementoblastic stage: a radiolucent area with radiopacities. Most lesions are discovered in this stage.

3. Mature stage: a radiopaque mass with a radiolucent rim.

Histologically

- Similar to other types of cemento-osseous dysplasias and the lesions can not be distinguished histologically.

Treatment

- Before the final maturation stage, surgical correction results in re-growth of the lesion and therefore should be avoided.
- Partial removal results in sequestration of the remaining bone and also should be avoided.
- Therefore, extensive resection and re-construction of the facial skeleton may be the best choice.

14.3 Benign Mixed Odontogenic Tumors

14.3.1 Ameloblastic Fibroma

Definition

A benign mixed odontogenic tumor in which ectodermal and mesenchymal tissues share in the production of the mass. The epithelium and connective tissue recapitulate the cap and bell stages of odontogenesis

Clinically

Race no racial predilection.
Sex no sex predilection.

Age below 20 years age.

Site mandibular molar area.

Features slowly growing, painless swelling.

X - Ray

- Well defined unilocular radiolucent area.
- Usually associated with an impacted tooth.
- Rarely appears as a multilocular radiolucent area.

Histologically

2 elements, epithelial and mesenchymal:

- The epithelial element consists of cords, strands, rosettes or follicles similar to that of ameloblastoma, each follicle consists of an outer layer of cuboidal cells and an inner mass of cells similar to stellate reticulum. Sometimes a zone of *juxta-epithelial hyaliniztion* about 30 microns wide is seen around the epithelial masses and is thought to be a collagenous material.
- Connective tissue element, consists of stellate or angular primitive fibroblasts with little collagen (similar to the primitive dental papilla).
- This picture is similar to the early stages of odontome.

Treatment

The lesion is well encapsulated and easily separated from the surrounding bone, hence simple enucleation is preferred and recurrence is rare

14.3.2 Compound Composite Odontome

Definition

A developmental malformation consists of multiple small denticles (miniature tooth-like structures). Compound and complex composite odontomes are considered to be developmental disturbances rather than being true neoplasms.

Clinically

Usually young age - mandibular molar area - usually associated with permanent dentition - the lesion is small and symptomless - rarely expands the jaw.

X - Ray

Numerous tooth like structures arranged in a haphazard fashion surrounded by a radiolucent margin.

Histologically

Enamel, dentin, cementum, and pulp tissue arranged in normal anatomical relationship to each other.

14.3.3 Complex Composite Odontome

Definition

A developmental malformation consists of one large gnarled mass of enamel, dentin, cementum, and pulp tissue arranged in abnormal anatomical relation to each other due to defective morphodifferentiation.

Clinically

As compound composite odontome.

X - Ray

A radiopaque mass surrounded by a radiolucent margin.

Histologically

Enamel, dentin, cementum, and pulp tissue arranged in an abnormal anatomical relationship to each other.

14.3.4   Ameloblastic Fibro-Odontome

Definition

A mixed odontogenic tumor consisting of an ameloplastic fibroma and a complex odontome. Compound odontome was also described in some reports. Some authors deny the existence of this tumor as a separate entity considering it to be a mature form of ameloblastic fibroma or a developing odontome.

14.3.5   Odonto-Ameloblastoma

(Ameloblastic Odontome)

Definition

A mixed odontogenic tumor consists of ameloblastoma and odontome

Clinically

Similar to ameloblastoma

X - Ray

A radiolucent area containing radiopacities, which may be a compound or complex odontome

Histologically

- Ameloblastoma like tissue, follicular or plexiform
- Primitive connective tissue identical to that of dental papilla
- Odontome, complex or compound

Table 14.2: Differential Diagnosis of Cemento-Osseous Dysplasias

Always Remember

lesion	Age	Race	Sex	Site	Solitary - Multiple	Etiology
Focal cemento-osseous dysplasia	30-50, mean 38	Whites	Females 90% of cases	Mandible, posterior region	Solitary	Unknown
Periapical cemento-osseous dysplasia	30-50	Blacks	Females 90% of cases	Mandible, anterior region	Multiple	Unknown
Florid cemento-osseous dysplasia	30-50	Blacks	Females 90% of cases	Mandible, posterior region, with or without maxilla, symmetrical	Multiple	Unknown
Familial gigantiform cementoma	First decade	Caucasians and blacks	No sexual predilection	Mandible and maxilla are affected equally, often both, posterior region	Multiple	Hereditary, autosomal dominant

Table 14.3: Differential Diagnosis of Facial Fibrous Dysplasia from Ossifying Fibroma

> **Always Remember**

Fibrous dysplasia	Ossifying fibroma
4–18 years age	20–40 years age
Maxilla > mandible	Mandible > maxilla
Diffuse or ill-defined	Well-defined
Self limiting	Continuous growth
May affect more than one bone	Single bone
Bone trabeculae are usually woven	Usually lamellar
Usually no osteoblastic rimming	Osteoblastic rimming
Surgical contouring	Enucleation or excision

Chapter 15
Malignant Odontogenic Tumors

Malignant odontogenic tumors are true neoplasms that my arise from a pre-existing benign tumor or arise de novo.

15.1 Malignant Ameloblastoma

- This term is used to describe a tumor that shows histologic features of classic ameloblastoma as a primary tumor associated with remote metastatic deposit.
- The ameloblastoma with metastatic potential is histologically indistinguishable from conventional ameloblastoma except for the presence of signs of malignancy.
- However, histologically the metastatic ameloblastoma usually does not show severe cytologic atypia or mitotic activity.
- Metastatic nodules develop in the lung (80%), cervical lymph nodes (15%), or extragnathic bones.
- Typically, the pulmonary metastases are multifocal and involve both lungs.
- Treatment:
    - ⋆ Surgical excision with safety margin
    - ⋆ Cervical metastasis is treated by neck dissection

- ★ Lung metastasis is treated by lobectomy
- ★ At surgery, more numerous pulmonary metastatic deposits often are identified than were apparent in diagnostic imaging studies.
- ★ Chemotherapy has been ineffective, but a short-term partial response is possible.

15.2 Ameloblastic Carcinoma

- This term should be applied to the cases in which squamous cell carcinoma occurs on the top of a pre-existing acanthomatous ameloblastoma (carcinoma ex ameloblastoma) or to those rare cases known as *"de novo ameloblastic carcinoma"* in which squamous cell carcinoma develops vague ameloblastomatous features such as plexiform or follicular patterns with peripheral palisaded cuboidal or columnar cells and central polygonal or angular cells.
- Metastatic deposits (secondary tumors) will show the histological picture of squamous cell carcinomatous structure.
- Ameloblastic carcinoma demonstrates greater cytologic atypia and mitotic activity than malignant ameloblastoma.
- Ameloblastic carcinoma is managed as a squamous cell carcinoma with attempted complete surgical excision, neck dissection, and postoperative radiation therapy.
- The prognosis is poor.

15.3 Odontogenic Carcinoma

The odontogenic carcinoma is an uncommon intraosseous epithelial malignancy that has features that are indicative of an odontogenic origin but not specific enough to relate it to a particular benign odontogenic tumor.

15.4 Primary Intraosseous Carcinoma of Jaw

- Primary intraosseous carcinoma (PIOC) is a squamous cell carcinoma that occurs in the jaw bone and developing from remnants of odontogenic epithelium that have undergone squamous metaplasia.
- It is called "primary" because it is not a secondary deposit from a distant tumor and arising from within the jaw.
- It is termed "intraosseous" because it develops centrally within bone; origin from surface stratified squamous or sinus epithelium must be ruled out.
- It lacks evidence of ameloblastic differentiation; otherwise it would be classified as an ameloblastic carcinoma.
- If the intraosseous carcinoma demonstrates mucous cells, then a diagnosis of central mucoepidermoid carcinoma is appropriate.
- The primary intraosseous carcinoma behaves like any other intraosseous malignancy, destroying larger areas of bone, resorbing roots of teeth, invading nerve trunks, and metastasizing regionally and to distant organs.

Primary intraosseous carcinoma of the jaw could be classified into the solid and the cystic primary intraosseous carcinomas:

15.4.1 Solid primary intraosseous carcinoma

This is a squamous cell carcinoma arising from remnants of odontogenic epithelium without the evidence of a preexisting cyst.

15.4.2 Cystic primary intraosseous carcinoma

- Is squamous cell carcinoma that shows a cystic lumen that contains fluid or keratin and a lining of stratified squamous epithelium that exhibits cytologic atypia.
- The most common odontogenic cyst to show carcinomatous changes is the dentigerous cyst.
- Odontogenic keratocysts can also give rise to squamous cell carcinoma but perhaps less frequently than dentigerous cysts.

15.5 Ghost cell odontogenic carcinoma

- Is an ameloblastic carcinoma that shows evidence of ghost cell keratinization.
- Ghost cells are immunoreactive for amelogenin which is a protein that is unique to enamel matrix.
- Therefore, the presence of ghost cells in jaw tumors represents evidence of ameloblastic differentiation.
- Ghost cell odontogenic carcinomas have a biologic behavior that is similar to that of an ameloblastoma or a low-grade ameloblastic carcinoma with a little metastatic potential.

15.6 Clear cell odontogenic carcinoma

- Is a low-grade carcinoma that is composed of cells that show uniform nuclei and clear cytoplasm.
- The tumor may show branching and anastomosing cords of polygonal epithelial cells that exhibit scanty eosinophilic cytoplasm and only focal clear cell features.
- Histologic differential diagnosis
    * Clear cell variant of calcifying epithelial odontogenic tumor, which produces amyloid and calcifications
    * Clear cell variant of mucoepidermoid carcinoma, which is positive for cytoplasmic mucicarmine.

15.7 Ameloblastic fibrosarcoma

- Ameloblastic fibrosarcoma may represent the malignant counterpart of ameloblastic fibroma.
- Histologically, it is a fibrosarcoma containing non-neoplastic odontogenic epithelium and occasionally hard dental tissues.
- When the tumor contains hard dental tissues such as dentin, cementum or enamel, it deserves the term ameloblastic fibrodentinosarcoma.

CHAPTER 16
DISEASES OF SALIVARY GLANDS

Salivary glands are exocrine glands that produce saliva through a system of ducts. There are three paired major salivary glands (parotid, submandibular, and sublingual) as well as many minor salivary glands scattered allover the oral cavity. Regarding to the type of secretion there are 3 types of salivary glands, serous, mucous or seromucous (mixed).

16.1 Classification of Salivary Gland Disorders

1. Functional disorders:
   (a) Xerostomia
   (b) Ptyalism (hypersalivation)
2. Developmental diseases:
   (a) Aplasia
   (b) Atresia
   (c) Aberrancy
3. Infections:
   (a) Bacterial:
      i. Acute suppurative parotitis
      ii. Chronic sialadenitis
      iii. Recurrent parotitis

iv. Auricultemporal syndrome

(b) Viral:

i. Mumps

ii. Uveoparotitis

iii. Cytomegallic Inclusion Disease

4. Obstructive diseases:

   (a) Sialolithiasis or salivary calculus

   (b) Salivary duct stenosis

5. Cysts: (mucocele)

   (a) Mucous retention cyst

   (b) Mucous extravasation cyst

   (c) Ranula

6. Degenerative (autoimmune):

   (a) Sjogren's syndrome

   (b) Mikulicz disease

7. Neoplastic:

   (a) Parenchymal tumors:

       i. Benign:

           A. Pleomorphic:
              - Pleomorphic adenoma

           B. Monomorphic:
              - Oncocytoma
              - Papillary cystadenoma lymphomatosum

       ii. Malignant:

           A. Malignant Pleomorphic Adenoma

           B. Mucoepidermoid Carcinoma

           C. Adenocystic Carcinoma

D. Acinic cell adenocarcinoma

   E. Polymorphous Low-grade Adenocarcinoma

   F. Salivary Adenocarcinoma, Not Otherwise Specified (NOS)

(b) Stromal tumors:

   i. Lipoma

   ii. Fibroma

   iii. Lymphoma. etc.

8. Tumor-like lesions:

   (a) Necrotizing sialometaplasia

   (b) Sialoadenosis (sialosis)

16.2 Functional Disorders of Salivary Glands

16.2.1 Xerostomia

Definition:

- Means dry mouth
- It may be temporary or chronic (persistent)
- Temporary xerostomia is of no clinical significance
- Persistent xerostomia is of grave consequences

Classification:

1. Primary, due to defective glands.
2. Secondary, due to defects outside the glands

Chapter 16. Diseases of Salivary Glands

Normal Salivary Flow:

1 – 2 ml / minute

Causes of Xerostomia:

- Sjogren's syndrome
- Irradiation
- Dehydration
- Fluid deprivation
- Hemorrhage
- Persistent diarrhea or vomiting
- Psychogenic
- Anxiety state
- Depression
- Drugs
- Diuretic overdose
- Atropine, ipratropium, hyoscine
- Tricyclic antidepressants
- Antihistamines

Oral Manifestations of Xerostomia:

- Sever dental caries
- Sever periodontal diseases
- Atrophied and ulcerated oral mucosa and tongue
- Superimposed infection, particularly candida albicans fungus due to changes in oral flora
- Difficulty in speech, mastication and swallowing

- Loss of taste
- Inability to wear dentures

Management:

- Remove the cause if possible
- Check for any associated drug treatment contributing to xerostomia
- Frequent small sips of water
- Prescribe saliva substitutes (artificial saliva)
- Suggest sugar-free gum
- Maintain good oral hygiene
- Chlorhexidine (0.2%) rinses
- Control caries
- Monitor for candidosis (antifungal drugs)
- Treat difficulties with dentures
- Observe regularly for possible ascending parotitis or chronic sialoadenitis

16.2.2 Ptyalism

(hypersalivation, Sialorrhoea)

Definition:

Is the condition of excess salivation

Types:

True ptyalism

- In which there is actual increase in the salivary flow and the swallowing mechanism is intact
- Increased salivary flow + Normal swallowing → no significant effect
- The condition is not a problem because any excess saliva can be swallowed
- Causes:
    1. Local reflexes
        (a) Oral infections e.g. ANUG
        (b) Oral wounds and ulcers
        (c) Dental procedures
        (d) New dentures
    2. Systemic e.g. nausea and toxicity e.g. iodine and heavy metal poisoning

False ptyalism

- In which the salivary flow is normal while the swallowing mechanism is defective resulting in saliva drooling from the mouth
- Normal salivary flow + Defective swallowing → saliva drooling
- Is more common and causes annoyance to the patient
- Causes:
    ★ Psychogenic
    ★ Bell's palsy (facial paralysis or paresis)
    ★ Parkinson's disease
    ★ Stroke

16.3 Infections of Salivary Glands

16.3.1 Bacterial infections

Acute Suppurative Parotitis

Definition

Acute suppurative inflammation of the parotid

Etiology

- Predisposing factors are xerostomia resulting from postoperative dehydration, irradiation or Sjogren's syndrome
- The causative organisms are staphylococci, streptococci and pneumococci
- The mode of infection is ascending i.e. via the duct and rarely blood born.
- The disease is now very rare due to the invention of antibiotics and proper post-operative care

Clinically

- Mainly affect the parotid gland.
- Painful swelling of the affected gland with uplifting of the ear lobe
- The overlying skin is red, shiny and tense
- In severe cases edema and difficulty in opening the mouth
- Purulent discharge or pus from the affected duct
- Fever and malaise

Chapter 16. Diseases of Salivary Glands

Histologically

Catarrhal inflammation followed by purulent one

Treatment

- Correction of the cause
- Antibiotics

Prognosis

Good and the condition end by resolution

Chronic Sialoadenitis

Definition

Chronic inflammation of salivary glands

Etiology

Usually results form chronic obstruction due to stones

Clinically

Painless or sometimes painful swelling of the affected gland which become worse at mealtime

Histologically

- Atrophy of the acini

- Ductal hyperplasia and dilatation.
- Lymphocytic infiltration.
- Fibrosis of the stroma

Treatment

- If possible remove the obstruction
- More often the gland has to be excised and biopsied to exclude the possibility of neoplasms

Recurrent Parotitis (Relapsing parotitis)

Definition

A condition of unknown nature thought to be allergic

Clinically

- Unilateral or bilateral recurrent enlargement of the parotid which becomes worse at mealtime
- The swelling is firm but not hot
- Usually, affecting children and sometimes adults
- There is a good oral hygiene

Sialography

Typically, sialography shows normal main ducts and punctate minor ducts. Sometimes there is dilation of salivary ducts

Auriculotemporal Syndrome (Frey's Syndrome)

- Is the flushing and sweating of the area of the skin supplied by the auriculotemporal nerve when tasting food
- There is also redness and anesthesia or hypo-aesthesia of the area
- The condition usually follows acute suppurative parotitis or surgery in the TMJ area
- The exact explanation of this condition is poorly understood.

16.3.2 Viral Infections

Mumps (Epidemic Parotitis)

Definition

Acute viral infection of the parotid.

Cause and pathogenesis

- The causative virus is a paramyxovirus which is RNA.
- The mode of infection is droplet infection.
- The virus reaches the gland through the duct or more commonly via blood.
- One attack produces permanent immunity.
- The incubation period is 2 – 3 weeks.
- The virus could be detected in saliva and blood (viremia) prior to the appearance of the disease by 2 – 3 days using complement fixing antibodies.

Clinically

- Fever and malaise.
- Enlargement of one parotid followed by enlargement of the other one within 2 – 3 days, rarely enlargement of both parotids occurs
- The enlargement is firm - painful - elevate the lobule of the ear and causing trismus
- No pus formation unless secondary infection occurs
- The disease is self limiting and spontaneous regression occurs after 2 – 3 weeks.

Complications

Usually in adults

- Extension to other salivary glands.
- Orchitis is a common complication in males which may lead to sterility.ovaritis is a less common complication.
- Hepatitis.
- Pancreatitis
- C.N.S. affection

Histologically

- Degeneration of the acini.
- Acute inflammatory cell infiltration.

Prevention

Vaccination with MMR.

Treatment

- Supportive treatment (analgesics & antipyretics)
- Plenty of fluids and soft diet
- Maintain good oral hygiene

16.4 Obstructive Diseases

16.4.1 Sialolithiasis, (Sialolith, Salivary Calculus)

- These are calcific bodies that can occur in the ducts of major salivary glands. Minor salivary glands are rarely affected.
- Occurs usually in adults.
- Occurs usually in submandibular gland more than parotid because the duct of the submandibular is more tortuous and the secretion is more viscous and. Also, the secretion flow of the submandibular gland is ascending (against the gravity) and not descending like that of the parotid.
- The condition is rare in edentulous mouths.
- Calcification occurs around a foreign body, bacteria or desquamated epithelial cell
- Calculus consists mainly of calcium carbonate and phosphate in addition to some trace minerals.
- Thus they could be detected in x ray as a radiopaque mass, however some cases may appear negative in X-ray films.
- The stone causes obstruction and secondary infection of the involved gland.
- Clinically there is tender enlargement of the gland and the duct become visible in the floor of the mouth.

16.4.2 Salivary Duct Stenosis

Salivary Duct Stricture

- Ductal stenosis or stricture formation accounts for almost 25% of cases of benign salivary obstruction and appears to have been an under recognized condition.
- The condition results from trauma to the duct wall. Such trauma may be the result of cheek biting, overextended denture flanges, damage during dental procedures, following surgery in the region or as a result of assaults or accidents
- Strictures more commonly affect parotid ducts and are typically found in the fourth, fifth or sixth decades, particularly in women.
- Until recently the only treatment for symptomatic strictures was adenectomy. This carried with the attendant risks of neurological damage and cosmetic deformity, which are important considerations in the management of benign disease. Balloon dilatation under fluoroscopic guidance and local anesthesia is now being used although it is not always possible to negotiate the stricture (63%-90%). However in those where it was possible post-operative sialographic examination showed partial or total elimination of the stricture in 96% of cases with an associated improvement in symptoms.

16.5 Cysts of Salivary Glands

16.5.1 (Mucoceles)

I- Mucous retention cyst

Definition

A cyst affecting minor salivary gland due to retention of mucous

Etiology

Partial obstruction of the duct by a stone or stenosis due to inflammation which will lead to slow build up of pressure behind the obstruction.

Clinically

- Usually occurs in the lip, tongue or buccal mucosa.
- Appears as a bluish small swelling which is fluctuant

Histologically

A pool of mucous surrounded by the acinar cells or the ductal cells.

II- Mucous Extravasation Cyst

Definition

A pseudocyst of salivary gland resulting from extravasation of mucous into the connective tissue due to torn duct

Etiology

Trauma to the duct

Clinically

As mucous retention cyst.

Histologically

A pool of mucous surrounded by compressed connective tissue with no epithelial lining (psuedocyst).

III- Ranula

Definition

Is a mucous retention or mucous extravasation cyst affecting major salivary gland usually submandibular or rarely sublingual

Etiology

Stone, stenosis or trauma of the duct.

Clinically

Large fluctuant, bluish swelling similar to frogs belly found in the floor of the mouth at one side of lingual frenum. May cause difficulty in eating, swallowing or speech

Histologically

A pool of mucous surrounded by acinar cells or ductal cells if it was a retention cyst or surrounded by compressed connective tissue if it was extravasation cyst

16.6 Degenerative (Autoimmune Diseases)

16.6.1 Sjogren's syndrome

Definition

An autoimmune disease affecting salivary gland

Etiology

- Autoimmune
- Retroviral infection, suspected but not proven yet.
- An autoimmune disease is that disease in which the body induces an immune reaction against one of its own tissues.
- Mikulicz Disease is postulated to be an expression of IgG4-related disease.
- IgG4-related disease comprises a group of lesions such as Mikulicz disease, inflammatory pseudotumor and some other inflammatory conditions.
- Serum concentrations of polyclonal IgG4 can measure up to 25 times greater than normal levels, although 20% to 40% of patients will have IgG4 levels within normal limits.

Types

1. Primary Sjogren's syndrome, Sicca Syndrome, Mikulicz Disease Benign Lymphoepithelial Lesion characterized by:
   - Dryness of the mouth **"xerostomia"**.
   - Dryness of the eyes **"xerophthalmia"**.
2. Secondary Sjogren's Syndrome characterized by:
   - Dryness of the mouth.
   - Dryness of the eyes.
   - Rheumatoid arthritis.
   - Other systemic diseases such as lupus erythematosis, polyarteritis nodosa or scleroderma.

Clinically

- **Age:** over 40 years.
- **Sex:** usually females.
- **Features:**
  - ★ Enlargement of lacrimal glands with keratoconguctivitis sicca
  - ★ Enlargement of salivary glands (particularly parotid) with xerostomia.
  - ★ Rhinopharyngiolaryngitis sicca.
  - ★ Any other autoimmune disease e. g. rheumatoid arthritis, lupus erythematosus or polyarteritis nodusa

Oral Manifestations

Are those of xerostomia:

1. Sever dental caries

2. Sever periodontal diseases
3. Atrophied and ulcerated oral mucosa
4. Superimposed infection
5. Difficulty in speech, mastication and swallowing
6. Inability to wear dentures

Histopathology

1. Atrophy of the acini.
2. Ductal hyperplasia forming masses of epithelial and myoepithelial cells called *epimyoepithelial islands*
3. Dense lymphocytic infiltration with or without germinal centers, thus the disease is described as a *lyphoepithelial lesion*.
4. 85 % of minor salivary gland show the same picture particularly those of the lip
5. The oral mucosa show signs of atrophy, parakeratosis and lymphocytic infiltration

Serologic Abnormalities

1. Antisalivary duct antibodies
2. Antinuclear factor
3. Hypergammaglobulinaemia
4. Rhaumatoid factor
5. Complement fixing antibodies
6. Increased sedimentation rate

Sialography

The injected material will escape from the ducts and produce radiopaque mass scattered within the salivary gland. This picture is called sialoectasis or snow storm appearance or branchless fruit laden tree.

Diagnosis

Depends on:

1. Labial gland biopsy
2. Sialography
3. Serological tests
4. Clinical picture

Differential Diagnosis

1. Malignant lymphoma: there is:
    (a) absence of epimyoepithelial islands
    (b) atypical lymphocytes
    (c) invasion of the connective tissue septa and the capsule
2. Papillary cystadenoma lymphomatosum

Treatment

No available treatment however management of xerostomia and xerophthalmia is essential.

Complications

- Malignant lymphoma in 6% of patients

- Squamous cell carcinoma is rare
- For these reasons treatment with immunosuppressive drugs e.g. corticosteroids is contraindicated

16.6.2 Mikulicz syndrome

Is the enlargement of salivary glands due to:

1. T.B.
2. Sarcoidosis
3. Leukemia
4. Lymphoma

16.6.3 Hashimoto's thyroiditis

Is similar to Sjogren's syndrome in:

1. Being autoimmune
2. Being lymphoepithelial in nature

16.6.4 IgG4-related diseases

See etiology of Sjorgren's syndrome and Mikulicz disease, page (418).

16.7 Salivary Gland Neoplasms

Salivary tumors are a particular challenge to pathologists. This is because of the complexity of the classification and that many tumors may show a broad spectrum of histological diversity. Furthermore, hybrid lesions may be seen, and histological diversity in individual lesions is so common as to be a characteristic feature of salivary tumors in general. Typical examples include adenoid cystic carcinoma, polymorphous low-grade adenocarcinoma and pleomorphic adenoma which can show such variable and similar features as to make a diagnosis on a small biopsy impossible. A diagnosis based on hematoxylin and eosin stained sections remains the gold standard in salivary gland pathology, but some recent developments in immunocytochemistry have been helpful and have a number of specific applications.

Although salivary gland neoplasms are characterized by diverse histopathology, accurate pathological diagnosis is essential. This is because accurate pathologic diagnosis greatly influences management, particularly when the recent anti-neoplastic modalities are to be used. Certain types of salivary gland tumors express growth factor receptors to which the newly developed receptor-targeted monoclonal antibodies are effective.

To know the salivary gland neoplasm terminology, it is essential to know the acini and the duct system of salivary glands, this is illustrated in figure ((16.1))

Features Suggestive of Benignancy

1. Slow growth
2. Long duration
3. No pain
4. No facial nerve palsy
5. Movable (except palate)
6. Unattached to skin or mucosa (except palate)
7. No ulceration of skin or mucosa unless by trauma

Features Suggestive of Malignancy

1. Rapid growth; rapid spurt

Chapter 16. Diseases of Salivary Glands

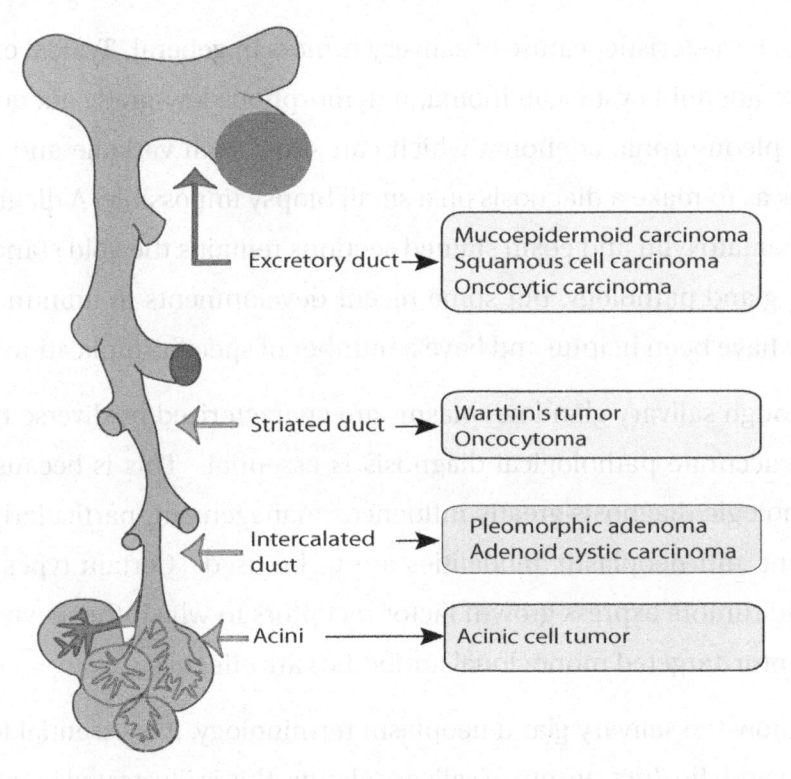

Figure 16.1: Salivary gland acini and duct system

- Excretory duct → Mucoepidermoid carcinoma, Squamous cell carcinoma, Oncocytic carcinoma
- Striated duct → Warthin's tumor, Oncocytoma
- Intercalated duct → Pleomorphic adenoma, Adenoid cystic carcinoma
- Acini → Acinic cell tumor

2. Short duration
3. Pain, often severe
4. Facial nerve palsy
5. Induration
6. Fixation to overlying skin or mucosa and to the underlying tissues
7. Ulceration of skin or mucosa

16.7.1 Benign Neoplasms

Pleomorphic Adenoma

(mixed tumor of the parotid)

Definition

Benign tumor of salivary glands characterized by variable histologic appearance. The histologic picture varies from one area to the other within the same tumor and from one tumor to the next.

Clinically

- **Frequency:** Is the most common neoplasm affecting salivary gland
- **Age:** Middle age.
- **Sex:** Females are more slightly affected than males
- **Site:** Major salivary gland more than minor. Among major salivary gland parotid is mostly affected. Among minor glands, palatal glands are mostly affected
- **Features:** swelling, firm, painless, slowly growing, not fixed to the surrounding structures, does not ulcerate unless by trauma and does not affect facial nerve if it occurs in the parotid.

Histologically

- Connective tissue capsule of varying thickness and completeness, some tumor cells lay inside and outside this capsule, this fact is responsible for the high recurrence rate of this tumor.
- Epithelial and myoepithelial cells arranged in solid masses or in a form of duct like structures. The ducts consist of double row of cells, the inner one is cuboidal or columnar and the outer layer consists of myoepithelial cells.
- Myoepithelial cells are either spindle shaped or plasma cell like (plasmacytoid).
- Squamous metaplasia may occur.

- Unusual matrix consists of mucoid, myxoid, chondroid, myxochondroid or rarely osseous tissues.
- Occasionally, the tumor may consists of almost entirely myoepithelial cells with no ductal elements. Such tumors often are called myoepitheliomas. Myoepitheliomas may represent one end of the spectrum of pleomorphic adenomas (see myoepithelioma).

Histogenesis

- Originally, it was supposed that the tumor is mixed. This postulate was introduced as an attempt to explain the unusual matrix of this tumor.
- Now it is believed that the tumor is not a true mixed tumor. It arises from the epithelial and myoepithelial cells of intercalated ducts.
- The unusual matrix is due to special forms of degeneration affecting epithelial or myoepithelial cells. Extensive accumulation of mucoid material produced by epithelial cells may occur between tumor cells, resulting in a myxomatous background. Vacuolar degeneration of cells in these areas can produce a chondroid appearance. The osseous tissues, if present are due to metaplasia of connective tissue cells.

Behavior

- Benign but there is high recurrence rate.
- Rare cases may progress into malignant pleomorphic adenoma (around 5% of cases).

Myoepithelioma

Definition

Myoepithelioma is a benign tumor of the myoepithelial cells. Myoepitheliomas may represent one end of the spectrum of pleomorphic adenomas.

Clinically

- Age: 30 – 80 with the mean age of 53 years
- Sex: No sex predilection
- Site: Most common in parotid and hard and soft palates
- Features: Slowly growing painless swelling

Histologically

- Fibrous capsule
- Sheets of myoepithelial cells which are either spindle shaped or plasmacytoid in shape. Approximately, 70% of cases contain spindle cells and approximately 20% of cases contain plasmacytoid cells. Sometimes both cell forms may be seen in the same lesion (10% of cases)
- Rarely, clear cells may dominate the histologic picture, leading to the designation of a "clear cell variant"
- Table (16.1) summarizes the differential diagnosis of myoepithelioma

Histogenesis

- The myoepithelial nature of tumor cells has been confirmed with immunohistochemistry.
- Tumor cells are positive with actin, cytokeratins and S-100 protein.

Chapter 16. Diseases of Salivary Glands

Table 16.1: Differential diagnosis of myoepitheloma and pleomorphic adenoma

> **Alawys Remember**
>
> **Myoepitheloma:**
> - Does not contain myxoid areas
> - Does not contain chondroid areas
> - Tumor cells are unable to form ducts (None, <5-10% or <1 duct/HPF)
> - Cells are spindle or plasmacytoid

Behavior

- Myoepithelioma has a slightly lower recurrence rate than mixed tumor, but complete surgical excision is indicated.
- The overall prognosis is excellent.

Oncocytoma

(Oxyphilic adenoma)

Definition

A benign tumor of salivary glands consists of oncocytes

Clinically

- **Age:** Old age
- **Site:** major salivary gland more than minor. Among major salivary gland parotid is mostly affected. Among minor glands, palatal glands are mostly affected

428

- **Features:** swelling - painless - slowly growing - not fixed to the surrounding structures - does not ulcerate unless by trauma - does not affect facial nerve if it occurs in the parotid.

Histologically

1. Connective tissue capsule
2. Connective tissue septa dividing the tumor into lobes
3. Connective tissue stroma
4. Oncocytes which forms solid masses or duct like structures. The cells are eosinophilic (oxyphilic) rounded or columnar, large, granular cytoplasm, pyknotic or vesicular nuclei.
5. Sometimes lymphocytic infiltration is found

Histogenesis

Arises from epithelial cells of striated ducts.

Oncocystosis (Nodular oncocytic hyperplasia)

- Is the proliferation of oncocytes within salivary gland tissue.
- It may mimic a tumor, both clinically and histologically.
- It may represent a metaplastic process rather than a neoplastic one.
- Oncyocytic metaplasia is the transformation of ductal and acinar cells to oncocytes. Oncocytes are rare before the age of 50; however, as people get older oncocytes become a common finding in salivary glands.
- Clinically, the condition usually affects the parotid gland and may be extensive enough to produce a multifocal and nodular swelling.
- The condition needs no treatment

Papillary Cystadenoma Lymphomatosum

(Warthin's tumor, Adenolymphoma)

Definition

Warthin's tumor is a unique neoplasm arising almost exclusively in the parotid gland and consists of two elements, epithelial and lymphoid

Clinically

- **Age:** Usually old ages (above forty years).
- **Sex:** Usually males
- **Site:** Parotid gland.
- **Features:**
  * Small slowly growing nodule occupying a superficial position just beneath the capsule of the gland.
  * The lesion feels soft and cystic to palpation.

Histologically

2 elements:

1. Epithelial element:
   - Consists of cystic cavities filled with mucin and lined by double row of epithelial cells.
   - The inner row is called the apical layer consists of tall columnar cells with palisading nuclei.
   - The outer row is called the basal layer consists of cuboidal cells. The epithelium projects into the cystic spaces in a papillary manner.

2. Lymphoid element:
   - Identical to that of lymph nodes.

Histogenesis

- It was suggested that the tumor arises from ectopic ductal epithelium (striated ducts) that has developed within intraparotid lymph nodes or entrapped in the periauricular lymph nodes. This theory is attractive, since it would account for the almost exclusive location in the parotid gland, which is the only salivary gland containing lymph nodes. Incorporation of the lymph nodes within the gland is felt to be a result of late encapsulation, which allows a lymph node to become trapped within the gland.
- It was also suggested that the epithelial cells incite a lymphocytic response which suggests a relationship between the epithelial and lymphoid tissues. This theory implies that the lymphoid tissue is recruited in the lesion by a yet unknown growth factor.
- Another theory suggests that these lesions are not true neoplasms but rather represent a hypersensitivity reaction. Unfortunately, recent immunohistochemical investigations of the lymphoid component have been inconclusive.
- There is a strong association with cigarette smoking. Smokers are at 8 times greater risk of developing Warthin's tumor than the general population.

Table (16.2) summarizes the key features of Warthin's tumor

16.7.2 Malignant Neoplasms

Table (16.3) shows a simplified biological classification of malignant salivary gland tumors.

Table 16.2: Key features of Warthin's Tumor

Warthin's Tumor

Warthin's tumor is unique in several ways:
- It contains lymphoid tissue
- Has a striking male predominance
- Is bilateral in 10
- Commonly has unilateral focal involvement
- Rare in black population

Table 16.3: Biologic classification of malignant salivary gland tumor

Malignant Salivary Gland Neoplasms

Low-grade malignancy
- Mucoepidermoid carcinoma (low-grade)
- Polymorphus low-grade adenocarcinoma
- Acinic cell carcinoma (low to intermediate-grade)
- Clear cell carcinoma
- Basal cell Adenocarcinoma

Intermediate-grade malignancy
- Mucoepidermoid carcinoma (intermediate-grade)
- Epimyoepithelial carcinoma
- Sebaceous adenocarcinoma

High-grade malignancy
- Mucoepidermoid carcinoma (high-grade)
- Adenoid cystic carcinoma
- Carcinoma ex-benign pleomorphic adenoma
- Salivary duct carcinoma
- Squamous cell carcinoma
- Oncocytic adenocarcinoma

Malignant Pleomorphic Adenoma

2 types exist:

1. Primary malignant pleomorphic adenoma:

    The tumor is malignant from the start, the malignant cells are the epithelial and myoepithelial cells and the metastasis in the remote area consists of both types of cells.

2. Malignant pleomorphic adenoma EX benign pleomorphic adenoma:

    Is the condition in which malignant transformation of a pre-existing benign pleomorphic adenoma occurs. In this condition the malignant cells are the epithelial cells and metastasis consists of epithelial cells only.

Clinically

Swelling - painful - rapidly growing - fixed to the surrounding tissues - ulcerative - cause facial nerve paralysis if the tumor occurs in the parotid

Histologically

Similar to the benign form except for the presence of signs of epithelial dysplasia

Mucoepidermoid Carcinoma

Definition

A malignant tumor of salivary gland consists of mucous, epidermoid and intermediate cells.

Clinically

- **Frequency:** Rare
- **Age:** Middle age
- **Site:** Major salivary gland more than minor. Among major salivary gland parotid is mostly affected. Among minor glands, palatal glands are mostly affected
- **Features:** Two grades have been described. The low grade malignancy type which resembles benign tumors. The high grade type which appears as a swelling - painful - rapidly growing - fixed to the surrounding tissues - cause facial nerve paralysis if the tumor occurs in the parotid. Tumors of intermediate behavior have been also described.

Histologically

1. Mucous secreting cells forming masses, sheets or duct like structures filled with mucin called primary cysts. Sometimes mucin is extruded into the connective tissue called secondary cysts. Mucous secreting cells are of pale cytoplasm and is best identified by mucicarmine stain.
2. Epidermoid cells which are polygonal in shape with basophilic cytoplasm forming masses or sheets, keratinization may occur
3. Sometimes intermediate cells which are basaloid in appearance are also found, they are undifferentiated cells considered to be the progenitor cells for mucous secreting and epidermoid cells.
4. The relative ratio of epidermoid to mucous cells determines the grade of the tumor: the greater the epidermoid component, the higher the grade and the worse the prognosis.

Histogenesis

The tumor arises from epithelial cells of the excretory ducts.

Central Mucoepidermoid Carcinoma

This is a rare situation in which mucoepidermoid carcinoma might occur centrally inside the bone. The origin of the lesion is from either:

1. Entrapment of retromolar mucous glands within the mandible.
2. Inclusion of the submandibular gland within the mandible (latent bone cyst).
3. Neoplastic transformation of mucous secreting cells (goblet cells) present in the wall of dentigerous cyst.
4. Neoplastic transformation of mucous secreting cells (goblet cells) present in the lining of the maxillary sinus.

Adenocystic Carcinoma

(Cylinderoma)

Definition

A malignant tumor of salivary gland characterized by formation of multiple cysts.

Clinically

- **Frequency:** Rare
- **Age:** Middle age

- **Site:** Minor more than major among the minor salivary gland palatal glands are mostly affected. Among the major salivary gland parotid is mostly affected.
- **Features:** Swelling - painful - rapidly growing - fixed to the surrounding tissues - can ulcerate - causes facial nerve paralysis if the tumor occurs in the parotid
- Tendency of the tumor to spread through perineural lymphatics thus early pain and tenderness is a constant feature of this tumor. The tumor is also characterized by late metastasis via blood.

Histologically

- Masses of malignant epithelial cells which may take the form or the combination of any of the following 3 patterns:
- Cribriform pattern: Consisting of masses of epithelial cells showing multiple cysts giving the characteristic Swiss chess, sieve-like or cylindrical appearance. These cells are basaloid in shape and show very little mitosis or pleomorphism.
- Tubular pattern: The epithelial cells take the form of tubules showing little cystification.
- Solid pattern: The epithelial cells form solid masses with minimal cystification. This form is the most aggressive one.
- Connective tissue stroma which is often hyalinized.

Behavior

The cribriform and the tubular patterns are of low grade malignancy, while the solid pattern is considered to be high-grade malignancy.

Histogenesis

Arises from epithelial cells of the intercalated ducts.

Acinic cell adenocarcinoma

(Acinic cell tumor)

Definition

ACA is a malignant tumor of salivary glands showing serous acinar differentiation. The tumor is considered to be of low-grade malignancy.

Clinically

- Frequency: Rare
- Age: Middle age
- Site: Major more than minor, among the major salivary gland parotid is mostly affected. Among the minor salivary gland, palatal glands are mostly affected.
- Features: Swelling - painful - rapidly growing - fixed to the surrounding tissues - can ulcerate - causes facial nerve paralysis if the tumor occurs in the parotid

Histologically

- Large cells with granular basophilic cytoplasm similar to serous cells. They contain cytoplasmic PAS-positive diastase digestion-resistant granules similar to those found in normal acinic cells.
- Arranged in masses or in acinar pattern.

Chapter 16. Diseases of Salivary Glands

- Scattered small round bodies (psammoma-like bodies) thought to be entrapped secretions are characteristic. Psammoma is an obsolete term for psammomatous meningioma or meningioma. Psammoma bodies are calcific bodies occurring in the meninges, choroid plexus, and in certain meningiomas; composed usually of concentric layers of meningocytes in various stages of hyaline change and mineralization; can also occur in benign and malignant epithelial tumors or with chronic inflammation.
- Areas of clear cells may be found (see table (16.4)).
- Scanty connective tissue stroma which may show hyalinization.

Histogenesis

- Arises from the acinar epithelial cells and it is believed that the acinic cells retain the potential for neoplastic transformation.
- It is also postulated that the tumor may arise from the intercalated duct reserve cells.

Salivary Adenocarcinoma, Not Otherwise Specified (NOS)

Definition

In spite of the wide variety of salivary gland tumors that have been identified and categorized, some tumors still defy the existing classification systems. These tumors are designated as salivary adenocarcinomas, not otherwise specified (NOS).

Clinical and Histological Features

- Because these tumors represent a diverse group of neoplasms, it is difficult to generalize about their clinical and histological features.

Table 16.4: The problem of clear cells in salivary gland tumors

Clear Cells in Salivary Gland Tumors

There are 2 salivary gland tumors that consist of cells showing clear cytoplasm; these are:

1. Clear cell carcinoma (due to accumulation of intracytoplasmic glycogen)
2. Epimyoepithelial carcinoma (due to accumulation of intracytoplasmic myofilaments)

There are 4 salivary gland tumors that, when poorly fixed, may have areas in which tumor cells exhibit clear cytoplasm as a result of autolysis; these are:

1. Adenoid cystic carcinoma
2. Oncocytoma
3. Acinic cell adenocarcinoma
4. Mucoepidermoid carcinoma

- However, the clinical and histological signs of malignancy could be detected in these lesions.
- Diagnosis is established by demonstration of infiltrative pattern and ruling out other types of adenocarcinomas of salivary glands.

16.8 Tumor-Like Lesions

16.8.1 Necrotizing Sialometaplasia

Definition

This is a tumor-like lesion usually affects minor salivary glands of the palate.

Etiology

Exact etiology is unknown; however the presumed cause is ischemia of the minor salivary glands resulting from infection, trauma, irradiation, or irritation caused by ill-fitting dentures.

Clinically

- Resembles carcinoma clinically and histologically and is readily mistaken for it.
- This condition most commonly develops in males in the form of a painless or painful deep, sudden ulcer of the hard palate usually opposite to the first molar. Once necrosis starts, the pain, if present, subsides.
- Lesions resolve without treatment within 6 to 10 weeks.

Histologically

- Biopsy is usually necessary to rule out squamous cell carcinoma or a minor salivary gland malignancy. Review of the tissue by a pathologist well versed in head and neck pathology is essential.
- Characteristic histologic findings include necrosis of the acini, ductal squamous metaplasia, and chronic inflammatory cell infiltration. The surface epithelium at the periphery of the lesion shows pseudoepithelomatous hyperplasia.

16.8.2 Sialoadenosis *(Sialosis)*

Definition

Sialoadenosis is a non-neoplastic, non-inflammatory enlargement of salivary glands, most usually affecting the parotids bilaterally.

Etiology

- Alcoholism
- Diabetes mellitus
- Drugs (sympathomimetics)
- Bulimia and obesity
- Endocrine disturbances
- Idiopathic

Histologically

- Hypertrophy of serous acini
- Edema of the interstitial connective tissue

CHAPTER 17
BONE DISEASES

Bone like reinforced concrete consists of 3 main elements and any defect in one of these elements will result in weakening of bone. These elements are:

1. Collagen fibers type I, which represent the steel bars of concrete. Arrangement of collagen fibers will determine the type of bone.

2. Ground substance, which represents the cement of concrete and consists mainly of osteocalcin and osteonectin. The collagen fibers together with the ground substance are sometimes termed osteoid tissue.

3. Hydroxyapatite crystals of calcium phosphates, which represents the stones (cobblestone or aggregates) of concrete.

17.1 Classification of bone diseases

1. Developmental diseases
    (a) Facial fibrous dysplasia
    (b) Cherubism, (Familial fibrous dysplasia)
    (c) Marble bone disease
    (d) Achondroplasia
    (e) Cleidocranial dysostosis
    (f) Oxycephaly
    (g) Osteogenesis imperfecta

(h) Hypophosphatasia

(i) Hypophosphatemia

2. Diseases of unknown etiology
   - Paget's disease of bone

3. Inflammatory
   (a) Periapical abscess
   (b) Periapical granuloma
   (c) Dry socket
   (d) Osteomyelitis
      i. Pyogenic osteomyelitis
         A. Acute pyogenic osteomyelitis
         B. Chronic pyogenic osteomyelitis
      ii. Chronic non-specific osteomyelitis
         A. Chronic osteomyelitis with proliferative periostitis (Garre's osteomyelitis)
         B. Diffuse sclerosing osteomyelitis
         C. Focal scelerosing osteomyelitis
      iii. Chronic specific osteomyelitis
         A. Tuberculous osteomyelitis
         B. Syphilitic osteomyelitis
         C. Actinomycotic osteomyelitis
   (e) Chemical necrosis of bones
   (f) Irradiation necrosis of bones (osteoradionecrosis)

4. Tumors of bone
   (a) Bone forming tumors
      i. Osteoma
      ii. Osteogenic sarcoma

       iii. Fibro-osteoma
- (b) Cartilage forming tumors
    - i. Chondroma
    - ii. Chondrosarcoma
- (c) Fibrous tissue forming tumors
    - i. Fibroma
    - ii. Ossifying fibroma
    - iii. Fibrosarcoma
    - iv. Giant cell tumor of bone
    - v. Giant cell granuloma
- (d) Marrow tumors
    - i. Ewing's sarcoma
    - ii. Lymphomas
    - iii. Myelomas
- (e) Tumors arising from entrapped cells
    - i. Odontogenic tumors
    - ii. Craniopharyngioma
- (f) Tumors of Langerhans histiocytes (Histocytosis X group)
    - i. Eosinophilic granuloma
    - ii. Hand - Schuller - Christian disease
    - iii. Letterer - Siewes disease
- (g) Metastatic Tumors of bone

5. Cystic (Refer to the chapter "Cysts & Cyst-Like Lesions", page (169)
6. Hormonal
    - (a) Hyperparathyroidism
    - (b) Hypoparathyroidism
7. Deficiency diseases

(a) Rickets

(b) Osteomalacia

8. Metabolic diseases

- Osteoporosis

17.2 Developmental Bone Diseases

17.2.1 Fibrous dysplasia (Maccune-Albright Syndrome)

Fibrous dysplasia[1] is a developmental fibro-osseous lesion. A fibro-osseous lesion is the lesion that consists of fibrous tissue intermingled with dysplastic bone trabeculae. Some controversy, still exists regarding the nomenclature of such lesions and their classifications.

Fibrous dysplasia of bone is of two types:

Monostotic

Affecting single bone, when affects one of the facial bones, it is called facial fibrous dysplasia

Polystotic

Affecting more than one bone and are further classified into two types:

1. Jaffe type (Jaffe-Lichtenstein syndrome): characterized by polystotic fibrous dysplasia and cafe au lait pigmentation of the skin.

---

[1] Unlike epithelial dysplasia, fibrous dysplasia is not a premalignant or precancerous lesion

2. Albright syndrome (Maccune-Albright syndrome): which in addition of the above, the patient shows sexual precocity particularly in females in addition to other endocrinopathy such as hyperthyroidism or pituitary adenoma.
3. Mazabraud syndrome, characterized by fibrous dysplasia and intramuscular myxomas.

17.2.2 Facial fibrous dysplasia

A developmental monostotic fibroosseous lesion, its growth stops with cessation of skeletal growth. Fibrous dysplasia of bone belongs to an arbitrary group of lesions known as fibro-osseous lesions. Fibro-osseous lesions could be defined as lesions that consist of fibrous tissue intermingled with bone, osteoid, cementum-like or other caclific tissues. For detailed classification of fibro-osseous lesions see table (17.1). For other types of fibro-osseous lesions, see Chapter "Benign Odontogenic Tumors" and tables (14.2) and (14.3).

Etiology

- Recent data reconfirm that the disease is not hereditary; very few convincing data are present to support the hereditary basis.
- The disease results form somatic mutation in the GNAS1 gene
- The mutation occurs post-zygotically and is lethal if it occurs in the single cell zygote (incompatible with life) and is compatible with life, only when it occurs in mosaic state (Happle hypothesis) i.e. other normal cells should coexist with the mutant cells for the latter to survive.
- The extent of the damage depends upon the stage at which the zygote was affected by such mutation. In the early stages, extensive involvement of the skeletal, skin and endocrine system will occur and vice versa.

Chapter 17. Bone Diseases

Table 17.1: Classification of Fibro-osseous Lesions

> **Always Remember**
>
> 1. Fibrous dysplasia
> 2. Cemento-osseous dysplasia (osseous dysplasia)
>   (a) Focal cemento-osseous dysplasia
>   (b) Periapical cemento-osseous dysplasia (periapical cemental dysplasia)
>   (c) Florid cemento-osseous dysplasia (florid cemental dysplasia)
>   (d) Familial gigantiform cementoma
> 3. Ossifying fibroma, cementifying fibroma and cemento-ossifying fibroma
> 4. Juvenile ossifying fibroma (Juvenile aggressive ossifying fibroma)
>
> Modified after Neville et al,[2]

- If the mutation occurs in one of the undifferentiated stem cells (embryonic stem cells) during early embryonic life, the osteoblasts, melanocytes and endocrine cells that represent the progeny of that mutated cell all will carry that mutation and express the mutated gene. The clinical presentation of multiple bone lesions, cutaneous pigmentation and endocrine disturbances would result. If the mutation occurs during postnatal life, the progeny of that mutated cells are essentially confined to one site, resulting in fibrous dysplasia affecting a single bone.

- The mutation affects the progenitor cell of the bone marrow –stromal stem cells–. These cells also termed (colony forming unit-fibroblastic, CFU-F) can differentiate into multiple phenotypes (cartilage, fat, bone, hematopoiesis-supportive stroma and fibrous tissue).

- This result in the formation of mutated fibroblasts, which will fail to form the supportive structure needed for hematopoietic tissue and fatty bone marrow formation, instead we will find abnormal fibrous tissue in place of the normal bone marrow. Also the mutated osteoblasts will fail to from the normal lamellar bone. The collagen fibers of the new bone are perpendicular to rather than collinear to the bone-forming surface.

Clinically

- Age: 4 – 18 years
- Sex: Female more than male
- Site: Maxilla more than mandible. Usually unilateral.
- Features: Start as a hard swelling distal to the canine causing buccal swelling, proptosis of the eye, maxillary sinus obliteration, nasal obstruction, and pushing the occlusal plain of the upper teeth downward resulting in malocclusion.

X- Ray

Three patterns have been described depending on the amount of formed lesional bone. The key feature of all patterns is that the margins merge faintly with surrounding normal bone. The 3 patterns are:

1. Orange peel pattern seen in intraoral films and ground glass appearance in extra-oral films
2. Ill defined radiolucent pattern in which few faint trabeculae are seen.
3. Smoke screen pattern.

Teeth

1. Faint or ill-defined lamina dura.
2. Reduced thickness of periodontal membrane space.
3. After extraction the socket is filled with dysplasia bone.

Histologically

- Resorption of the original bone and replacement by fibrous tissue with many blood vessels.
- Then, trabeculae of osteoid are laid down and are equidistant form each other. These trabeculae are Chinese letter shaped or U, C, and W shaped.
- Osteoblastic rimming is usually absent or minimal, and peritrabecular clefting (artifactual retraction of the stroma from the bony trabeculae) is common.
- Calcification of osteoid occurs and formation of woven bone is complete. In less active lesions lamellar bone may be found.

Complications

- Rarely neoplastic changes.
- Deformity of the orbit.
- Obliteration of the maxillary sinus.

Treatment

- Plastic surgery after 20 years of age.
- Surgical correction may be required to alleviate the severe deformity before the age of 20 years

17.2.3 Cherubism (Familial fibrous dysplasia)

This is a developmental intraosseous fibrous swelling, its growth stops with cessation of skeletal growth. The term cherubism is derived from the word cherub, which means a child with a beautiful and chubby (rounded and plump) face similar to an angel. In theology cherub is a member of the second order of angels, often represented as a beautiful rosy-cheeked child with wings. The term Cherubism is given because of the bilateral involvement of the maxilla and or mandible, which result in the chubby and rounded appearance of the face. The term –familial fibrous dysplasia should be avoided because cherubism has no relationship to fibrous dysplasia of bone.

Etiology

- Hereditary, autosomal dominant. Penetrance in males is 100% while penetrance in females is only 50 to 70%.
- The Cherubism gene was mapped to 4p16.3. The responsible gene was named SH3-binding protein (SH3BP2). The onset of the abnormalities of Cherubism and their organ-restricted characteristics may be related to dental developmental processes in children, when signals unique to the mandible and maxilla are transmitted through the extracellular matrix, triggered by the eruption of secondary teeth.

Clinically

- Age: 2 –4 years of age.
- Sex: Males are affected more than females in a ratio of 2:1.
- Site: Mandible more than maxilla, bilateral more than unilateral. Cases were also described in which both mandible and maxilla were involved.
- Features: Bilateral firm swelling at the angle of the mandible or in the maxilla or both. When the disease occurs bilaterally in the maxilla, there is an "upward look to heaven" or "eyes upturned to heaven" appearance that is due to a wide rim of exposed sclera resulting from downward stretching of the lower eye lid by the swelling. Failure of eruption of teeth in the affected site is a common finding.

X- Ray

Well defined multilocular radiolucent area.

Histologically

Cherubism is a central giant cell lesion, it consists microscopically of:

1. Loose vascular connective tissue stroma containing mononuclear cells and areas of hemorrhage.
2. Multinucleated giant cells.
3. Little amount of bone trabeculae.
4. This picture is identical to any other giant cell lesion.

Treatment

- Plastic surgery after 20 years age.
- Surgical correction may be required to alleviate the severe deformity before the age of 20 years

17.2.4 Marble bone disease

(osteopetrosis, Albers-Schönberg disease)

Definition

- Developmental bone disease characterized by decreased osteoclastic resorption of bone resulting in increased bone density.
- There are two main forms of the disease, the infantile and the adult types

Infantile osteopetrosis (malignant osteopetrosis)

- Autosomal recessive inheritance
- Congenital or starts in early childhood
- The most severe form
- Brittle bones with multiple bone fracture
- Marrow failure resulting in anemia, thrombocytopenia, leucopenia and granulocytopenia
- Compensatory hepatosplenomegaly
- Evidence of cranial nerve compression such as blindness, deafness and facial paralysis are common
- Increased susceptibility to infection
- Facial deformity, broad face, hypertelorism, snubs nose and frontal bossing
- Delayed or failure of eruption of teeth
- Difficult extraction of teeth
- Dry socket and osteomyelitis are the most common complication after dental extraction
- Delayed formation of sequestrum is the most common feature of osteomyelitis
- The prognosis is bad and the disease is fatal within the first decade of life
- Less severe variants exist and have been termed intermediate osteopetrosis

Adult osteopetrosis (benign osteopetrosis)

- Autosomal dominant inheritance
- Starts later in adult life

- Less severe than the infantile osteopetrosis
- Usually affects the axial skeleton and rarely affects long bones
- 40% of cases are asymptomatic and discovered by routine dental radiographs
- The disease is usually associated with long-term survival

Histologically:

- Replacement of spongy bone with dense compact bone
- Reduced marrow spaces
- Osteoclasts lack normal Howship's lacunae

X- Ray

- Increased radiopacities of bone to the degree that outlines of teeth are obliterated.
- Dental radiographs are useful in diagnosis due to the contrast between the shadows of teeth and bones

Treatment

- Bone marrow transplantation is the treatment of choice with a success rate of about 45%
- Because of the unavailability and risk of marrow transplantation, the following modalities may be useful
- Calcitriol
- Parathromone
- Corticosteroids
- Antibiotics

- Hyperbaric oxygen

Dental Management

- Extraction of teeth should be the last resort, conservative treatment is preferred
- Extraction, if performed should be atraumatic as possible with saucerization and suturing of sockets. The use of prophylactic antibiotics is recommended
- Osteomyelitis of the jaw needs rapid intervention to minimize bone loss
- Osteomyelitis requires pus drainage, surgical debridement, bacterial culture with sensitivity test and appropriate antibiotics
- The infection often requires prolonged antibiotic therapy with fluoroquinolones and lincomycin being most effective
- Hyperbaric oxygen is useful in promoting healing

17.2.5 Craniosynostosis

- Craniosynostosis is a generic term denoting early ossification of one or more of the cranial sutures resulting in abnormal head shape
- Skull deformity occurs due to retarded skull growth perpendicular to the affected suture associated with increased growth along the same direction that the suture follows
- Craniosynostosis is classified into primary and secondary
- Primary craniosynostosis results form abnormal suture biology and is further classified into syndromic and non-syndromic (isolated)

- Syndromic craniosynostosis occurs as a result of many syndromes, the major ones are: Crouzon syndrome, Apert syndrome, Pfeiffer syndrome and Carpenter syndrome
- Most of these syndromes show autosomal dominant inheritance
- Most of theses syndromes are due to mutations in one of the FGFR genes
- Non-syndromic (isolated form) is of unknown etiology
- Secondary craniosynostosis shows normal biology of sutures but there is abnormal internal or external forces resulting in early closure of sutures
- Secondary craniosynostosis usually results from failure of brain growth and thus results in micorcephaly
- No medical treatment exists to stop an early ossification of a cranial suture. Infants may require a series of surgical procedures to reduce the intracranial blood pressure or for cosmetic or other functional reasons

17.2.6 Achondroplasia

Developmental disease characterized by defective growth of bones developed in cartilage.

Etiology

Hereditary, autosomal dominant. Although this condition can be inherited in an autosomal dominant manner, 80% of cases are due to new, sporadic mutations. Mutations involve the gene encoding fibroblast growth factor receptor 3 (FGFR3), situated on chromosome 4. Most commonly, a point mutation causes the substitution of arginine for glycine in the transmembrane region of the receptor. There is growing evidence that mutations of FGFR3 confer a

–gain of function–. It is proposed that the normal function of FGFR3 is to slow down the formation of bone by inhibiting the proliferation of chondrocytes. Hence, the FGFR3 acts as a negative regulator of bone growth. The mutation increases the activity of FGFR3, severely limiting bone growth. This theory is supported by the knock-out mouse model in which the receptor is absent, and so the negative regulation of bone formation is lost. The result is a mouse with excessively long bones and elongated vertebrae, resulting in a long tail. Achondroplastic mouse models will be a useful tool in developing potential treatments.

Clinically

- Short legs, arms and fingers
- The trunk is of normal length
- Saddle nose
- Small maxilla (midfacial hypoplasia)
- Normal mandible
- Intelligence is normal and the patient is strong taking wrestling as a profession

17.2.7 Osteogenesis Imperfecta

A hereditary condition resulting from abnormality in the type I collagen, which most commonly manifests as increased fragility of bones. Four types of OI exist, based on the classifications of Sillence et al.

Etiology

- Hereditary, more than one mode of inheritance, most cases are autosomal dominant, autosomal recessive inheritance was also reported.

- The basic defect lies in the gene coding for collagen type I
- Mutations in the loci (COL1A1 on band 17q21 and COL1A2 on band 7q22.1, respectively) cause osteogenesis imperfecta
- Type I collagen fibers are found in bones, organ capsules, cornea, sclera, and meninges
- Qualitative defects (abnormal collagen I molecule) and quantitative defects (decrease in production of normal collagen I molecules) both exist

Clinically

- Dentinogenesis imperfecta in types II and III and in around 50% of patients with types I and IV
- Patients most commonly present with bone fragility.
- Prenatal ultrasound during second trimester shows bowing of long bones, fractures and limb shortening.
- Repeated fracture after mild trauma.
- Deafness (50% by age 40 years)
- Blue sclera
- Mild short stature

Histologically and histochemistry

- Decreased trabecular bone volume and thin cortices
- Reduced calcification rates and smaller apatite crystals
- Decreased collagen fibril diameter

17.3 Bone Diseases of Unknown Etiology

17.3.1 Paget's disease of bone (Osteitis Deformans)

Overview

- First diagnosed by Sir James Paget in 1877, Paget's disease of bone, or osteitis deformans is a disease characterized by increased deossification associated with dysplastic reossification.
- In this disorder, the osteoclasts become abnormally activated, possibly by viral infection, and produce an irregular and distorted pattern of resorption, to which there is usually an intense osteoblastic response with irregular new bone formation often in the form of woven bone. Thus, in Paget's disease there may be increased bone density, but because of the irregular architecture, bone strength is decreased and pathologic fractures may occur. Paget disease also has a genetic component that may be linked to an osteosarcoma tumor suppressor gene. This could account for the increased risk of osteosarcoma in patients with Paget disease.

Pathology of Paget's Disease

- The initial abnormality in Paget's disease is a dramatic increase in the rate of bone resorption at areas of heightened bone remodeling.
- Pagetic osteoclasts are abnormal – approximately five times larger than normal containing an average number of 20 nuclei per cell compared with three to four nuclei in normal adult osteoclasts.
- The osteoblasts are not apparently affected, however. the extreme difference in size between the two cell types causes the intensely elevated rate of bone resorption.

- Because bone resorption triggers bone formation, the rate of bone resorption is matched by a rapid rate of bone formation. The new bone is structurally disorganized, however, resulting in an overall decrease in bone strength and an increase in susceptibility to bowing and fractures.
- In addition, the abnormal bone is marked by a high level of vascularity and an excess of fibrous connective tissue in the marrow.

Etiology

- The exact etiology of Paget's disease is obscure. Historically, the postulated etiologies of Paget's disease could be described as follows:
- Paget's view was that the disease is inflammatory due to hotness and redness of the mucosa covering the affected bone.
- Disturbance of bone vascularity was also postulated as the cause of Paget's disease.
- Viral etiology was proposed by others. Osteoclasts in Paget's disease are markedly increased in number and size, have increased numbers of nuclei per multinucleated cell, and demonstrate increased resorption capacity and increased sensitivity to 1,25-(OH)2D3, the active form of vitamin D. These cells also contain nuclear inclusions, reminiscent of those seen in paramyxovirus-infected cells, which cross-react with antibodies to measles virus nucleocapsid (MVNP) antigen.
- Hereditary background was also postulated to account for the increased incidence in certain families and or population groups.
- In about 40% of familial cases and 8% of sporadic cases, germline mutations in the sequestosome 1 gene (SQSTM1) (known as p62) have been identified. Patients with SQSTM1 mutations tend to have more severe disease than those without such mutations. SQSTM1 activates osteoclasts via the nuclear factor-kappa B (NF-κB) signaling pathway.

- Studies suggest that increased bone resorption in Paget's disease may result from increased vitamin D receptor binding affinity among osteoclasts.
- It was suggested that there is increased responsiveness of osteoclast precursors to RANKL (receptor activator of nuclear factor kappa B ligand) and decreased inhibition of RANK signaling.
- Some studies suggest that underlying defects may reside not only in osteoclasts but also in osteoblasts.

Clinically

- Age: Over 40 years.
- Sex: Male affected more than female.
- Race: More common in Anglo-Saxon ancestry. The highest rates are in the United Kingdom.
- Site: Most cases are polystotic (more than one bone is affected). Rarely the disease is monostotic (limited only to one bone). Bones usually affected are legs, vertebral column, sacrum, pelvis, skull, maxilla and mandible.
- Features: Bending of legs, kyphosis, progressive enlargement of head, enlargement of face, deafness, blindness, facial neuralgia (due to compression of cranial nerves).

Oral Manifestations

See complications of the disease.

Blood Chemistry

- Increase of alkaline phosphatase, the normal level is 3 – 13 King Armstrong units, 1.5–5 Bodansky units.
- In Page's disease of bone the level of alkaline phosphatase can reach above 200 King Armstrong units and above 250 Bodansky units.
- Normal levels of blood calcium and phosphorus.
- In patients with mild disease, total serum alkaline phosphatase may be normal. In such cases, it may be helpful to assess specialized markers:
    1. For bone formation, serum N-terminal *propeptide* of type 1 collagen.
    2. Or for bone resorption e.g., urinary N-terminal *telopeptide* of type 1 collagen.

X- Ray

1. Osteolytic stage
    (a) Osteoporosis and definite radiolucent areas.
    (b) Loss of lamina dura.
    (c) Resorption of the roots of teeth.
2. Osteoblastic stage
    (a) New bone is laid down in a form of dense sclerotic patches giving the characteristic *cotton wool appearance*.
    (b) Hypercementosis of roots.

Histologically

- In the osteoclastic phase (bone resorption phase)
    ★ Resorption of bone and replacement of marrow by highly vascular connective tissue.

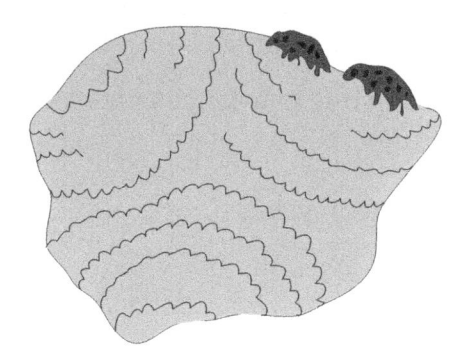

Figure 17.1: Diagrammatic representation of mosaic appearance resulting from repeated resorption of bone or cementum by osteoclasts and cementoclasts and apposition by osteoblasts or cementoblasts.

- ★ The osteoclasts are larger than normal with increased number of nuclei.
- ★ Masses of bone which show many reversal lines giving *mosaic appearance* due to repeated resorption and apposition, see figure ((17.1)).
- ★ Mosaic appearance of roots is also found.
- In Osteoblastic phase (sclerotic phase)
    - ★ Large masses of dense bone trabecule with many reversal lines
    - ★ Fibrous bone marrow

Complications

1. Heart failure due to multiple arteriovenous shunts.
2. 2 % of cases develop osteosarcoma.
3. Pathological fracture of bones.
4. Spacing of teeth.
5. Delayed sequestration.

6. Frequent remaking of dentures.
7. Difficult extraction due to hypercementosis.
8. Hemorrhage.
9. Dry socket and osteomyelitis.
10. Sever neuralgia.

Treatment

- The disease is partially controlled with calcitonin and Bisphosphonates, however the following measures should be followed:
- Good oral hygiene is mandatory to avoid complications.
- Frequent remaking of dentures to avoid bone necrosis.
- Extraction should be the last resort. Surgical extraction with minimal trauma may be necessary to avoid post-extraction complications. Suturing of extraction wounds is preferred to prevent hemorrhage and infection.
- Antibiotics before extraction.

17.4 Inflammatory Bone Diseases

17.4.1 Dry socket (Alveolar Osteitis)

(*Fibrinolytic Alveolitis*)

A localized osteitis affecting the lamina dura lining the tooth socket. Dry socket may be defined as that socket in which the blood clot disintegrates or fails to form, with production of foul dour without pus formation. It is the most common painful complications of dental extractions. The exact etiology of dry socket is not clear.

Predisposing factors

Many factors are blamed:

1. Infection, before, during or after extraction (active or recent history of acute ulcerative gingivitis or pericoronitis).
2. Trauma, use of excess force during extraction.
3. Local analgesia: Could be attributed to the effect of local vasoconstrictor used.
4. Contamination of the socket with food, saliva and bacteria.
5. Excessive rinsing after extraction.
6. Curettage of the socket after extraction.
7. Use of oral contraceptives.
8. Paget's disease and marble bone disease.
9. General diseases as diabetes and leukemia.
10. Pathological conditions as cysts of the jaw.
11. Immunocompromized patients.
12. Table (17.2) summarizes the risk factors responsible for developing dry socket.

Pathogenesis

- The initial event is destruction of the clot which may be due to:
  ★ Bacterial proteolytic enzymes.
  ★ Excessive local fibrinolytic enzymes (more accepted). The alveolar bone and other oral soft tissues in particular have a high content of fibrinolytic activators (plasmin) which are released when bone is traumatized. The estrogen component of oral contraceptives enhances serum fibrinolytic activity and hence is associated with increased incidence of dry socket.

Table 17.2: Risk factors associated with dry socket

> **Risk factors associated with dry socket**
>
> - Previous experience of dry socket
> - Deeply impacted mandibular third molar
> - Poor oral hygiene
> - Active or recent history of acute ulcerative gingivitis or pericoronitis associated with the tooth to be extracted
> - Smoking (especially >20 cigarettes per day)
> - Use of oral contraceptives
> - Immunocompromised individuals

Note

- Clot destruction leaves an open socket in which infected food and other debris accumulates in direct contact with bone which become necrotic (particularly the lamina dura)
- The necrotic bone lodges bacteria which proliferate freely, protected form leukocytes unable to reach them through this avascualr material.
- Dead bone gradually becomes separated by granulation tissue with osteoclasts and sequestra are usually shed in tiny fragments.
- Healing is by granulation tissue from the base and walls of the socket.
- The cause of pain could be attributed to the presence and formation of kinin locally in the socket. It has been shown that kinins activate the nerves, which may have already been presensitized by other inflammatory mediators.
- Plasmin is also involved in the conversion of kallikreins to kinins in the alveolar bone marrow. Thus, the presence of plasmin may give a possible explanation for the two most characteristic features of AO, namely neuralgic pain and disintegrated blood clot.

Clinically

- Three main features:
    1. Presence of bare bone
    2. Presence of pain starting 1–3 days after extraction
    3. Foul odor
- It is highly unlikely for dry socket to occur before the first postoperative day, because the blood clot contains anti-plasmin that must be consumed by plasmin before clot disintegration can take place.
- The duration of dry socket varies to some degree, depending on the severity of the disease, but it usually ranges from 5–10 days.
- Dry socket is common in the mandible than maxilla because blood supply of the mandible is lesser than that of maxilla and mandibular teeth are difficult in extraction when compared with the maxillary teeth.
- The incidence of dry socket has been reported as 3–4% following routine dental extractions and ranges from 25% to 30% after the removal of mandibular third molars.

Prevention

- Alveolar osteitis is usually unpredictable.
- Since excessive bone trauma seems to be an important predisposing factor, extraction should be atraumatic as possible.
- The prophylactic use of antibiotics is questionable and their use in routine dental extractions cannot be justified.

Treatment

- Irrigation with saline solution.

- Packing the socket with zinc oxide eugenol pack, Alvogel or similar dressings.
- See table (17.3) for further measures used to prevent dry socket

Complications

Osteomyelitis is the most common complication.

17.4.2 Delayed Healing of tooth socket

- Dry socket
- Irradiation on the site of extraction
- Presence of malignant tumor in the site of extraction
- Paget's disease of bone
- Marble bone disease
- AIDS
- Diabetes mellitus

17.4.3 Acute Pyogenic Osteomyelitis

(Derived from Greek words osteon, meaning bone, myelo- meaning marrow, and -itis meaning inflammation)

Is the inflammation of bone and bone marrow that includes the production of pus. It is thus distinct from an osteitis such as alveolar osteitis, which is the inflammation of bone only. Also it should be differentiated from sclerosing osteomyelitis, which is characterized by proliferation of bone without pus formation.

Table 17.3: A summary of measures to prevent the risk of dry socket

> **Always Remember**
>
> - Use of sound surgical practice.
> - Extractions should be performed with minimum trauma.
> - Confirm presence of blood clot subsequent to extraction (if absent, scrape alveolar walls gently)
> - Wherever possible preoperative oral hygiene measures to reduce plaque levels to a minimum.
> - Encourage the patient to stop or limit smoking in the immediate postoperative period.
> - Advise patient to avoid vigorous mouth rinsing for the first 24 h post extraction.
> - For patients taking oral contraceptives extractions should ideally be performed during days 23 through 28 of the menstrual cycle.

Causative Organisms

- Anaerobic bacteria e.g. bacteroids are the usual etiologic factor.
- Sometimes Gram negative bacteria are also encountered.
- Rarely Gram positive bacteria particularly staphylococci or streptococci in contrary to osteomyelitis of long bones in which staphylococcus aureus is the most common cause.

Mode of Infection

- Dental infection, which is the most common cause e. g. periapical abscess, pericoronitis, periodontal abscess.
- Compound fracture.
- Hematogenous i. e. blood born infection as in pyemia
- Irradiation.

Pathogenesis

- Inflammation of bone will result in edema.
- As bone cannot swell, edema will occur on the expense of the blood vessels leading to collapse of these vessels (self-strangulation) and stasis of blood stream with thrombosis.
- Necrosis of the affected area will start.
- A line of separation consists of granulation tissue will appear around the necrotic area on the expense of vital bone as an attempt to localize the infection.
- Once the necrotic area is separated from the normal bone it is termed sequestrum.
- Pus, formed by liquefaction of necrotic soft tissue and inflammatory cells may escape through multiple sinuses called cloacae.
- The sequestrum will undergo gradual resorption.
- New bone will occur under the periostium and is termed involucrum.
- Where bone has died and been removed, healing is by granulation tissue which is gradually replaced by new bone.
- The sequestrum is porous, light in weight and color.

Clinically

- Rise of temperature, particularly in the early stages.
- Severe, throbbing, deeply-seated pain
- The affected area is swollen due to inflammatory edema.
- Numbness of the lower lip may occur if the inflammation spread to the inferior alveolar nerve.
- Teeth are tender and may become loose with pus may ooze from an open socket or gingival margins.

- When pus is formed it discharges through multiple sinuses into the mouth or the skin. Once pus is formed acute osteomyelitis is termed chronic osteomyelitis.
- Regional lymphadenopathy occurs.
- Osteomyelitis is common in the mandible more than the maxilla due to its poorer blood supply and due to the fact that the bone of the mandible is denser than that of maxilla.
- Osteomyelitis of maxilla is rare and is usually due to surgical interference in acute sinusitis, severe maxillo-facial injury or irradiation.

Histologically

- Dead bone (sequestrum) is recognized histologically by lacunae empty of osteocytes.
- The periphery of the sequestrum show eroded outline due to osteoclastic resorption.
- Sequestrum is surrounded by granulation tissue heavily infiltrated with acute and chronic inflammatory cells with areas of pus formation.

Blood Picture

In acute stage there is leukocytosis (increase in white blood cells).

X-Ray

- In the first two weeks no changes could be detected in the radiographic films.
- Later on irregular radiolucent areas indicating bone resorption and formation of separating lines are evident. Such radiolucent lines are usually described as moth-eaten appearance or worm eaten appearance.

Subperiosteal bone formation may be seen. The sequestrum is slightly more radiopaque than normal bone, probably due to over-calcification caused by the long standing inflammatory condition (dystrophic calcification).

Complications

- Numbness of lower lip.
- Pathological fracture.
- Ankylosis of TMJ.
- Pyaemia or septicemia is rare now except in immunocompromised patients.

Treatment

- Antibiotics.
- Drainage of pus.
- Remove the source of infection such as remaining roots or foreign body.
- Monitoring good oral hygiene.
- Extraction of loose teeth.
- Removal of sequestrum when it is completely separated.
- Hyperbaric oxygen is useful in persistent cases.

17.4.4 Chronic Pyogenic Osteomyelitis

- Chronic osteomyelitis may develop without any apparent acute episode (de novo) and may be due to an exceptionally low-grade infection or high local resistance. The infection is localized but persistent because bacteria growing in dead bone are inaccessible to the host defenses.

Clinically and radiographically it is similar to acute osteomyelitis in its terminal stages. There is bone destruction and granulation tissue formation with little suppuration.

- Chronic osteomyelitis is subdivided into secondary chronic osteomyelitis (SCO) and primary chronic osteomyelitis (PCO), depending on the severity of the initial symptoms. SCO is defined as chronic osteomyelitis that develops secondary to acute symptoms and PCO is defined as chronic osteomyelitis that starts insidiously, with no acute phase.
- It is difficult, however, to differentiate existent lesions according to the severity of the initial symptoms. The borderline between SCO and PCO is vague and cannot be determined objectively.

17.4.5 Chronic Non-pyogenic Osteomyelitis

Chronic non-pyogenic osteomyelitis is characterized by bone formation resulting in the increased density of bone (sclerosis). Figure (17.2) illustrates the basic differences between the 3 types of chronic non-pyogenic osteomyelitis.

Chronic Osteomyelitis with Proliferative Periostitis

(Garre's osteomyelitis, Periostitis Ossificans)

- This is a rare reaction, usually to periapical infection in young patients.
- Young individuals are more prone to be affected because of their high resistance, increased local blood supply, and greater bone regenerative capabilities.
- The newly formed bone is deposited under the periosteum on the surface of the affected bone.
- A non-tender or rarely tender bony swelling will appear usually in the mandible.

Chapter 17. Bone Diseases

> **Always Remember**
>
> Different types of chronic osteomyelitis shown diagrammatically, Garres osteomyelitis (left) the reaction is subperiosteal. Focal sclerosing osteomyelitis (middle) the reaction is central and is limited to a single tooth. Diffuse sclerosing osteomyelitis (right) the reaction is central and involves several teeth.

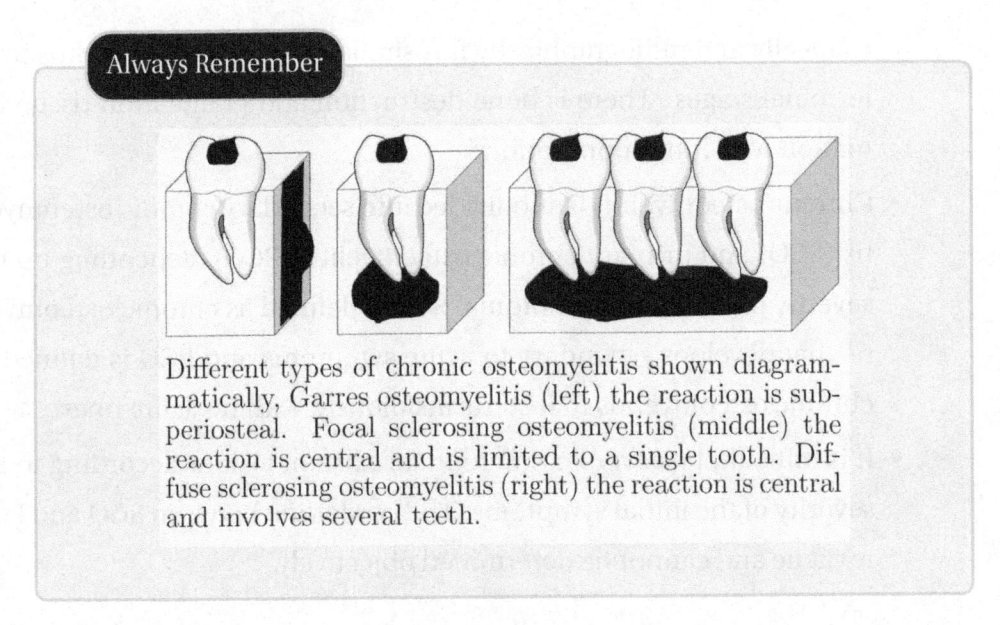

Figure 17.2: The 3 basic types of chronic non-pyogenic osteomyelitis

- Radiographically is characterized by the presence of lamellae of newly formed periosteal bone outside the cortex, giving the characteristic appearance of *"onion skin"*.
- Treatment of the causative infection will result in resolution.

Diffuse Sclerosing Osteomyelitis

- A condition in which intrameullary bone proliferation occurs resulting in sclerosis
- The condition is of obscure nature and probably results from low-grade non-pyogenic infection. *Actinomyces* combined with *Eikenella corrodens* are accused as being the causative agents. These organisms are normal inhabitants of the oral flora, they become pathogens upon gaining an entry into bone. Their portal of entry may be via spread from severe periodontal disease.

- The condition shows some similarities to gigantiform cementoma and hence it was thought to be a variant of the latter. However, as the condition is usually associated with severe periodontal disease, the infective nature is postulated.
- **Clinically**, persistent *intense pain*. Mild expansion of the mandible, and even soft tissue swelling "active exacerbation,". The mandible is usually affected more than the maxilla and mostly in the body, angle, and ramus area. The mandible may be tender to palpation, particularly at the buccal cortex. No suppuration is noted.
- **Radiographically**, it shows areas of diffuse or nodular sclerosis resembling the cotton wool appearance of Paget's disease of bone.
- **Microscopically**, shows masses of bone with many reversal lines (mosaic appearance) and infiltration with many chronic inflammatory cells and fibrosis of the marrow.
- Treatment is by removal of the source of infection and antibiotics for long period of time. Patients may relapse from an antibiotic-induced remission because the bone sclerosis limits drug penetrance.

Focal sclerosing osteomyelitis

- This is a rare form of bone reaction to periapical infection and may cause mild pain.
- The condition thus represents a localized form of the diffuse sclerosing osteomyelitis.
- The reaction is basically proliferation of bone in response to mild bacterial infection leading to bone formation rather than destruction. It is usually seen as a sclerotic area related to the apex of a dead tooth in a young patient. Mandibular teeth are affected more than maxillary teeth.

- Extraction or root canal treatment of the infected tooth should lead to resolution of the infection.
- Microscopically, there is a dense mass of bony trabeculae with minimal marrow.

17.4.6 Medication-related Osteonecrosis of the Jaw

(Antiresorptive-related Osteonecrosis, (ARONJ))

- Medication-related osteonecrosis of the jaw is the bone necrosis which results from one of the following antiresorptive medications:
    1. Bisphosphonates medication
    2. Antiangiogenic therapy
    3. Monoclonal antibody designed to prevent osteoclastic maturation.
- These medications are used to treat osteoporosis or various malignancies that involve bone e.g. multiple myeloma, metastatic breast carcinoma, and prostate carcinoma. Less frequent uses include treatment for Paget's disease, osteogenesis imperfecta, rheumatoid arthritis, and giant cell tumors of bone.
- The majority of cases of osteonecrosis occurs in the jaw bone. Extragnathic bones are affected but to a far lesser extent. Cases have been reported in the ear and femur. The exact cause for such a phenomenon is not known and might be related to the selective deposition of the drugs in the skeleton.
- The majority of cases results from the intravenous use (94%), while the remaining 6% of cases results in patients taking the drug orally.
- Risk factors that can aggravate the incidence of osteonecrosis are:
    1. Use of antiresorptive drug combination
    2. Smoking
    3. Age older than 65

4. Corticosteroids
5. Alcohol
6. Poor oral hygiene
7. Diabetes
8. Chemotherapy

- The mandible is involved in 65% of cases, the maxilla in 27%, and both jaws in 8%.
- In patients with exposed bone, 16% were asymptomatic, 84% were painful.
- In some cases the necrosis can lead to development of a cutaneous or mucosal sinus or pathologic fracture.
- It should be noted that the clinical, radiographic and histopathological features of all medication-related osteonecrosis are very similar.
- **Radiographically:**
    1. In early stages, increased radiopacity of the crestal portions of each jaw (particularly the alveolar ridges), with a more normal appearance of the bone away from tooth-bearing portions.
    2. In advanced stages, moth-eaten and ill-defined radiolucency with or without central radiopaque sequestra (a feature that mimics osteomyelitis).
- **Histopathological feature:**
    1. Biopsy of vital bone reveals irregular trabeculae of pagetoid bone, with adjacent enlarged and irregular osteoclasts that often demonstrate numerous intracytoplasmic vacuoles.
    2. Specimens of severely affected areas reveal trabeculae of sclerotic lamellar bone, with loss of osteocytes from their lacunae and frequent peripheral resorption with bacterial colonization. Although the peripheral bacterial colonies often resemble actinomycetes, the infection is not supportive of a diagnosis of invasive cervicofacial actinomycosis.

Bisphosphonates Bone Necrosis (BON)

- Bisphosphonates are a class of drugs that prevent the loss of bone density, used to treat osteoporosis and similar diseases. They are the most commonly prescribed drugs used to treat osteoporosis.
- The drug is also used in the treatment of Paget's disease of bone, bone metastasis, multiple myeloma, primary hyperparathyroidism, osteogenesis imperfecta, fibrous dysplasia, and other conditions that exhibit bone loss.
- This drug may lead to surgical complication in the form of impaired wound healing following oral, periodontal surgery or endodontic therapy.
- The majority of cases appear to result from intravenous bisphosphonate therapy (94%). Only the remaining 6% of cases arose in patients taking bisphosphonates orally.
- In the serum, 50% of bisphosphonates is cleared rapidly by the kidneys with the remainder going to bone.
- The mode of action is not yet completely understood, it is hypothesized that the condition is related to a defect in jaw bone physiologic remodeling or wound healing. The strong inhibition of osteoclast function precipitated by bisphosphonate therapy can lead to inhibition of normal bone turnover. Because bisphosphonates are preferentially deposited in bone with high turnover rates, it is possible that the levels of bisphosphonate within the jaw are selectively elevated.
- A diagnosis of bisphosphonate-associated osteonecrosis of the jaw relies on three criteria:
    ★ Current or history of bisphosphonate medication.
    ★ Area of exposed bone in the jaw persisting for more than 8 weeks.
    ★ No history of radiation therapy to the head and neck.

- There is presently no known prevention for bisphosphonate-associated osteonecrosis of the jaw.
- **Precautions:** Similar to that of osteoradionecrosis. See page (480)

Antiangiogenic therapy bone necrosis

- A correlation was found between the use of antiangiogenic therapy and osteonecrosis of the jaw.
- The antiangiogenic agents are prescribed for a variety of malignancies and include tyrosine kinase inhibitors and monoclonal antibodies directed against vascular endothelial growth factor.
- This risk is increased if these agents are combined with bisphosphonates.

Monoclonal antibody against osteoclastic maturation

- It was found that there is a correlation between the use of monoclonal antibody designed to prevent osteoclastic maturation (denosumab) and the incidence of osteonecrosis of the jaw.
- Denosumab is a monoclonal antibody that reduces osteoclastic function, but it does this by inhibiting osteoclastic differentiation. This medication quickly reduces osteoclastic activity by 85% with maximal reduction occurring within 1 month of an injection.
- The medication is not deposited in bone and has a half-life of 24.5 days, with complete clearance in 4 to 5 months.

17.4.7 Irradiation Necrosis

(Osteoradionecrosis)

Is the necrosis or decreased vitality of bone due to irradiation.

Etiology

Historical: In luminal dial painters. Nowadays the most usual cause is radioactive isotopes used in the treatment of malignancy without good protective measures.

Pathogenesis

Irradiation will result in:

1. Endarteritis obliterans.
2. Death of osteoblasts and osteocytes.
3. This will result in necrosis of bone or at least decreased vitality, which allow easy infection.

Clinically

Similar to pyogenic osteomyelitis but there is prolonged course with delayed sequestration.

Irradiation also will result in:

- Delayed eruption of teeth or exfoliation of tooth germs.
- Stunted teeth.
- Asymmetry of face duo to affection of the mandibular growth centers.

Precautions

- Improvement of dental health to prevent future procedures that disrupt bone; this includes elimination of foci of infection and removal of partially impacted teeth, loose teeth and remaining roots.
- Conservative treatment of teeth is preferred in irradiated jaws.

- Extraction or surgery is contraindicated unless special preparation of the patient is done. These preparation includes antibiotic prophylaxis starting one day before and extending 3 days after any invasive dental procedure.

17.5 Tumors of Bone

17.5.1 Compact and Cancellous Osteoma

See chapter "Benign Non-Odontogenic Tumors & Tumor-Like Lesions", page (268)

17.5.2 Osteoid Osteoma

See chapter "Benign Non-Odontogenic Tumors & Tumor-Like Lesions", page (269)

17.5.3 Ossifying Fibroma

Ossifying fibroma and its related disorders (cementifying, cemento-ossifying fibroma) are discussed in the chapter "Benign Odontogenic Tumors", page (379)

17.5.4 Central Giant Cell Granuloma

(Central giant cell reparative granuloma)

A lesion of unknown nature, it may represents unusual reaction of bone against unknown irritant. It was thought that the lesion is a local reparative process, hence the name reparative was proposed.

Clinically

- Appears clinically as a slowly growing painless swelling.
- Age: Usually below 20 years of age.
- Site: Mandible is affected more than maxilla. Usually in the molar region.

X-Ray

Multilocular radiolucent area.

Histologically

Similar to any giant cell lesion it consists of:

- Loose vascular connective tissue rich in mononuclear cells thought to be fibroblasts.
- Multinucleated giant cells which are found usually around areas of hemorrhage. They are formed by fusion of neighboring cells or by division of the nucleus without division of the cytoplasm. The origin of these cells is thought to be histiocytes, osteoclasts or stromal cells.
- Little amount of bone trabeculae.

Treatment

- Surgical enucleation
- In recurrent or aggressive cases, more radical surgery
- Intralesional injection of corticosteroids (particularly, triamcinolone acetonide) weekly for 6 weeks
- Systemic calcitonin by intradermal injection or by intranasal spray daily for 12 months

- Interferon alpha was also tried with variable success rate

17.5.5 Giant Cell Tumor of Bone (Osteoclastoma)

A tumor of bone of variable clinical behavior, some cases are of low-grade malignancy with no metastasis while others are of high-grade malignancy and do metastasize to the lungs.

Clinically

- The lesion affects old age groups usually at 40 years of age.
- It occurs at the ends of long bones and very rarely in the jaws (epiphysis). This lesion appears clinically as a painful rapidly growing swelling that destroys the affected bone and can metastasize to remote areas (about 15% of cases).

X - Ray

Radiographically giant cell tumor of bone appears as an aggressive radiolucent area.

Histologically

The microscopic picture of giant cell tumor of bone is similar to any giant cell lesion except for the presence of abnormal mitosis, nuclear pleomorphism and hyperchromatic nuclei. The lesion consists of:

1. Loose vascular connective tissue stroma rich in mononuclear cells thought to be fibroblasts. The cells are plump shaped showing criteria of malignancy.

2. Multinucleated giant cells which are more large than those of giant cell granuloma.
3. No or very little bone formation.

Treatment

Hemiresection, yet recurrence is common unless the tumor is adequately removed during surgery.

17.5.6 Tumors of Langerhans Cell Histiocytes

(Histocytosis X group)

This group of lesions commonly involves bone, although it is not primarily a tumor of bone. The cell of origin of this group of lesions is believed to be the Langerhans cell of the surface epithelium. This cell is of bone marrow origin and is a member of the mononuclear phagocystic system MPS. The cell is S-100 protein positive. An alternative name of Langerhans histiocytosis was proposed for this group of lesions instead of the older term histiocytosis X.

This group of lesions contains 3 known diseases includes eosinophilic granuloma, Hand–Schüller–Christian disease and Letter–Swie disease.

The pathogenesis is unknown. An ongoing debate exists over whether this is a reactive or neoplastic process.

Arguments supporting the reactive nature of this disorder include
- The occurrence of spontaneous remissions
- The failure to detect aneuploidy, metaphase or karyotypic abnormalities
- The good survival rate in patients without organ dysfunction.

support for the neoplastic origin for this proliferation

- The infiltration of organs by aberrant cells
- A possible lethal evolution
- Successful treatment using cancer-based modalities

Eosinophilic granuloma

Eosinophilic granuloma represents the most benign form of epidermal cell Langerhans histiocytosis.

Clinically

- Eosinophilic granuloma affects young age, usually below 10 years.
- The lesion is usually solitary, rarely multiple. Flat bones are commonly affected rarely long bones or soft tissues. In the jaws eosinophilic granuloma appears as a painful swelling associated with inflammation of the area and looseness of the teeth.

X- Ray

Radiographically eosinophilic granuloma appears as an area of complete radiolucency (*punched out radiolucent area*).

Histologically

The microscopic picture of eosinophilic granuloma is a mass of granulation tissue with eosinophils and histiocytes.

Treatment

Curettage.

Prognosis

The prognosis of this lesion is very good.

Hand–Schüller–Christian Disease

Hand–Schüller–Christian disease represents the moderate form of Langerhans cell histiocytes group.

Clinically

- This lesion is common in young age - below 10 years.
- It consists of triad of symptoms that includes:
    1. Exophthalmos because the lesion occurs behind the eye and displace the eyeball.
    2. Diabetes insipidus, because the lesion occurs in the sella tursica and then replace the posterior pituitary which secretes the antidiuretic hormone.
    3. Multiple affection of bones and if the jaw bones are affected it produces painful swellings with inflammation and loose teeth.

X- Ray

The radiographic picture of Hand–Schüller–Christian disease is similar to that of eosinophilic granuloma.

Histologically

Microscopically the lesion is composed mainly of granulation tissue, histiocytes, eosinophils and foam cells. The presence of foam cells is diagnostic for this disease.

Treatment

No effective treatment.

Prognosis

The prognosis of this disease is bad.

Letterer-Swie Disease

Letterer–Swie's disease represents the most dangerous form of Langerhans cell histiocytes.

Clinically

- This lesion is common in infants below 2 years of age. It is a multiple disease affecting many bones.
- Hepatomegally, splenomegally, enlargement of lymph nodes, anemia and thrombocytopenia are common clinical signs of this disease. The patient might complain of erythematous skin rashes.

Histologically

The lesion appears microscopically as granulation tissue with histiocytes replacing the normal tissues.

Prognosis

The prognosis of this disease is bad, it is usually fatal.

17.6 Hormonal bone diseases

17.6.1 Hyperparathyroidism

(Von-Recklinghausen's disease of bone, Osteitis fibrosa cystica)

Is the over secretion of parathromone (parathyroid hormone).

Types

1. Primary: Which is due to adenoma or hyperplasia of the gland.
2. Secondary: Which is due to renal failure.
3. Rarely, occurs as a part of some inherited syndromes, e.g. multiple endocrine neoplasia type 1 or type 2a, or hyperparathyroidism–jaw tumor syndrome. In the latter condition, affected patients develop multiple jaw lesions that histopathologically are consistent with central ossifying fibroma with increase risk of developing parathyroid carcinoma.

Action of parathormone

The action of parathormone is to elevate calcium level of the blood through:

1. Activation of osteoclastic activity.
2. Decrease phosphate reabsorption in the kidney.
3. Increase calcium reabosrption in the kidney.

Blood Chemistry

- Serum calcium level is increased.
- Serum phosphorus level is decreased.

- Alkaline phosphatase is increased.
- Urinary output of calcium is increased.

Clinically

- Sudden cardiac arrest might occur due to hypercalcemia.
- Renal failure due to multiple renal stones.
- Hypertension and heart failure due to renal failure.
- Pain in the back and extremities.
- pathological fracture of bones.

Pathogenesis

Generalized resorption of bone and replacement by new bone poorer in calcium. Sometimes, a failure of bone formation occurs instead, granulation tissue with multinucleated giant cells is formed. This granulation tissue appears radiographically as radiolucent masses and hence the term *osteitis fibrosa cystica* was given.

X- Ray

1. Generalized osteoporosis with ground glass appearance best seen in the jaw because teeth are used as a marker.
2. Loss of lamina dura.
3. Sometimes areas of complete radiolucency appear and are termed *osteitis fibrosa cystica*. At the time of the operation, these areas appear brown due to excess hemosiderin pigments and are termed *brown nodes of hyperparathyroidism*.

Histologically

- The bone marrow is replaced by granulation tissue.
- Brown nodes are similar to any giant cell lesion and consist of spindle shaped cells with many multinucleated giant cells and areas of hemorrhage.

Treatment

- Primary hyperparathyroidism, the treatment is partial or total parathyroidectomy.
- Secondary hyperparathyroidism, the treatment is kidney transplant.

17.7 Deficiency Diseases

17.7.1 Rickets

Is a deficiency disease that occurs between 6 months and 2 years and the changes persist throughout life.

Etiology

Deficiency of calcium, phosphorus or vitamin D. Other rare cause of rickets is the excess fluorides in drinking water. The excess fluorides can interfere with the proper formation of bone and teeth

Blood Chemistry

Low phosphorus level, low calcium level and elevated serum alkaline phosphatase.

Clinically

Rickets is characterized clinically by deformity of long bones, delayed closure of fontanels, thin and flat cranial bones (*craniotabes*), delayed eruption of teeth, enamel and dentin hypocalcification and open bite.

Histologically

Osteoblasts continue to lay down excess soft bone matrix with deficient calcification.

Treatment

- Adequate diet rich in calcium and phosphorus such as milk.
- Calcium, Phosphorus and vitamin D supplementation.

17.7.2 Osteomalacia

Is the adult form of rickets and occurs usually in women associated with pregnancy and lactation due to increased demand for calcium.

Blood Chemistry

Low Phosphorus level, low calcium level and elevated serum alkaline phosphatase.

Clinically

Osteomalacia is characterized clinically by Deformity of legs and pelvis, deformity of vertebral column leading to pain due to compression of the spinal nerves. The jaws are rarely affected, however cases have been described in which increased mobility of teeth occurring during pregnancy were noticed in the absence of any inflammatory gingivitis or periodontitis. Such mobility may be attributed to the softness of the alveolar bones supporting the teeth due to marginal deficiency of calcium associated with pregnancy.

Treatment

As in the cases of rickets.

17.8 Metabolic Bone Diseases

17.8.1 Osteoporosis

Definition

Is defined as low bone mass with a normal ratio of mineral to osteoid (the organic matrix of bone). Bone mass increases until approximately age 30 and then gradually declines. Both men and women experience an age-related decline in bone mass density (BMD) starting in midlife. Women experience more rapid bone loss in the early years following menopause. Diagrammatic representation of osteoporosis is illustrated in figure ((17.3))

Classification

Osteoporosis can be classified into primary and secondary:

1- Primary Osteoporosis

- Primary osteoporosis is the most common metabolic disorder of the skeleton.
- Can be classified into type 1, or postmenopausal osteoporosis, and type 2, or senile osteoporosis.
- However, recent studies have suggested that estrogen deficiency is important for the pathogenesis of both types of osteoporosis and in both men and women.
- Primary osteoporosis can occur in both genders at all ages but often follows menopause in women and occurs later in life in men.
- Primary osteoporosis is often called the "*silent disease*" because bone loss occurs without symptoms. People may not know that they have osteoporosis until their bones become so weak that a sudden pathological bone fracture occurs.
- The loss of bone mass and strength can be contributed to:
    1. Failure to reach an optimal peak bone mass as a young adult.
    2. Excessive resorption of bone after peak mass has been achieved.
    3. Decreased bone formation during remodeling.
- The rate of bone formation is inadequate to replace the bone lost by resorption. This could be because of a defect in osteoblast function. The defect in osteoblast function could be the consequence of cellular senescence, or a decrease in the synthesis or activity of systemic and local growth factors.

2- Secondary Osteoporosis

- Secondary osteoporosis occurs as a result of prolonged corticosteroid therapy, hypogonadism, and immobilization (prolonged recumbency).

Osteoporosis and alveolar bone loss

Chapter 17. Bone Diseases

- It has been confirmed that there is decreased thickness of the mandibular alveolar process in the first premolar region.
- Studies have also shown that age-related bone loss is greater in women than men after the age of 50 years.
- These findings may possibly explain the findings in several surveys of dental health that women tend to lose their teeth earlier.

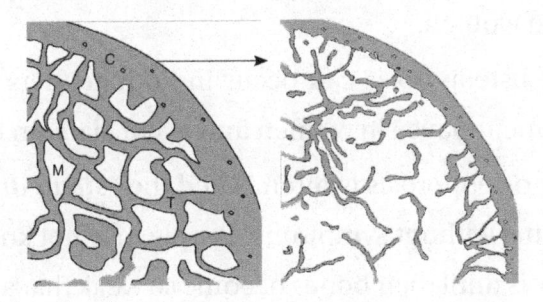

Figure 17.3: Diagrammatic representation of osteoporosis. Left panel represents normal bone structure while the right panel represents the osteoporotic bone with thin bone trabeculae (T), cortex (C) and wide marrow spaces (M).

Chapter 18
INFECTIONS OF THE ORAL AND PARA-ORAL TISSUES

Infections of the oral cavity are common. They might be caused by viruses, bacterial or fungi.

18.1 Classification of infectious agents

1. Metazoa
   - Multicellular organisms, complex life cycle, multiple hosts.
   - Classified initially according to external morphology e.g.:
     (a) Tapeworms (Cestodes) (platyhelminths)
     (b) Roundworms (nematodes)
     (c) Flatworms (*trematodes*) (Flukes): e.g. *Schistosoma* (the agent of bilharziasis) and *Fasciola hepatica* (the agent of liver fluke).

2. Protozoa
   - Single cell eukaryotes (i.e. nuclear is enclosed within a nuclear membrane)
   - Classification according to methods of locomotion and reproduction:
     (a) Flagellates: Trichomonas, Gardia, Leishmania, Trepansoma.
     (b) Amoeba: e.g. Entamoeba.

(c) **Sporozoa:** (have cycles of sexual and asexual reproduction): e.g. Plasmodium malaria, Toxoplasma, Cryptospora, Isospora, Coccidia and Babesia.

(d) **Unclassified:** e.g. Pneumocystis *Jiroveci* (the agent causing *Pneumocystis Carinii* pneumonia now termed *Pneumocystis Jiroveci* pneumonia), currently classified as yeast-like fungus.

3. Fungi
   - Eukaryotes, rigid continuous cell walls.
   - Classified morphologically into:

     (a) **Moulds:** Multicellular, filamentous, spore forming, grow in the form of branching tubules called hyphae (mycelia). Hyphae are further classified into septate and non-septate and branch under varying angles. These morphologic features are essential for the microscopic diagnosis of fungal organisms.

     (b) **Yeasts:** Unicellular, rounded or oval, reproduce by binary fission or budding. As an example of yeasts are *Candida albicans*. Budding in *Candida Albicans* can form chains termed as pseudohyphae. Pseudohyphae are yeast cells with a bud that remain attached to the parent cell, then elongate and bud again. Pseudohyphae which are a hallmark of *C. albicans*, resemble true hyphae, but a slight constriction remains where each but begins.

     (c) **Dimorphic:** Unicellular or multicellular, grow as moulds or yeasts, depending upon the cultural condition. In tissues, in exudates and in medium incubated at 37 °C, dimorphic fungi appear as yeasts. In culture media incubated at 25 °C, dimorphic fungi appear as moulds. Conversion to the yeast form appears to be essential for the pathogenicity of dimorphic

fungi. Table (18.1) summarizes the morphologic classification of medically important fungi.

4. Bacteria
   - Unicellular prokaryotes (have no nuclear membrane). They lack mitochondria. Bacteria reproduce by binary fission.
   - Classification:
     (a) Filamentous bacteria (higher bacteria): e.g. Actinomyces, Mycobacteria, Corynebacteria and streptomyces.
     (b) True bacteria (Eubacteria): Are classified into:
         i. Cocci: e.g. *Streptococcus, Staphylococcus, Neisseria* and *Veillonella*; see classification of streptococci (table18.2).
         ii. Bacilli: Which is further classified into:
             A. Gram-positive spore forming bacilli e.g. *Clostridia*.
             B. Gram-positive non-spore forming bacilli e.g. *Lactobacilli* and *Listeria*.
             C. Gram-negative bacilli e.g. *Pseudomonas, Coliform bacilli* (*E. coli*), *Hemophilus, Brucella* and *bacteroids*.
     (c) Vibrios and spirilla: e.g. *Vibrio cholerae.*
     (d) Spirochaetes: Are classified into:
         i. *Borrelia*
         ii. *Treponema*
     (e) *Mycoplasma*: Which lack rigid cell wall.
     (f) *Rickettsiae* and *Chlamydia*: Which are strict intra-cellular parasites. *Rickettsia* species are transmitted by numerous types of arthropod, including chigger, ticks, fleas, and lice, and are associated with typhus.

5. Viruses

- Consist of DNA or RNA (never both) and enclosed in a protein shell known as capsid. Sometimes the nucleocapsid may be enclosed in a lipoprotein envelope largely derived from the host.
- A simple classification of important viruses that are involved in human disease is shown in Table (18.3).

6. Prions
    - A tiny proteinaceous particle, having no genetic component
    - Thought to be the infectious agent in bovine spongiform encephalopathy (BSE "mad cow syndrome"). The human equivalent disease is Creutzfeldt-Jakob disease, and similar encephalopathies.

Table 18.1: Morphologic Classification of Medically Important Fungi

Medically Important Fungi

Filamentous fungi (moulds)	Zygomycetes
	Dermatophytes (caustive of all types of tinea except tinea versicolor)
	Malassezia furfur (caustive of tinea versicolor)
	Aspergillus species
Yeasts	Candida species
	Cryptococcus neoformans
Dimorphic fungi	Histoplasma capsulatum
	Blastomyces dermatitides
	Coccidiodes imitis
	Paracoccidiodes brasiliensis

Table 18.2: Classification of Streptococci

> **Always Remember**
>
> 1. Classification according to culture characteristics
>   (a) α hemolytic: Produces a narrow zone of partial hemolysis and green discoloration around the colony e.g. streptococcus viridans associated with dental caries and endocarditis
>   (b) β hemolytic: Produces a wide clear translucent zone of complete hemolysis around the colony e.g. streptococcus pyogenes
>   (c) γ hemolytic (non-hemolytic): are usually not pathogenic
> 2. Classification according to serology (Lancefield classification):
>   A serologic classification dividing hemolytic streptococci into groups (A to O) depending upon group-specific substances in the cell wall, that are carbohydrate in nature; not all are equally important as human pathogens
>   (a) Group A: Includes the important human pathogen streptococcus pyogenes
>   (b) Group B: Contains one species, streptococcus agalactiae associated with a variety of human infections, especially those of the urogenital tract
>   (c) Group C: Pathogenic in animals
>   (d) Group D: Includes the enterococci (streptococcus faecalis)

18.2 Bacterial Infections

Bacterial infections of the oral and para-oral cavity are numerous and it is not possible to mention them all in this chapter; only the more clinically important infections are to be mentioned herein.

18.2.1 Acute Necrotizing Ulcerative Gingivitis, ANUG

Definition

- This is an acute necrotizing inflammation of the marginal gingiva and interdental papilla.
- ANUG is a part of what is known as necrotizing oral diseases which include: Necrotizing ulcerative gingivitis, Necrotizing ulcerative periodontitis, Vincent angina and necrotizing stomatitis (noma, maxillofacial gangrene).

Etiology

The etiology is multifactorial, 2 factors play a role:

- The causative organisms: *fusispirochetal* infection, which consists of a Gram negative *fusiform bacilli* (*fusobacterium fusiforms, fusobacterium necrophorum*) and the spirochete *borellia vincenti*, (both fusiform bacilli and borellia vincenti are called Vincent organisms). Vincent organisms are members of the normal oral flora (oral commensal).
- Decreased tissue resistance due to:
    1. Local factors e.g. calculus, plaque or poor oral hygiene.
    2. Psychological or physiological stresses e.g. students during examinations or soldiers at wartime so the disease was termed trench mouth.
    3. Immunosuppression

Clinically

- Rarely there is mild general malaise or slight fever, however, when the disease progress, the fever becomes worse.

- Necrosis and ulceration of the marginal gingiva and interdental papilla. The ulcers are covered by grayish pseudomembrane which can be wiped off leaving a red bleeding surface. The interdental papillae are eroded giving the characteristic *crater* shaped appearance.
- The attached gingiva is normal or show redness and edema.
- There is bleeding and foul odor.
- No significant regional lymphadenopathy.
- Extension of infection may occur to produce Vincent angina or Noma.

Histologically

Non-specific, necrosis of surface epithelium and infiltration of the connective tissue with inflammatory cells.

Treatment

- Removal of the local irritating factors, plaque or calculus.
- Antibiotics: Metronidazol (Flagyl) 200 mg taken by mouth, after food 3 times a day for 3 days.

18.2.2 Vincent Angina

Vincent angina is the sever form of ANUG, usually occurring in immunocompromised patients. There is extension of infection to the throat with necrosis, edema and formation of pseudomembranes with regional lymphadenopathy. The disease responds well to metronidazol but shows poor response if penicillin is to be used alone.

18.2.3 Maxillofacial Gangrene (Noma, Cancrum Oris)

Overview

- Noma is an overwhelming severe necrotizing inflammation of the orofacial region.
- Was common among starving prisoners in Nazi concentration camps.
- Noma has disappeared from developed countries and for decades the disease has been ignored.
- However it becomes widespread again in sub-Saharan Africa as to become a subject for international and World Health Organization concern. This results from the widespread expansion of political unrest, poverty, malnutrition, poor oral hygiene and debilitating diseases as AIDS.

Clinically

- Noma starts within the oral cavity from an acute necrotizing ulcerative gingivitis associated with extensive edema, but extends outwards rapidly destroying soft tissues and bone.
- The gangrene starts as a painful, small reddish-purple spot or indurated papule which ulcerates. The ulcer spreads to involve the adjacent mucosa, skin and bone associated with diffuse edema of the face. As the overlying tissues become ischemic, the skin turns blue-black. The gangrenous area becomes sharply demarcated and ultimately sloughs away. As the slough separates, the bone dies with sequestration and exfoliation of teeth. A gaping facial defect is left.
- The disease is fatal if inadequately treated

Etiology

1. Causative organisms:
   - The main bacteria are anaerobes including Fusobacterium necrophorum and spirochaetes. Fusobacterium necrophorum is a commensal in the gut of herbivores and also a cause of necrotizing infections in animals.
   - It has been suggested that Fusobacterium necrophorum plays an important role in noma in Africa as a result of patients living in close proximity and often sharing drinking water with cattle.
2. Predisposing factors:

   Are usually severe malnutrition, poor oral hygiene, poor general hygiene, AIDS and debilitating diseases.

Treatment

- Correction of the predisposing factor, if possible
- A combination of penicillin or an aminoglycoside and metronidazole will usually control the local infection.
- Debridement of the necrotic tissues is also required.
- Reconstructive surgery is needed to correct the deformity.

18.2.4 Acute Streptococcal Gingivitis

Definition

Acute inflammation of the gingiva usually as a result of spread from acute streptococcal tonsillitis.

Etiology

Hemolytic streptococci, group A.

Clinically

- Malaise and fever.
- Redness, edema and bleeding of the gingival
- No ulceration or necrosis.
- Regional lymphadenopathy.

Treatment

Penicillin or erythromycin - Should be treated as soon as possible to avoid post-streptococcal complications (rheumatic fever and glomerulonephritis).

18.2.5 Pericoronitis

Introduction

- The term pericoronitis refers to inflammation of the gingiva in relation to the crown of a partially erupted tooth.
- It occurs most frequently in the mandibular third molar area. It may be acute subacute or chronic

Clinical Features

- The partially erupted or impacted mandibular third molar is the most common site of pericoronitis. The space between the crown of the tooth and overlying gingival flap is an ideal area for the accumulation of food debris and bacterial growth, see figure (18.1).

- In patients with no clinical signs or symptoms, the gingival flap is often chronically inflamed and infected, with various degrees of ulceration along its inner surface.
- Acute inflammatory involvement is a constant possibility. Acute pericoronitis is identified by various degrees of involvement of pericoronal flap and adjacent structures, as well as systemic complication. Edema and cellular exudates results in increase in the bulk of the flap which interferes with complete closer of mouth.
- The flap is traumatizes by contact with the opposing teeth, and the inflammatory involvement is aggravated. The clinical picture is that of markedly red, swollen, suppurating lesion that is tender, with radiating pains to ear, throat and floor of mouth.
- Pain, a foul taste and inability to close the jaw. Swelling of the cheek in the region of the angle of the jaw and lymphadenitis are common findings. The patient may also have toxic systemic complication such as fever, leukocytosis and malaise.
- Figure (18.1) illustrates the clinical appearance of pericoronitis.

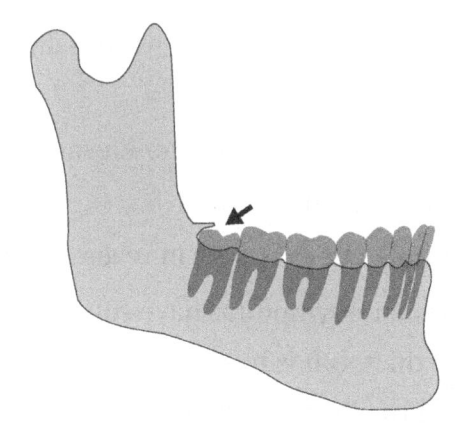

Figure 18.1: Diagrammatic representations of pericoronitis; note the operculum, which is the soft tissue that partially cover the third molar. Food debris will accumulate under the operculum initiating an inflammatory response.

Complications

- The involvement may become localized in the form of periodontal abscess. It may spread posteriorly into the oropharyngeal area & medially to the base of the tongue, making it difficult for the patient to swallow.
- Depending on severity and extent of the infection, there is involvement of the submaxillary, posterior cervical, deep cervical, and retropharyngeal lymph nodes.
- Peritonsillar abscess formation, cellulitis, and Ludwig's angina are infrequent potential sequelae of acute pericoronitis.

Treatment

- The treatment of pericoronitis depends on the severity of the inflammation and the decision of retaining the involved tooth. Persistent symptomless pericoronal flaps should be removed as a preventive measures against subsequent acute involvement.
- The treatment of acute pericoronitis is consist of
    1. Gently flushing the area with warm saline to remove debris & exudate.
    2. Swabbing with antiseptic after elevating the flap gently from the tooth with a scalar.
    3. Antibiotic can be prescribe in severe cases.
    4. After the acute symptoms have subsided, a decision is made as to whether the tooth is to be retained or extracted. This decision is governed by the possibility of further eruption into a good functional position.
- The following points may be considered to decide whether the tooth is to be retained or not.

1. stage of eruption of tooth. If a possibility that the tooth will erupt further into a good functional position, it is advisable to retain the tooth.
2. impacted 3rd molar. If the tooth is impacted, it is better to extract the tooth as soon as the acute symptoms have subsided.
3. position of tooth. Very often the tooth may be buccally placed with no attached gingiva on the buccal aspect. It may also be placed very much distally making it difficult to remove the gingival tissue adequately to create an environment which could be maintained plaque free.

- If it is decided to retain the tooth, the pericoronal flap is removed using periodontal knives.
- It is necessary to removed the tissues distal to the tooth as well as the flap on the occlusal surface.
- Incising only the occlusal portion of the flap leaves a deep distal pocket, which invites recurrence of acute pericoronal involvement. After the tissue is removed, a periodontal pack is applied.
- The pack may be retained by bringing it forward along the facial & lingual surface into the interproximal space between the second & third molar. The pack is removed after one week.

Conclusion

It is the most common type of pericoronal infection found mostly in mandibular third molar. Clinical features include red, swollen suppurating lesion along with the pain which may radiate to the surrounding tissues. Proper & immediate management is necessary to prevent its complication.

18.2.6 Periodontal Abscess

Definition

A periodontal abscess is a localized collection of pus in the periodontium communicating with the oral cavity through the gingival sulcus and/or other periodontal sites (and not arising from the tooth pulp).

Etiology

The abscess probably forms by occlusion or trauma to the orifice of a periodontal pocket, resulting in the extension of infection from the pocket into the supporting tissues. These events might result from impaction of food such as a fish bone, or of a detached toothbrush bristle, or compression of the pocket wall by orthodontic tooth movement or by unusual occlusal forces.

Normally the abscess remains localized in the periodontal tissues, and its subsequent development depends on:

- the virulence, type and number of the causative organisms
- the health of the patient's periodontal tissues
- the efficiency of the specific and non-specific defense mechanisms of the host.

Clinical features

1. Onset is sudden, with swelling, redness and tenderness of the gingiva overlying the abscess.
2. Pain is continuous or related to biting and can be elicited clinically by percussion of the affected tooth.
3. There are no specific radiographic features, although commonly associated with a deep periodontal pocket.

4. Pus from the lesion usually drains along the root surface to the orifice of the periodontal pocket; in deep pockets pus may extend through the alveolar bone to drain through a sinus which opens on to the attached gingiva.
5. Because of intermittent drainage of pus, infection tends to remain localized and extraoral swelling is uncommon.
6. Untreated abscesses may lead to severe destruction of periodontal tissues and tooth loss.

Microbiology

Endogenous, subgingival plaque bacteria are the source of the microorganisms in periodontal abscesses; infection is polymicrobial, with the following bacteria being commonly isolated:

- Anaerobic Gram-negative rods, especially the black pigmented *Porphyromonas* and *Prevotella* spp., and *fusobacteria*
- *Streptococci*, especially *haemolytic streptococci* and *anaerobic streptococci*
- Others, such as *spirochaetes, Capnocytophaga* spp. and *Actinomyces* spp.

Treatment

1. Make a thorough clinical assessment of the patient, including a history of systemic illnesses (e.g. diabetes).
2. If the prognosis is poor, owing to advanced periodontitis or recurrent infection, and it is unlikely that treatment will achieve functional periodontal tissues, then extract the tooth. If the abscess is small and localized, extraction may be carried out immediately; otherwise extraction should be postponed until acute infection has subsided.

3. Drainage should be encouraged and gentle subgingival scaling performed to remove calculus and foreign objects.
4. Irrigate the pocket with warm 0.9% sodium chloride solution and prescribe regular hot saline mouthwashes.
5. If pyrexia or cellulitis is present, antibiotics should be prescribed: penicillin, erythromycin or metronidazole are the drugs of choice.

18.2.7 Scarlet Fever

Definition

This is an acute pharyngitis accompanied by skin rash.

Etiology

- Hemolytic streptococci, Group A.
- Produces erythrogenic exotoxins that attacks the blood vessels and produces the characteristic skin rash.

Clinically

- Incubation period 2–3 days.
- Fever and malaise.
- The lesions are painful and consists of:
- Erythematous skin rash with the characteristic circumoral pallor, which is an area of pallor around the mouth corresponding to the anatomy of orbicularis oris muscle.
- Edema of the pharynx and oral mucosa
- The tongue shows a white coating through which only the fungiform papillae can be seen giving the characteristic *strawberry tongue*

18.2.8 Diphtheria

Acute necrotizing inflammation of the pharynx usually in children

Etiology

Corynebacterium diphtheria, which is *Gram-positive bacilli*. The organisms elaborate a potent exotoxin which causes severe systemic manifestations on the heart and nervous tissue.

Clinically

- High fever.
- Necrotic lesions in the pharynx covered by grayish white pseudomembrane which may extend to the mouth.

18.2.9 Anthrax

This is a disease caused by **bacillus anthracis** affecting usually herbivores (cattle and sheep). The disease is rare in man usually affecting farmers, veterinarians and butchers.

Etiology

Gram +ve *bacillus anthracis* - a soil organism.

Clinically

- Cutaneous lesions: necrotic lesions surrounded by edema and erythema.

- Mucous membrane lesions: necrotic lesions surrounded by edema and erythema.
- Pulmonary lesions: pneumonia, which is often fatal.

Treatment

Penicillin - Vaccination in high risk individuals.

18.2.10 Syphilis

Definition

A chronic specific granulomatous inflammation.

Etiology

The spirochete ***Treponema Pallidium***, could be detected by dark field illumination.

Types

Classified into:

1. Congenital (prenatal)
2. Acquired (postnatal)

This classification is misleading since the congenital syphilis is acquired during embryonic life.

Acquired syphilis, 3 stages

Primary stage

- Characterized by the formation of chancre.
- Occurs at the site of introduction of the *treponema pallidium.* In the oral cavity, the lips and tip of the tongue are the most extra-genital affected site.
- Appears as a painless nodule, which soon ulcerates forming an indurated ulcer.
- Regional lymphadenopathy, unilateral, rubbery and discrete.
- Highly contagious.
- The incubation period is 2–3 weeks.
- Heals with minimum scar formation after 2–3 weeks.
- Diagnosis is by smear from the chancre to detect the organisms by dark field illumination.
- Biopsy shows non-specific inflammation with perivascualr infiltration.

Secondary stage

- Characterized by the formation of mucous patches.
- Appears 6–8 weeks after disappearance of chancre.
- Appears as irregular painless ulcers covered by grayish pseudomembrane which when removed leaves a raw red surface. Neighboring ulcers coalesce producing the typical snail track appearance.
- The lesion is highly contagious.

Tertiary stage

- Appears 2–3 years later.

- Oral manifestations consists of:
    1. Gumma: Which may occur in the palate leading to perforated palate, or may occur in the tongue or bone.
    2. Diffuse syphilitic glossitis: which is multiple gumma occurring in the tongue producing multiple ulcers and fibrosis accompanied by endarteritis obliterans resulting in atrophy of the tongue papillae giving the characteristic bold tongue appearance which may be followed by leukoplakia and malignancy.
    3. Diffuse syphilitic osteitis: See bone diseases.

Congenital syphilis

Oral manifestations are:

1. Hutchinson's teeth which is a part of Hutchinson's triads (interstitial keratitis, 8th cranial nerve involvement resulting in deafness and Hutchinson's incisors)
2. Moon's molar
3. Mulberry molar
4. Enamel hypoplasia
5. Rhagedes: which are linear fissures or scars radiating from mouth corners.
6. Perforated palate.

18.2.11 Leprosy (Hansen's disease)

Definition

A chronic specific granulomatous inflammation of low infectivity caused by the acid-fast *Mycobacterium Leprae*. Leprosy is only moderately contagious;

transmission of the disease requires frequent direct contact with an infected individual for a long period.

Route of infection

1. By inhalation of droplet infection
2. Through intact skin by direct contact

When infection develops in the skin, the initial lesion is the indeterminate macule. Thereafter two major clinical forms may develop:

A. Lepromatous leprosy

- This occurs in patients with low cell-mediated immunity to the organism and produces widespread infection.
    1. Skin involvement
        - Papules
        - Nodules covered by greasy skin
        - Diffuse thickening, e.g. leonine facies
        - Loss of hair
        - On histology the skin shows
            - Dermal granulomata rich in histiocytes
            - *Mycobacterium leprae* in large numbers within histiocytes. These can be best demonstrated using the Ziehl-Neelsen method without acid differentiation.
    2. Nerve involvement
        - Edema and ischemic necrosis
        - Progressive fibrosis
        - Peripheral neuritis which is symmetrical

Chapter 18. Infections of the Oral and Para-Oral Tissues

- ★ Anesthesia may lead to neuropathic arthropathy (Charcot's joints) and trophic ulcers

3. Mucous membranes
   - ★ Nasal blockage and epistaxis
   - ★ Ulceration of the nasal septum
   - ★ Ulceration and stenosis of the larynx

4. Eyes
   - ★ Keratitis
   - ★ Iritis
   - ★ Corneal ulceration

5. Testes
   - ★ Testicular atrophy leading to sterility and gynecomastia

6. Death may result from
   - ★ Respiratory infection; pneumonia, tuberculosis
   - ★ Septicemia from chronic osteomyelitis following infection of bone marrow
   - ★ Renal failure due to chronic glomerulonephritis or amyloidosis

- **Oral manifestations**

Multiple non-caseating granulomas are present in the connective tissue. Ziehl–Neelsen staining shows acid-fast lepra bacilli.

B. Tuberculoid leprosy

- This develops when there is a high cell-mediated immunity and the infection is limited to skin and nerves and the lesions contain very few organisms.

    1. Skin lesions

Scattered hypopigmented, anesthetic areas showing anhidrosis

2. Nerve involvement

  - ★ Destruction by granulomata
  - ★ Repair by fibrosis with consequent thickening
  - ★ Anesthesia, muscle wasting
  - ★ On histology these lesions show:
    - * A mass of lymphocytes and epithelioid cells
    - * Langhans-type giant cells
    - * Very few organisms
    - * Skin involvement extending through the dermis and epidermis
    - * Caseous necrosis, sometimes within nerve lesions
    - * Many of these features resemble those found in tuberculosis.

- **Oral manifestations**

  Nodules can form in the tongue or lips which usually ulcerate.

- **Treatment**

  Multi-drug therapy, dapsone, rifampin and minocycline

18.2.12 Tuberculosis of the Oral Cavity

Definition

- A chronic specific granulomatous disease characterized by caseation.
- The incidence of tuberculosis is increasing and multiple drug-resistant strains are becoming widespread.

Etiology

- *Mycobacterium tuberculosis*
- *Mycobacterium bovis*

Clinically

- Tuberculosis of the oral cavity is rare. This may be attributed to the protective effect of saliva or due to the natural resistance of the oral tissues.
- Tuberculosis of the oral cavity occurs usually secondary to pulmonary tuberculosis. Figure (18.2) illustrates the natural history of tuberculosis in man.
- Tuberculosis of the oral cavity occurs in the oral mucosa or the jaw bones. Tuberculous lymphadenitis may also affect submandibular or cervical lymph nodes.

1. **Tuberculosis of the oral mucosa:**
   - The most common site is the lip and the tip of tongue.
   - The lesion consists of granulating ulcers, which are punched out.

2. **Tuberculous lymphadenitis (Scrofula):**
   - May be presented to the dentist and he should be aware of its features and management.
   - May appear as one or two large nodes, indurated and fixed with a suspicion of fluctuation due to necrosis. Others will present as several smaller, firm nodes that are freely movable.
   - Best line of treatment is excision with anti-tuberculous drugs for at least 9 months.
   - For details, see table (18.4).

3. **Tuberculous osteomyelitis of the jaws:**

- Tuberculosis of bone is usually secondary to pulmonary TB.
- It is common in the vertebrae (Pott's disease) and rare in the jaws.

Clinically

- Pain is not a feature.
- There is a swelling, which is first firm, then softens and discharge pus.

Histopathology

The lesion consists of multiple tubercles each consists of:

1. Central area of caseous necrosis.
2. Surrounded by granulation tissue containing epithelioid cells, Langhans giant cells and chronic inflammatory cells.
3. In bone, the lesion is osteolytic. There is bone resorption and replacement by multiple tubercles.

Treatment

- Incision and drainage is best avoided
- Anti-tuberculous drugs
- In bone, removal of sequestra when formed

18.2.13 Actinomycosis

A type of chronic specific granulomatous infection, which usually occurs at the soft tissues at the angle of the mandible. Involvement of other soft tissues exists, although is uncommon.

Chapter 18. Infections of the Oral and Para-Oral Tissues

Etiology

The causative organisms are usually *actinomyces bovis* and / or *actinomyces Israeli*. These organisms were considered to be fungi because of their filamentous nature and hence named "*ray fungus*" but now classed as bacteria. The organisms are anaerobic Gram positive filaments. They are members of the normal oral flora. Infection only occurs when there is an abrasion, wound or extraction socket. Decreased body resistance is the most predisposing factor for the infection.

Histologically

Multiple granulomas each consists of:

1. The organisms in the center. The organisms consists of hyphae which are hematoxyphilic and Gram positive situated in the center and club shaped terminations which are eosinophilic and Gram negative being situated at the periphery.
2. Surrounded by granulation tissue containing chronic inflammatory cells with macrophages and occasionally multinucleated giant cells.
3. Fibrosis at the periphery.

Clinically

Two types of actinomycosis can be distinguished:

1. **Peripheral actinomycosis:**
    (a) Cervicofacial, the most common site is in the soft tissues at the angle of the mandible (lumpy jaw).
    (b) Tongue.
    (c) Palate.

In the peripheral type there is a diffuse firm swelling which becomes nodulated them soften and discharge pus through multiple sinuses.

This pus contains sulfur granules, which are the colonies of the microorganisms. Lymph nodes are enlarged only when there is secondary infection.

2. **Central actinomycosis:**
   - This is a very rare type of actinomycosis. The mandible is affected more than maxilla.
   - In the central type the lesion runs a chronic course with multiple sinuses discharging pus. Appears in X-ray as a radiolucent area.

Diagnosis

Any inflammatory swelling persists for more than 6 weeks or more without evidence of dental pathology or osteomyelitis should arouse suspicion of actinomycosis. Culture should be taken by incising a non- ruptured nodule to avoid secondary infection, which destroys sulfur granules.

Treatment

- Sensitivity test and giving the most appropriate antibiotic, which is usually penicillin
- Penicillin should be continued for 4–6 weeks or sometimes longer as surviving organisms may persist in the depth of the lesions to cause relapse.
- Abscesses should be drained surgically as they form.

18.2.14 Orofacial Granulomatosis

Overview

- Orofacial granulomatosis comprises a group of lesions characterized by orofacial swellings associated with non-caseating and non-infective granulomas.
- Although there in no convincing evidence that these lesions are infective diseases and their exact etiology is still unknown, they are mentioned herein for their relevance to the subject of granulomatous infections.
- These diseases may respond to systemic or intralesional injections of corticosteroids.
- The term orofacial granulomatosis should not be confused with midfacial granulomas (midline lethal granuloma) which are lethal diseases.
- These lesions include:
    1. Cheilitis granulomatosa
    2. Melkersson Rosenthal syndrome
    3. Sarcoidosis
    4. Oral lesions of Crohn's disease

18.2.15 Sarcoidosis

Definition

A multi-system granulomatous disease of unknown etiology which can affect lungs, eye, spleen, kidney, lymph nodes, skeleton or nervous tissues

Etiology

Unknown, the following causes were postulated:

1. Unidentified infectious agent
2. Autoimmunity
3. Allergy
4. Genetic factors

Oral manifestations

1. Salivary glands enlargement, particularly causing parotid swelling
2. Intraoral submucosal nodules
3. Submandibular lymph node enlargement
4. Heerfordt's syndrome which includes (uveoparotid fever):
   (a) Uveal tract inflammation
   (b) Lacrimal gland enlargement
   (c) Parotid enlargement
   (d) Facial palsy
   (e) Fever

Laboratory findings

1. Immunological:
   (a) Positive to Kveim antigen (Kveim test is an intradermal test for sarcoidosis in which an antigen prepared from the lymph nodes or spleen of human sarcoidosis patients is injected intracutaneously. The test is positive when an infiltrated area, papule, nodule, or superficial necrosis appears around the site of injection. If the pa-

tient has been on treatment (e.g. glucocorticoids), the test may be false negative.

    (b) Skin biopsy yields typical tubercles and giant cell formations upon histological examination.

    (c) Anergy (negative test) to tuberculin.

    (d) Raised serum immunoglobulin, rheumatoid factor and antinuclear antibody.

2. Biochemical: Hypercalcemia due to increased sensitivity to vitamin D
3. Anemia, leucopenia, eosinophilia and raised ESR

Histopathology

Non-caseating granuloma consists of:

- Multinucleated giant cells (Langhans cells), epithelioid cells and lymphocytes
- Presence of *astroid bodies* which are eosinophilic star shaped cytoplasmic inclusions seen within the cytoplasm of multinucleated giant cell (also present in tuberculoid leprosy).
- Presence of *Schaumann bodies* (conchoidal[1] bodies) which are concentric lamellated calcified bodies seen within the cytoplasm of multinucleated cells. See figure.
- No central caseation
- While this picture is frequently seen, these findings are not specific to sarcoidosis.

[1] Shaped like a shell; having alternate convexities and concavities on the surface.

18.2.16 Crohn's Disease (Regional ileitis)

Definition

A granulomatous disease affecting any part of the gastrointestinal tract from the mouth to the anus but typically affects the ileum. The disease is characterized by diarrhea, cramping, loss of appetite and weight with local abscesses and scarring.

Etiology

Unknown, the following causes were postulated:

1. Autoimmunity
2. Infective etiology due to Escherichia coli or viruses.

Oral manifestations

1. Recurrent aphthous ulcers
2. Diffuse swellings of lips, cheek or gingiva
3. Cobblestone swellings of the oral mucosa with fissuring and hyperplastic growths
4. Mucosal tags

Treatment

- Oral lesions may resolve when intestinal Crohn's disease is controlled with corticosteroids or sulfasalazine
- Alternatively, oral lesions may respond to oral sulfasalazine or to intralesional injections of corticosteroids

18.3 Mycotic (Fungal) Infections

18.3.1 Moniliasis (Candidiasis)

Definition

- This is a fungal infection of the oral mucosa.
- Oral candidiasis and oral candidosis are synonyms.

Etiology

- The causative fungus is *candida albicans* which is a yeast fungus.
- It is one of the normal oral flora. Candida species are opportunistic pathogens, which may cause disease mostly when there are changes in oral ecology or when the host defenses have been compromised, hence the epithet "candidosis is the disease of the diseased".
- The predisposing factors may be local or systemic:
  - ⋆ Local predisposing factors:
    - ∗ Loss of integrity of the oral mucosa as in thin or ulcerated epithelium, resulting from an ill-fitting denture, or after anticancer chemotherapy or head and neck radiotherapy, ect., allows for candida to adhere on the epithelial cells, penetrate the mucosa, and cause infection.
    - ∗ Heavy smoking, leukoplakia and other oral mucosal diseases make oral mucosa prone to the development of candidal infections.
    - ∗ Xerostomia result in decreased flushing action and in reduced antifungal components of saliva, thus enhancing the development of candidosis.

- Topical corticosteroids, via local immunosuppression, also promote oral candidosis.
- Excessive moisture, particularly at mouth corners.
★ Systemic predisposing factors:
  - Immunodeficiency and immunosuppression are important host factors, especially in view of the increasing numbers of patients with acquired immune deficiency syndrome/AIDS and of individuals who receive immunosuppressive or cytotoxic treatment (organ and bone marrow transplant recipients, patients with malignant disease, patients with autoimmune disorders).
  - Corticosteroid therapy due to immunosuppression.
  - Broad-spectrum antibiotics due to disruption of the local ecology.
  - Pregnancy.
  - Dietary factors, such as poor nutrition, iron and vitamin deficiencies as they can alter the integrity of the oral mucosa, promoting the development of candidosis.
  - Endocrine disorders, such as diabetes mellitus, hematologic dyscrasias, malignant diseases, age (neonatal, elderly) also enhance candidosis.

Clinical Spectrum (Classification)

Oral candidosis may present with a variety of clinical patterns or forms. Some patients may exhibit more than one clinical form of candidosis and in more than one oral site, thus presenting with multifocal candidosis. Oral candidosis is, in most cases, endogenous and most often remain superficial and localized in the oral mucosa. Regional extension and systemic or deep-seated candidosis may occur, but it is relatively rare. Although no satisfactory classification of candidiasis exists, the following classification can be considered (see also figure 18.3):

1. Acute candidiasis
   (a) Acute pseudomembranous candidiasis (Thrush)
   (b) Acute erythematous candidiasis (Acute antibiotic stomatitis)
   (c) Angular cheilitis (angular stomatitis, perleche) common to all types of oral candidosis
2. Chronic candidiasis
   (a) Chronic erythematous candidosis (denture stomatitis, denture sore mouth, chronic atrophic candidiasis)
   (b) Chronic hyperplastic candidosis (candidal leukoplakia)
   (c) Angular cheilitis (angular stomatitis, perleche) common to all types of oral candidosis
   (d) Median rhomboid glossitis (Central papillary atrophy)
   (e) Chronic mucocutaneous candidosis syndromes: 4 types:
       i. Localized form
       ii. Diffuse form (candidal granuloma)
       iii. Familial form (endocrine candidosis syndrome)
       iv. Thymoma associated (late onset mucocutaneous candidosis)

Acute Candidiasis

Acute pseudomembranous candidiasis (Thrush)

- Any part of the oral mucosa may be affected especially the tongue, palate and buccal mucosa, mucobuccal folds, oropharynx and tongue.
- The lesion appears as white creamy patches similar to milk curds that can be wiped off leaving a raw red bleeding surface. Pseudomembra-

nous candidosis is rarely painful, however, some cases complain of burning sensation.

- Extension of infection to the area of the oral commissures may occur and is known as angular stomatitis or perleche (see later).

Acute erythematous candidiasis

(Acute antibiotic stomatitis, antibiotic glossitis)

- Persistence of acute pseudomembranous candidiasis may eventually result in loss of the pseudomembrane with presentation a more generalized red lesion known as acute erythematous candidiasis. Remnants of the pseudomembrane may be noted in some areas. There are also multiple erosions and intense inflammation associated with burning sensation.
- This form of candidiasis was known as antibiotic stomatitis because of its association with broad-spectrum antibiotic treatment.
- Withdrawal of the antibiotic, if possible and institution of oral hygiene lead to improvement.

Chronic Candidiasis

Chronic candidiasis is the persistence of candidal infection, either due to:

- Persistence of the predisposing factors
- Or immune deficiency

Chronic erythematous candidiasis

(Denture stomatitis, denture sore mouth, chronic atrophic candidiasis)

- This form usually occurs in patients who wear complete upper dentures. There is a distinct predilection for the palatal mucosa as compared with the mandibular alveolar arch. Chronic low-grade trauma resulting from poor denture fit and failure to remove the denture at night may contribute to the development of this condition.
- Clinically, the lesion appears as a bright red, somewhat velvety surface with little keratinization.

Chronic hyperplastic candidiasis

(Candidal leukoplakia)

- A hyperplastic tissue response against chronic candidal infection.
- It occurs in adults with no apparent predisposition to infection by candida albicans and it is believed by some clinicians to represent a premalignant lesion.
- When occurring in the retro-commissural area, the lesion resembles speckled leukoplakia and in some classifications is known as candidal leukoplakia.
- Papillary Hyperplasia of the Palate is considered as a subtype of chronic hyperplastic candidiasis. These are individual nodules or papules measuring 2 to 3 mm in diameter on an erythematous background found usually under ill-fitting upper dentures. For further details see the chapter of "Benign Non-Odontogenic Tumors & Tumor-Like Lesions.
- Differential diagnosis of candidal leukoplakia and leukoplakia on the basis of clinical picture only is difficult. Differentiation between the two conditions should therefore depends on:
    1. Finding PAS positive hyphae in histological smears or in tissue sections.
    2. High candidal antibody titer in serum and saliva.

Angular cheilitis

(Perleche, Angular stomatitis)

- Angular stomatitis is typically caused by leakage of candida infected saliva at the angles of the mouth.
- It can be seen in infantile thrush, in denture wearers or in association with chronic hyperplastic candidiasis.
- Hence, angular cheilitis can associate other types of candidiasis and is a characteristic feature of candidal infection.
- The condition may occur in patients wearing denture with deep overbite resulting form loss of vertical dimensions of dentures.
- Saliva will accumulate in the skin folds at the oral commissures and is subsequently colonized by candidal yeasts associated sometimes with staphylococcus aureus.
- Clinically, the lesions are somewhat painful, fissured, eroded and encrusted.
- In acute pseudomembranous candidiasis, extension of infection may occur to the area of the oral commissures.
- Treatment of intra-oral candidal infection alone causes angular stomatitis to resolve. If there is co-infection with staphylococcus aureus, local application of topical antibiotics may be required.

Median rhomboid glossitis

(Central papillary atrophy)

- Median rhomboid glossitis is a developmental disturbance of the tongue which sometimes may be secondarily infected with candida albicans.
- Since median rhomboid glossitis is never seen in children, its developmental etiology is denied by some authors.

- The role of candida albicans as the primary etiology of the condition is still controversial because of the fixed site and shape of the lesion.
- Therefore, the etiology of median rhomboid glossitis remains speculative.

Chronic mucocutaneous candidiasis

- Chronic mucocutaneous candidiasis is a persistent candidal infection of the skin and mucous membranes secondary to defective immune response.
- Four forms have been recognized:
    1. Localized form: Persistent candidiasis of the oral mucosa, vaginal mucosa, nails and skin. This form begins early in life (first decade) as pseudomembranous candidiasis and is soon followed by nail and skin involvement. Lesions are resistant to treatment with only temporary remissions following the use of standard antifungal drugs.
    2. Diffuse form: Is similar to the localized form but there is diffuse and widespread involvement of the oral mucosa, vaginal mucosa, pharyngeal mucosa, skin and nails. This form was known as "candidal granuloma" because of the extensive disfiguring warty overgrowths on the skin. However, there is no granuloma formation microscopically, instead, there is extreme epithelial proliferation.
    3. Familial form (also termed familial chronic mucocutaneous syndrome, endocrine candidosis syndrome, candidosis endocrinopathy syndrome): A rare autosomal recessive disorder in which the cause and effect relationship between the candidosis and the endocrine deficiency is unknown. The condition is characterized by:

(a) Candidal infection which may precede the onset of the endocrine deficiency by as long as 15 years but occasionally the sequence is reversed.

(b) Hypothyroidism

(c) Hypoparathyroidism

(d) Diabetes mellitus

(e) Addison's disease (adrenal cortex insufficiency)

(f) Hypoplastic dental defects are frequently present

4. Thymoma associated (late onset mucocutaneous candidosis): This syndrome has a clear immunological basis, in that there is a persistent defect in the T-cell mediated immunity produced by a thymoma. The condition is characterized by:

(a) Candidal infection.

(b) Thymoma.

(c) Myasthenia gravis (a disease characterized by progressive weakness of voluntary muscles without atrophy or sensory disturbance and caused by an autoimmune attack on acetylcholine receptors at neuromuscular junctions).

(d) Red cell aplasia.

Histological Features

- Destruction of the surface epithelium and replacement by the pseudomembrane which consists of masses of monilial organisms, bacterial, desquamated epithelial cells and fibrin.
- Destruction of the epithelium may be due to the combined effects of toxins and enzymes (lipases and proteases) produced by the monilial organisms.

- Polymorph nuclear leukocyte aggregation and chronic inflammatory cell infiltration of the connective tissue.
- Pseudohyphae are best demonstrated using **PAS** or Grocott methenamine silver stains.
- Epithelial atrophy is a characteristic feature of chronic erythematous candidiasis.
- Epithelial hyperplasia is a characteristic feature of chronic hyperplastic candidiasis.

Treatment

- Correction of the predisposing factors, if possible.
- Mild cases, topical application of nystatin.
- Severe cases, ketoconazole 400 mg daily in a single dose by mouth.

18.3.2 Systemic Mycoses

The Systemic mycoses are that type of infection which involve deep viscera with wide dissemination. It is more common in immunocompromised patients. Clinically most of the systemic mycoses can cause oral lesions. Oral lesions are usually nodular granulomas with ulcerations which can be tumor-like in appearance. The most interesting systemic mycoses include histoplasmosis, blastomycosis, mucormycosis, coccidioidomycosis, paracoccidioidomycosis and cryptococcosis.

18.4 Parasitic Diseases

18.4.1 Leishmaniasis

Overview

- Leishmaniasis is a zoonotic[2] infection caused by the protozoa belonging to the genus *Leishmania*
- It is named for Leishman, who first described it in London in May 1903
- Leishmaniasis is transmitted by sandflies (Phlebotomus species), and, in the human host, *Leishmania* are intracellular parasites that infect the mononuclear phagocytes
- Many animals act as reservoir hosts, particularly dogs and rodents, hence leishmaniasis is a zoonosis
- The spectrum of human disease ranges from self-healing localized ulcers to widely disseminated progressive lesions of the skin, mucous membranes, and the entire reticuloendothelial system

Cutaneous Leishmaniasis (Oriental Sore)

- Most frequent on the extremities.
- Head and neck involvement does occur.
- Papules which undergo ulceration with crust formation (1–3 cm).
- Ulcers may heal completely, but usually leave permanent scars.
- Histologically, the lesion shows hyperplasia with or without hyperkeratosis and acanthosis. Rarely epithelial atrophy and ulcerations occur. The underlying connective tissue shows multiple non-caseating granulomas. The connective tissue contains a large number of lymphocytes,

---

[2]Zoonosis and as zoonotic diseases are infectious diseases caused by bacteria, viruses and parasites that spread between animals and humans.

histiocytes, plasma cells and eosinophils with occasional presence of multinucleated giant cells. The blood vessels are usually abundant and dilated, however, areas of necrosis is seen in some cases. Macrophages are typically loaded by the **amastigotes** known as **Leishman-Donovan** bodies which appear as a small 2–4 μm rounded or ovoid bodies within the cytoplasm. Some of the amastigotes could be seen free outside macrophages and in the epithelium. The amastigotes (also known as Leishman-Donovan) bodies are one of the phases of parasite. It may be difficult to detect parasites in older lesions.

- Treatment is with pentostam.
- Special stains for leishmaniasis: The leishmania organisms are typically intensely positive with Giemsa stain where they stain blue on paraffin embedded sections.
- Differential diagnosis of leishmaniasis histopathology: Histoplasmosis –The organisms are of a similar size to leishmania but stain readily with silver stains, show narrow-based budding, and a peri-organism halo.

Mucocutaneous Leishmaniasis (Espundia)

- Involves macrophages of the skin around the mucous membranes.
- The disease starts with a cutaneous lesion that enlarges to involve the mouth, nose, and soft palate leading to severe tissue destruction.
- Lesions are papules which ulcerate and often become secondary infected.
- Diagnosis is by biopsy which reveals granulomas with typical intracellular parasites inside macrophages best stained with Giemsa stain. For differential diagnosis of mucocutaneous leishmaniasis see table (18.5).
- **Treatment** with pentostam.

Visceral Leishmaniasis

- Also known as kala azar - is characterized by irregular bouts of fever, substantial weight loss, swelling of the spleen and liver, and anemia (occasionally serious).
- If left untreated, the fatality rate in developing countries can be as high as 100% within 2 years.

18.5 Viral diseases

18.5.1 Introduction

Viral Structure

- A virus (virion) consists of a nucleic acid core surrounded by a protein coat (capsid).
- Some viruses have an additional protective layer, the envelope.
- Viruses without an envelope are known as naked viruses.
    1. Nucleic acid core
        * Known as viral genome and contains either DNA or RNA.
        * Can exist as a single strand (as in the case of most RNA viruses, except reoviruses) or double strand (the case of most DNA viruses, except parvoviruses).
        * Most viruses have a linear genomes, with the exception of papovaviruses which have a circular genomes.
    2. Viral capsid
        (a) Functions:
            i. Protects the nucleic acid core.

　　　　ii. Responsible for viral adsorption and penetration of host cells throught interaction with host cell membrane receptors.

　(b) Composition:
　　　★ Viral capsids are composed of varying numbers of capsomeres each of which is made up of one or more polyppide chains known as protomeres.

3. Viral envelope
★ The envelope is derived from the host cell membrane and is acquired by the virus during the late stages of budding.
★ The envelope consists of a lipid bilayer (derived from host cell) and viral coded glycoproteins, which are inserted into the lipid bilayer and projects to the outer surface. Its serve two basic functions:
　* Promote interaction with nucleocapsid proteins essential for the final stages of viral assembly.
　* Mediate attachment to the host cell receptors essential for infectivity of the virus.

Table (18.6) summarizes the most important viral infections that can affect the oral mucosa

Table 18.6: Summary of Viral Infections of the Oral Mucosa

Viral Infections of the Oral Mucosa

Virus Type	Primary Infection	Reactivation
Herpes simplex	Primary herpetic gingivostomatitis	Herpes labialis, Recurrent intra-oral herpes
Herpes zoster	Chickenpox	Shingles
Epstein-Barr	Infectious Mononucleosis	Many: Burkitt's lymphoma, nasopharyngeal carcinoma, Oral hairy leukoplakia
Coxsackie group	Herpangina, Hand, foot and mouth disease	No Known disease
Human papilloma virus	Squamous cell papilloma, Verruca vulgaris, Condyloma accuminatum	Squamous cell papilloma, Verruca vulgaris, Condyloma accuminatum
Pox virus	Molluscum contagiosum	No known disease
Paramyxovirus	Mumps, measles	No known disease

18.5.2 Herpes Simplex I (Labialis)

There are 2 types of herpes simplex virus, the first one is called herpes simplex type I (herpes simplex libialis) which affects the upper part of the body and the second is called herpes simplex II (herpes simplex genitalis) which usually affects the lower part of the body. Herpes simplex infection occurs in two forms. The first form which occurs as a result of the primary attack by the virus and is known as primary herpetic gingivostomatitis, after which the virus remains latent in the sensory ganglia or epithelial cells waiting for the chance of decreased body resistance and then reactivates and produce the secondary attack known as recurrent herpes labialis which is the second form of the disease. Herpetic whitlow refers to viral infection of fingers.

Primary Herpetic Gingivostomatitis

Definition

This is the primary attack of *herpes simplex* virus.

Clinically

- Usually occurs in infants or young children.
- Fever and malaise. Then vesicles appear in the oral cavity. These vesicles rupture forming painful ulcers.
- The disease is self limiting and heals in 10–14 days.

Histologically

- Intraepithelial vesicles, which result from edema (hydropic degeneration) of epithelial cells.
- Nuclei of epithelial cells show viral inclusion bodies (Lipschutz bodies).
- Infiltration of the underlying connective tissue by PNL, lymphocytes and plasma cells.

Treatment

- Symptomatic and includes administration of antipyretic drugs and mild sedation at bedtime. The general supportive measures used in the management of oral viral infections are listed in table (18.7)
- Plenty of fluids and soft diet.
- Acyclovir 20 mg/kg body weight every 8 hours iv for 10 days. Is recommended only in immunocompromised patients.
- The efficiency of topical acyclovir ointments has not been proven.

- Newer concepts of using antiviral drugs even in normal none immuno-compromised patients have been advocated to decrease the viral load in the population.

Complications

Encephalitis and/or memingitis.

Table 18.7: Supportive Measures Used in Infections with Herpes Viruses.

> **Always Remember**
>
> 1. Adequate intake of fluids
> 2. Antipyretic medication (e.g. paracetamol)
> 3. Analgesics (e.g. paracetamol)
> 4. Topical agents for the prevention of plaque build-up (e.g. 0.2
> 5. The patient should be advised to avoid (if possible) contact with fingers, genitalia and eyes to prevent inoculation of these areas
>
> *Note*

Recurrent Herpetic Infection

- Usually called recurrent herpes labialis
- Although rare, recurrent intra-oral herpes may occur and usually affected hard palate or attached gingiva

Definition

This is the secondary attack by the herpes simplex virus. The disease is usually confined to the mucocutaneous junction of the lip and rarely occurs in the oral cavity.

Etiology

The predisposing factors for reactivation of the latent virus are usually influenza (so the disease is sometimes called cold sores), stresses or other diseases lowering the body resistance.

Predisposing Factors

- Upper respiratory tract infection
- Common cold
- Ultraviolet light over exposure
- Mechanical trauma
- Menstruation and pregnancy
- Stress and emotional upset
- Immunosuppression
- Genetic factors

Clinically

- Numbness or pain in the site of the subsequent eruptions.
- Followed by appearance of multiple small vesicles.
- Vesicles rupture forming painful ulcers covered by a crust.
- The disease is self limiting and disappears within 7–10 days.

Treatment

- Is recommended only in immunocompromised patients.
- Acyclovir 400 mg 4 times daily for 5 days given by mouth, otherwise no treatment is needed as the disease is self limiting.

- Newer concepts of using antiviral drugs even in normal none immunocompromised patients have been advocated to decrease the viral load in the population.

18.5.3 Varicella - Zoster Virus

The primary attack of the virus causes varicella (chicken pox) while the secondary attack causes herpes zoster infection.

Chicken Pox (Varicella)

- Occurs usually in childhood.
- Mild fever, followed by vesicles on the skin and / or rarely on oral mucosa which rupture forming ulcers.
- Treatment
    * Is indicated only in immunocompromised patients. Acyclovir at the dose of 20 mg/kg body weight (800 mg maximum), 4 times daily by mouth for 5 days.
    * Newer concepts of using antiviral drugs even in normal none immunocompromised patients have been advocated to decrease the viral load in the population.

Herpes Zoster Infection (Shingles)

- This is the secondary attack of *herpes zoster* virus.
- After the primary attack (chicken pox) the virus remains latent in the cells of the sensory ganglia. Decreased body resistance produces reactivation and migration of the virus to affect the skin and mucous membrane supplied by the affected nerve.

- When the mandibular or maxillary branches of the trigeminal nerve are affected, oral lesions may appear as a grouped vesicles which rupture forming painful ulcers occurring on the skin and oral mucosa supplied by the affected nerve.
- Treatment
    ⋆ Acyclovir 20 mg/kg body weight (800 mg maximum), 4 times daily by mouth for 7–10 days.
    ⋆ Newer concepts of using antiviral drugs even in normal none immunocompromised patients have been advocated to decrease the viral load in the population.

Ramsay-Hunt Syndrome

Definition

This is a special form of herpes zoster affecting the facial nerve via the geniculate ganglion.

Clinically

1. Predromal stage:
    - Headache, malaise and fever
    - Sometimes, pain localized to the ear or radiating to the jaws and neck
2. Herpetic oticus:
    - Vesicles on the tragus of the ear, on the external auditory canal or on the tympanic membrane
3. Oral manifestations:
    - Localized pain affecting the anterior two thirds of the tongue and soft palate

- Vesicles which soon rupture forming painful ulcers
- Facial palsy
- Loss of taste sensation
- Xerostomia in some cases
- Deafness on the affected side

Treatment

- Acyclovir 20 mg/kg body weight (800 mg maximum), 4 times daily by mouth for 7–10 days.
- Corticosteroid therapy may be used in addition to acyclovir. Prednisone, 60 mg/daily with gradually withdraw in 10 days.

18.5.4 Hand-Foot and Mouth Disease

Definition

Highly contagious disease caused by Coxsackie virus type A16 (belonging to the family of picornaviruses).

Clinically

- Fever and malaise.
- Appearance of vesicles, which rupture forming painful ulcers on the palms, soles and oral mucosa.
- The disease lasts only for few days (self limiting) and complications are rare.

Treatment

Symptomatic.

18.5.5 Herpangina

Definition

Highly contagious disease caused by Coxsackie virus type A10 (belonging to the family of picornaviruses).

Clinically

- Fever and malaise and sometimes headache, nausea and vomiting.
- Appearance of vesicles, which rupture forming painful ulcers. Ulcers characteristically affect the soft palate near the tonsils. The rarity of involvement of the anterior buccal mucosa or the gingiva helps differentiate herpangina from herpes simplex. Herpangina also differs from herpes simplex by its brief evolution, the lesions last only 2–4 days, while herpes lesions lasts 7–10 days.

Treatment

Symptomatic and complications are rare.

18.5.6 Measles (Rubeola)

Definition

- Rubeola is an infection produced by a virus in the family *Paramyxovirus*

- The virus is associated with significant lymphoid hyperplasia that often involves sites such as the lymph nodes, tonsils, adenoids, and Peyer's patches.

Clinical Features

- There are three stages of the infection, with each stage lasting 3 days and justifying the designation nine-day measles.
- The first 3 days are dominated by the three Cs: Coryza (runny nose), Cough (typically brassy and uncomfortable), and Conjunctivitis (red, watery, and photophobic eyes). Fever typically accompanies these symptoms. During this initial stage, the most distinctive oral manifestation, *Koplik's spots*, is seen.
- *Koplik's spots* are multiple areas of mucosal erythema on the buccal and labial mucosa, and less often on the soft palate; within these areas are numerous small, blue-white macules.
- These pathognomonic spots represent foci of epithelial necrosis and have been described as *"grains of salt"* on a red background.
- As the second stage begins, the fever continues, the Koplik's spots fade, and a maculopapular and erythematous rash begins. The face is involved first, with eventual downward spread to the trunk and extremities. Ultimately, a diffuse erythematous maculopapular eruption is formed, which tends to blanch on pressure.
- Abdominal pain secondary to lymphatic involvement is not rare.
- In the third stage, the fever ends. The rash begins to fade and demonstrates a similar downward progression with replacement by a brown pigmented staining. Ultimately, desquamation of the skin is noted in the areas previously affected by the rash.

Complications

- Otitis media, pneumonia, persistent bronchitis, and diarrhea. Acute appendicitis occasionally is seen secondary to vascular obstruction created by the swelling of Peyer's patches.
- Encephalitis develops in approximately 1 in 1000 cases, often resulting in death or permanent brain damage and mental retardation.
- Measles in immunocompromised patients can be serious, with a high risk of complications and death. Most of these patients exhibit either an atypical rash or no exanthem.

Oral Manifestations

- *Koplik's spots* are not the only oral manifestation that may be associated with measles.
- Candidiasis, necrotizing ulcerative gingivitis, and necrotizing stomatitis may occur if significant malnutrition also is present.
- Severe measles in early childhood can affect odontogenesis and result in pitted enamel hypoplasia of the developing permanent teeth. Enlargement of accessory lymphoid tissues such as the lingual and pharyngeal tonsils also may be noted.

Mode of Infection

- Droplet infection
- The incubation time is from 10–12 days
- Affected individuals are infectious from 2 days before becoming symptomatic until 4 days after appearance of the associated rash.

Histopathologic Features

- *Koplik's spots* represent areas of focal hyperparakeratosis in which the underlying epithelium exhibits spongiosis, intercellular edema, dyskeratosis, and epithelial syncytial giant cells.
- The number of nuclei within these giant cells ranges from three to more than 25.
- Close examination of the epithelial cells often reveals pink-staining inclusions in the nuclei or, less commonly, in the cytoplasm.
- Examination of hyperplastic lymphoid tissue during the prodromal stage of measles often reveals a similar alteration.
- In 1931, Warthin and Finkeldey, in two separate publications, reported an unusual finding in patients who had their tonsils removed within 1 to 5 days of the clinical appearance of measles. Within the hyperplastic lymphoid tissue, there were numerous multinucleated giant lymphocytes.
- These multinucleated cells subsequently have been termed **Warthin-Finkeldey** giant cells and were thought for a time to be specific for measles. Since that time, similar-appearing cells have been noted in a variety of lymphoproliferative conditions such as lymphoma, AIDS-related lymphoproliferative conditions.

Diagnosis

- The diagnosis of typical measles in an epidemic situation usually is based on the clinical features and history.
- Laboratory confirmation usually is established through a demonstration of rising serologic antibody titers.
- The antibodies appear within 1 to 3 days after the beginning of the exanthem and peak in about 3 to 4 weeks.

Treatment and Prognosis

- In healthy patients with measles, fluids and non-aspirin antipyretics are recommended for symptomatic relief.
- Immunocompromised patients also may be treated with ribavirin; however, immunoglobulin, interferon, and vitamin A also are being used.

Prevention

Vaccination with MMR (Mumps, Measles, Rubella Vaccine)

18.5.7   German Measles (Rubella)

Definition

- Rubella is a mild viral illness that is produced by a virus in the family Togavirus, genus Rubivirus.
- The greatest importance of this infection lies not in its effects on those who contract the acute illness, but in its capacity to induce birth defects in the developing fetus.

Clinical Features

- A large percentage of infections are asymptomatic; the frequency of symptoms is greater in adolescents and adults.
- Prodromal symptoms may be seen 1 to 5 days before the exanthem and include fever, headache, malaise, anorexia, myalgia, mild conjunctivitis, coryza, pharyngitis, cough, and lymphadenopathy.
- The lymphadenopathy may persist for weeks and is noted primarily in the suboccipital, postauricular, and cervical chains.

- The most common complication is arthritis, which increases in frequency with age and usually arises subsequent to the rash.
- The exanthematous rash is often the first sign of the infection and begins on the face and neck, with spread to the entire body within 1 to 3 days.
- The rash forms discrete pink macules, then papules, and finally fades with flaky desquamation.
- **Oral lesions**, known as **Forchheimer's sign**, have been reported to be present in about 20% of the cases. These consist of small, discrete, dark-red papules that develop on the soft palate and may extend onto the hard palate. This enanthem arises simultaneously with the rash, becoming evident in about 6 hours after the first symptoms and not lasting longer than 12 to 14 hours. Palatal petechiae also may occur.

Mode of Infection

- Droplet infection
- The incubation time is from 14 to 21 days
- Infected patients are contagious from 1 week before the exanthem to about 5 days after the development of the rash.
- Infants with a congenital infection may release virus for up to 1 year.

Diagnosis

- The diagnosis of rubella depends mainly on laboratory tests because the clinical presentation of the acquired infection is typically subclinical, mild, or nonspecific.
- Although viral culture is possible, serologic analysis is the mainstay of diagnosis.

Prevention

Vaccination with MMR (Mumps, Measles, Rubella Vaccine)

Treatment and Prognosis

- Rubella is mild, and therapy usually is not required.
- Non-aspirin antipyretics and antipruritics may be useful in patients with significant fever or symptomatic cutaneous involvement.
- Passive immunity may be provided by the administration of human rubella immunoglobulin.
- If immunoglobulin is given within a few days of exposure, it decreases the severity of the infection. This therapy typically is reserved for pregnant patients who decline abortion.

18.5.8 Infectious Mononucleosis

(Glandular Fever, Benign Lymphoadenosis)

Definition

- An acute febrile illness caused by the Epstein-Barr virus, a member of the Herpesviridae family.
- Infectious mononucleosis is the primary infection of EBV seen usually in children and young adults.
- The virus remains latent for years (possibly for life) in the B lymphocytes of infected individuals.

Pathogenesis

- The incubation period is 30–50 days.
- The mode of infection is by droplet infection (contaminated saliva).
- EBV receptors (CD21 molecule) are expressed on mature resting B lymphocytes and stratified squamous epithelium of the oropharynx and salivary glands.
- In the host, the virus invades and replicates within epithelial cells of salivary glands and nasopharynx and then invade B-lymphocytes which possesses receptors for the virus.

Clinically

- The infection is usually subclinical in children, but symptomatic in young adults.
- Fever and malaise with headache and sweating.
- Sore throat and pharyngitis which may be severe and accompanied by a grayish white membrane and gross tonsillar enlargement.
- Pinpoint petechiae in the palate.
- Cervical lymphadenopathy which may become generalized, often with splenic enlargement and tenderness.
- Mild hepatomegaly in some cases and clinical jaundice in 5–10 %.
- The illness can last several weeks.

Diagnosis

- Complete blood picture reveals atypical lymphocytes.
- Epstein-Barr virus-specific antibody test.

Complications

- Are rare but some are serious.
- Acute air way obstruction may occur as a result of the lymphoid enlargement and edema which usually respond well to corticosteroid therapy and rarely needs emergency tracheostomy.
- Splenic rupture is also rare.
- Neurological complications include meningitis and encephalitis.

Treatment

- Supportive treatment.
- Acyclovir therapy does reduce EBV shedding in acute infections and may be used in immunocompromised patients.

Other EBV-associated diseases, tumors and immunodeficiency

- EBV is associated with an increasing number of diseases, including malignant tumors some of which are listed in table (18.8).
- The role played by EBV in each of these in not entirely clear in all cases.
- Cellular immunodeficiency states lead to lack of control over the proliferate phase of EBV infection and a risk of development of lymphomas.
- In some situations as in African Burkitt's lymphoma, EBV infection at an early age associated with chronic immunosuppression due to endemic malaria proceeds to a highly aggressive tumor.

Table 18.8: Diseases Associated with EBV

EBV Associated Diseases

Disease	Cells Infected	Link
Infectious mononucleosis	B lymphocytes and nasopharyngeal epithelium	Causal; acute primary infection
Oral hairy leukoplakia	Differentiated epithelium along edge of the tongue	Causal; productive recurrence in immunocompromized host
Nasopharyngeal carcinoma	Undifferentiated nasopharyngeal epithelium	100% EBV-positive cells; cofactor(s) + genetic risk
Burkitt's lymphoma	Monoclonal B cell tumor	100% EBV-positive; immunocompromized by malaria
Hodgkin's lymphoma	Hodgkin and Reed-Sternberg cells	30–90% EBV-positive cells
T-cell lymphoma	T lymphocytes	30–90% EBV-positive cells

18.5.9 AIDS

Definition

AIDS is the acquired immunodeficiency syndrome.

In AIDS, there is severe $CD4^+$ lymphocyte depletion (less than 200 $CD4^+$ lymphocytes per μl of blood). The normal $CD4^+$ lymphocyte count is between about 550 and 1000 lymphocytes /μl blood.

Etiology

- The disease is caused by the retrovirus known as human immunodeficiency virus (HIV), which belong to the family of lentiviruses.

- HIV is a retrovirus that primarily infects components of the human immune system such as $CD4^+$ T cells, macrophages and dendritic cells. It directly and indirectly destroys $CD4^+$ T cells.
- Two types of HIV have been characterized: HIV-1 and HIV-2. HIV-1 is the virus that was originally discovered. It is more virulent, more infective, and is the cause of the majority of HIV infections globally.
- HIV-2 is of lower infectivity as compared to HIV-1. Being less prevalent than HIV-1 and is largely confined to West Africa.

Pathogenesis

The virus binds to the $CD4^+$ receptor on T lymphocytes and thus produces elimination of the entire population of $T4^+$ cells (helper T lymphocytes).

Transmission

1. Sexual
2. Parenteral
    (a) Blood transfusion
    (b) Shared needles in drug addicts
    (c) Accidental needle stick
3. From mother to fetus (vertical transmission)

Incubation Period

3–7 years

Clinically

1. An acute viral like illness in 50% of patients

2. Persistent generalized lymphadenopathy with mild illness
3. AIDS related complex consists of: Persistent fever, Weight loss, Diarrhea
4. Full blown AIDS: Appear after 5–7 years and consists of:
   - Opportunistic infections e.g. *pneumocystis carinii*[3] *pneumonia*
   - Multiple malignancies
   - Neurologic involvement:
     * Encephalopathy
     * Dementia

Diagnosis

- Most people infected with HIV develop specific antibodies (i.e. seroconvert) within three to twelve weeks of the initial infection.
- Detection of antibodies can be done by the routine test known as enzyme-linked immunosorbent assay (ELISA) or by Western blot test which is more accurate.
- Confirmation is done by detecting the virus particles by PCR.
- Diagnosis of primary HIV before seroconversion is done by PCR.
- Detection of the antibodies in the oral fluids is possible. The oral test uses a collector specially designed to obtain a sample of transudate through the oral mucosa. Oral fluid testing has been approved as a test that can be done by people at home. A positive oral test is confirmed by a blood test.
- HIV testing is an important means of controlling HIV infection by allowing infected individuals to be treated and as a result, their viral load and potential infectivity are decreased.

---

[3] *In the new classification the organism is termed pneumocystis jirovecii. The organism is a yeast-like fungus.*

Prevention

Pre-exposure

- Routine HIV screening is an important mean for controlling HIV Infection by allowing infected individuals to be identified and treated.
- Treating people with HIV whose CD4$^+$ count ≥ 350 cells / μL with antiretrovirals protects 96% of their partners from infection.
- Pre-exposure prophylaxis (PrEP) with a daily dose of the medications tenofovir, with or without emtricitabine, is effective in a number of groups including men who have sex with men, couples where one is HIV positive, and young heterosexuals in Africa.

Post-exposure

- A course of antiretrovirals administered within 48 to 72 hours after exposure to HIV-positive blood or genital secretions is referred to as post-exposure prophylaxis (PEP).
- The duration of treatment is usually four weeks and is frequently associated with adverse effects such as nausea, fatigue, emotional distress and headaches.
- The use of the single agent zidovudine reduces the risk of a HIV infection five-fold following a needle-stick injury.
- As of 2013, the prevention regimen recommended in the United States consists of three medications –tenofovir, emtricitabine and raltegravir –as this may reduce the risk further.

Vaccination

There is currently no effective HIV vaccine.

Prognosis

With full blown AIDS, the 5 year survival is 85%.

Oral Manifestation

- Moniliasis: in 70% of cases.
- Viral infections: *Herpes simplex, Herpes zoster.*
- Bacterial infections: gingivitis and periodontitis.
- Deep mycosis: *Histoplasmosis, Cryptococcosis.*
- Tumors: Kaposi's sarcoma, Non-Hodgkin's lymphoma.
- Hairy leukoplakia: Is a type of leukoplakia occurring in AIDS patients characterized by presence of a keratinous hair like projections from its surface and occurring at the lateral border of tongue.
- Miscellaneous: Multiple aphthous ulceration.

Chapter 18. Infections of the Oral and Para-Oral Tissues

Table 18.3: Principle Types of Virus Causing Human Disease

> Always Remember

Type of virus	Examples
RNA viruses:	
Orthomyxoviruses	Influenza A, B, C, viruses
Paramyxoviruses	Parainfluenza viruses
	Mumps virus
	Measels virus
	Newcastle disease virus
	Respiratory syncytial virus
Rhabdoviruses	Rabies virus
Arenaviruses	Lassa virus
Filoviruses	Ebola virus
Togaviruses	Rubella virus
Flaviviruses	Yellow fever virus
	Dengue virus
	Japanese encephalitis virus
Coronaviruses	OC42
Calciviruses	Hepatitis E virus
Picoranviruses	Poliovirus
	Coxsakie virus
	Hepatitis A virus
	Rhinoviruses
Retroviruses	HIV 1
	HIV 2
	Human T-lymphotropic virus
Reoviruses	Rotaviruses
DNA viruses:	
Poxviruses	Variola (smallpox), vaccinia
	Molluscum contagiosum virus
Herpesviruses	Herpes Simplex type 1 and 2
	Varicella-Zoster virus
	Cytomegealo virus
	Epstein-Barr virus
Adenoviruses	Many serotypes
Polyomaviruses	Papillomavirus
Hepadnaviruses	Hepatitis B virus
Parvoviruses	B19 virus

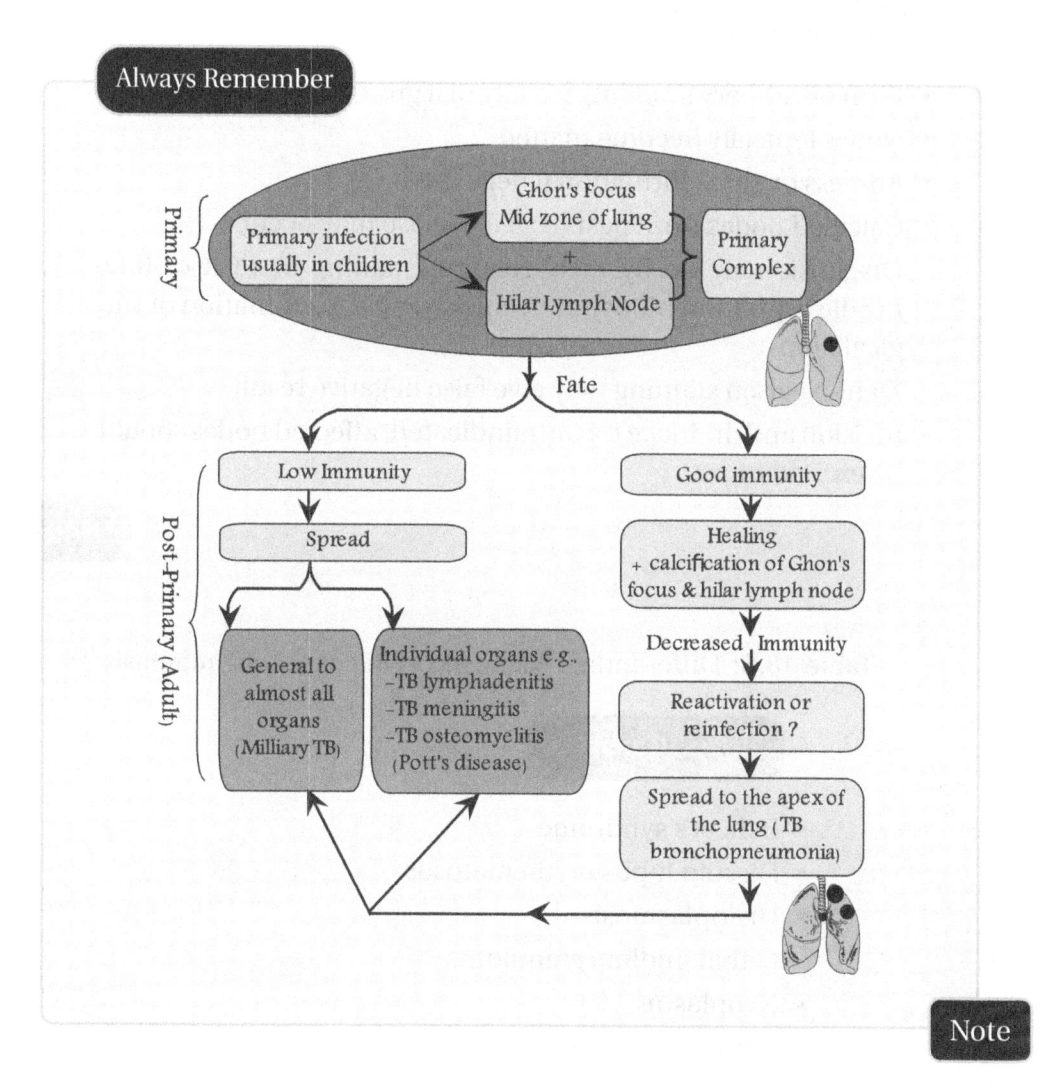

Figure 18.2: Natural History of TB. For intestinal tuberculosis resulting from mycobacterium bovis, the sequence of events is nearly the same but with the initial focus in the tonsils or in the gut associated lymphoid tissues.

Table 18.4: Clinical Features of Tuberculous Lymphadenitis

> **Always Remember**
>
> - Firm or rubbery swelling, usually of a group of nodes
> - Nodes typically become matted
> - Abscess or sinus formation if neglected
> - Calcified nodes from past healed disease may occur
> - Diagnosis may be by Ziehl-Neelsen staining or PCR of fine-needle aspiration biopsy or by microscopic examination of surgical biopsy
> - Ziehl-Neelsen staining may give false negative result
> - Incision and drainage is contraindicated, affected nodes should be excised intact
>
> *Note*

Table 18.5: Differential Diagnosis of Mucosal Leishmaniasis

> **Always Remember**
>
> - Behcet's syndrome
> - Discoid lupus erythematosus
> - Histoplasmosis
> - Lethal midline granuloma
> - Neoplasms
> - Paracoccidioidomycosis
> - Rhinoscleroma
> - Sarcoidosis
> - Syphilis
> - Tuberculosis
> - Wegener's granulomatosis
>
> *Note*

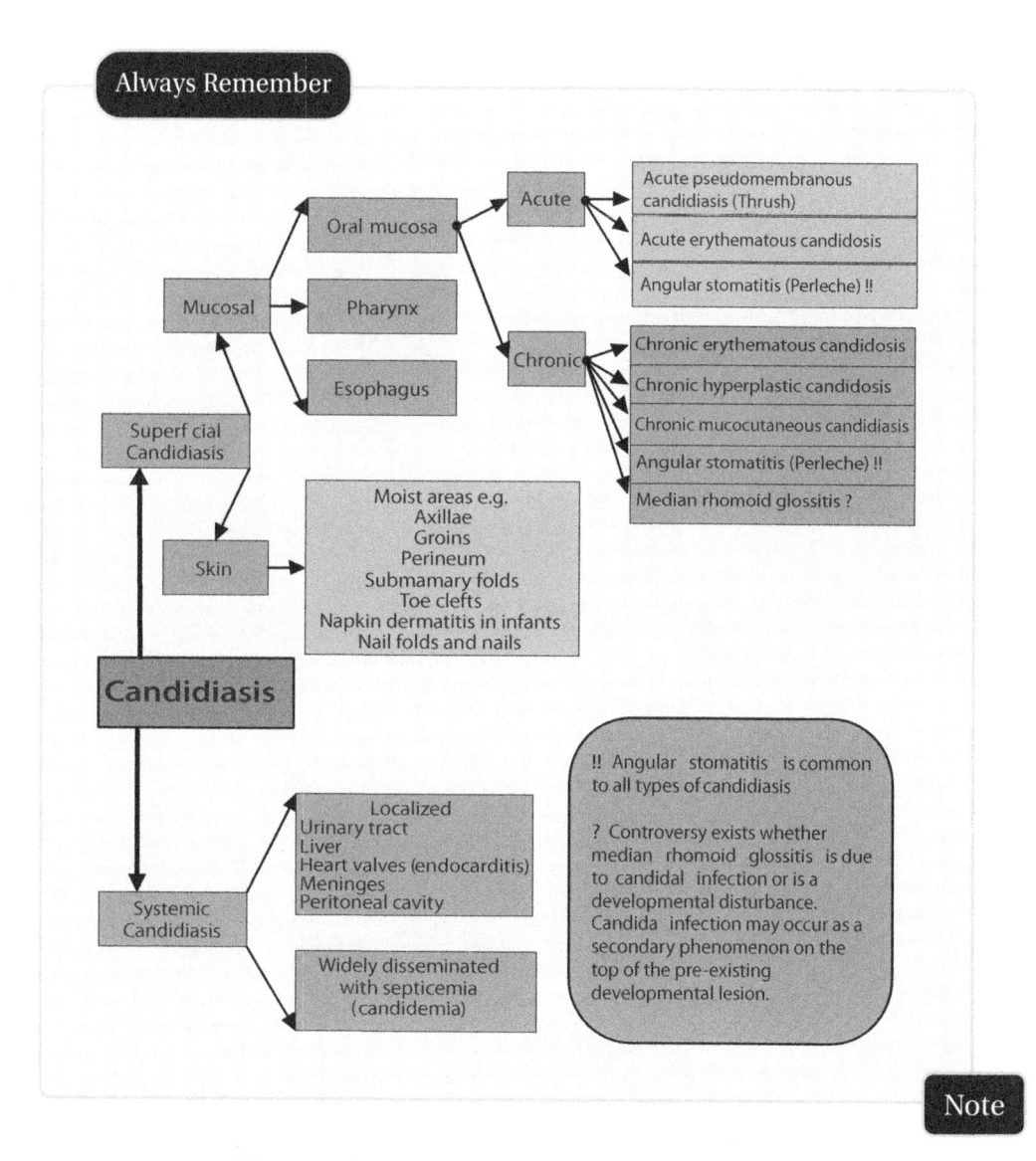

Figure 18.3: Clinical Spectrum of Candidiasis

CHAPTER 19
DISEASES OF THE MAXILLARY SINUS

Maxillary sinus or "Antrum of Higmore" is a bilateral pyramidal bony cavities found in the skull at the sides of the nose and above the maxillary teeth. The maxillary sinus is part of a group of paranasal sinuses, which includes the ethmoid, frontal, and sphenoid sinuses. The maxillary sinus is the largest of all sinuses and opens in the middle meatus of the nasal cavity with single or multiple openings.

19.1 Anatomy

- The maxillary sinus shows significant variation in size, shape, and position between individuals and even between the right and left sides in the same individual. See figure (19.1)
- The sinus is pyramidal in shape with a base, an apex, and four walls:
    ⋆ The base is the lateral wall of the nasal cavity
    ⋆ The apex is towards the zygomatic process of the maxilla
    ⋆ The 4 walls are:
        1. The anterior wall is the facial surface of the maxilla
        2. The posterior wall is the infratemporal surface of the maxilla
        3. The roof is the floor of the orbit
        4. The floor is the alveolar process of the maxilla

Chapter 19. Diseases of the Maxillary Sinus

- The sinus communicates with the middle nasal meatus through an opening that is known as ***ostium maxillare***. It is about 3–6 mm in diameter and is found in a recess called ***hiatus semilunaris***.
- The average volume of the maxillary sinus ranges from about 15–20 ml.
- Growth of the maxillary sinus occurs by the process of bone remodeling, referred to as ***pneumatization***, which is carried out by resorption of the sinus internal walls (except the medial wall) at a rate that slightly exceeds the growth of the maxilla.
- In old age, pneumatization may result in the phenomenon that the roots of the upper molars may protrude into the sinus cavity, a condition that may result in complications during teeth extraction or endodontic treatment.

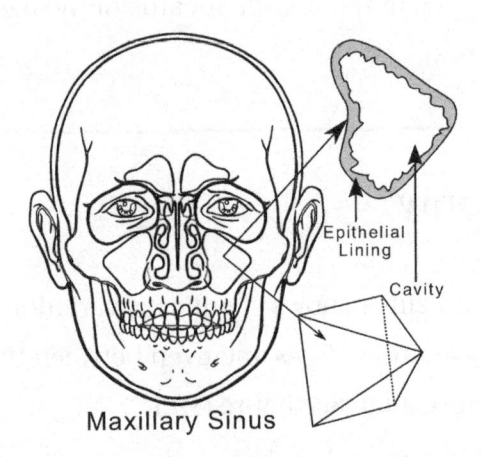

Figure 19.1: Diagrammatic representation of the maxillary sinus with its pyramidal shape.

19.2 Histology of the maxillary sinus

The maxillary sinus is lined by a mucous membrane, which is more lax and thinner than that of the nasal mucosa. The mucous membrane consists of two layers, an epithelial layer and a connective tissue layer that lies beneath the epithelium.

1. The epithelial lining:

    Consists of pseudostratified columnar ciliated cells with many goblet cells. The goblet cells are unicellular gland; it is mucous secreting cells. It resembles an inverted wine glass with a short narrow basal end that contains the nucleus and a swollen apical end containing mucin. It is an apocrine gland, i.e., it pours its secretion through the rupture of its apical cell membrane that gets regenerated. So it has all the criteria of the synthesizing and secreting cells.

2. The connective tissue:

    Consists of fibroblasts, collagen bundles, and few elastic fibers. It is moderately vascular. It contains many minor salivary glands, which are mostly mixed, i.e., serous and mucous acini with myoepithelial cells. These minor salivary glands can contribute to the formation of many antral cysts, which will be discussed in the chapter on the cysts of the oral and para-oral cavity.

19.3 Dental Relevance

1. Nerves that supply maxillary sinus are those that supply the maxillary teeth; this may account for dental pain from healthy teeth arising from maxillary sinusitis.

Chapter 19. Diseases of the Maxillary Sinus

2. The floor of the sinus can be the bone surrounding the apex of some maxillary teeth. Thus periapical infection of maxillary teeth can spread to the maxillary sinus. The reverse can occur with maxillary sinus infection being perceived as originating from maxillary teeth.
3. Pain from carious lesions or other insults to the dental pulp may be referred to the sinus and vice versa.
4. Communication between the oral cavity and the sinus may occur during tooth extraction or surgical intervention leading to an oroantral fistula.
5. Roots of posterior maxillary teeth may be in close relationship to the floor of the maxillary sinus. Teeth that are in close approximation to the sinus are in the following order: first molar, second premolar, second and third molars, first premolar, and rarely the canine.
6. The anatomical relationship of the maxillary sinus with maxillary teeth is shown in figure ()

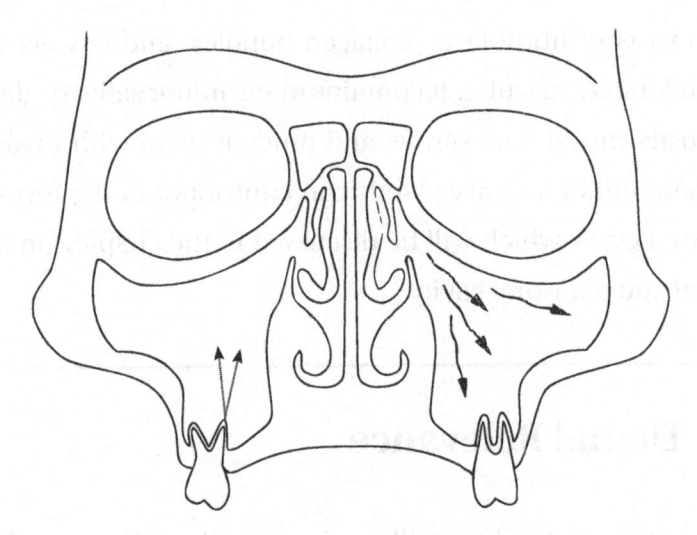

Figure 19.2: Anatomical relationship of the maxillary sinus with maxillary teeth.

19.4 Sinus Diseases

19.4.1 Infections

Viral Infection

Viral infection of the maxillary sinus is a common sequela of viral upper respiratory tract infection such as influenza and the common cold. This viral infection is usually self-limiting and resolves spontaneously; however, it may act as a predisposing factor for a bacterial infection to start and complicate the condition. Viral upper respiratory tract infections predispose the maxillary sinus to bacterial infection because of the interference with mucociliary function and narrowing of the ostium due to edematous sinus mucous membrane.

Bacterial Infection

Sinusitis is also termed rhinosinusitis because the condition usually involves nasal mucosa. The main signs and symptoms of sinusitis are:

- Facial pressure pain which is usually described as a dull and localizing pressure pain in the upper cheek
- Continuous headache on the same side of the involved sinus
- The decreased smell which may be partial or total
- Reduced taste sensation
- Nasal congestion
- Rhinorrhea (running nose) with a thick yellow mucus discharge (Purulent nasal discharges)
- Postnasal discharge
- Foul odor (fetid smells)

Sinusitis could be classified into acute, subacute, and chronic according to the duration of the involvement.

1. Acute Sinusitis

    Symptoms which lasts for less than 4 weeks.

2. Subacute Sinusitis

    Symptoms persist between 4 and 8 weeks despite treatment with medications.

3. Chronic Sinusitis

    Symptoms persist for more than 8 weeks despite treatment with medications.

Etiology:

Bacterial sinusitis is typically described as a polymicrobial infection, with predominantly anaerobic bacteria. Anaerobic *Peptostreptococcus* and *Prevotella spp.* are found in more than 75% of cases. Aerobic *Staphylococcus aureus* and *Streptococcus pneumonia* (*S. pneumonia*) and methicillin-resistant *Staphylococcus aureus* is found in 10–12% of patients.

Odontogenic Maxillary Sinusitis

Odontogenic maxillary sinusitis is the sinusitis resulting from odontogenic or dental causes. Exact and accurate diagnosis of odontogenic origin is necessary to avoid the long-term use of inappropriate antibiotics or unnecessary surgical interference.

About 10–12% of sinusitis cases can be attributed to odontogenic infections. Teeth most commonly involved are in the following order, first molar (22.51%), the third molar (17.21%), and the second molar (3.97%). The premolar region is involved in 5.96%, followed by the canine in 0.66% of cases. The signs and symptoms are similar to that of non-odontogenic sinusitis.

Etiology:

1. Periapical infection e.g., dentoalveolar abscess
2. Odontogenic cysts
3. Impacted teeth
4. Iatrogenic[1] causes e.g., over instrumentation during endodontic treatment, induction of oroantral fistula during dental extraction, and introduction of filling material or other medications during the endodontic or surgical treatment.

Diagnosis:

1. Thorough nasal and dental examination
2. CT, MRI and cone beam computed tomography (CBCT)

Fungal Infection

Mucormycosis and aspergillosis are the most common fungal diseases that can affect the maxillary sinus. Usually, they affects immunocompromised patients.

Fungus Ball

- Fungus ball (also, called mycetoma) is a fungal mass that is usually bilateral and often occurs in the maxillary sinus
- It Usually occurs in immunocompromised patient
- The causative organisms are usually *Aspergillus*
- Symptoms are similar to chronic rhinosinusitis but with a prolonged course, which are unresponsive to medical management. Patients may

---

[1] Iatrogenic means diseases or adverse effects resulting from errors induced by healthcare individuals

complain of facial pain and pressure, congestion, foul odor (fetid smells), or report blowing a "gravel-like" substance from their nose

- Radiographically, complete or subtotal opacification of the involved sinus
- Histopathologically, the sinus fungal ball consists of a dense accumulation of fungal hyphae

Treatment of Sinus Fungal Diseases:

Fungal sinus is treated by:

1. Surgical intervention

    Surgery is performed to reestablish sinus aeration and to promote improved sinus access for medical therapy

2. Medical therapy

    (a) Antifungal drugs

    (b) Immunotherapy, is important to lengthen time between, or even prevent, recurrences

19.4.2 Tumors

Sometimes, the Neoplasms can originate from any of the tissues that form the architecture of the maxillary sinus. These include the mucosa, minor salivary glands, mesenchymal tissues, blood vessels, remnants of ontogenic tissues, and bone. They are rare tumors. Many of these pose significant diagnostic challenge requiring a high degree of histopathological expertise. Tumors of the maxillary sinus affect a wide age range from children to the elderly, and some have either sex predilection. Lesions such as fibrous dysplasia tends to stabilize, but others are slowly progressive. Most of these tumors are discussed in their relevant chapters.

The most common tumors that can affect the maxillary sinus are:

1. Papillomas
2. Salivary gland tumors (pleomorphic adenoma, oncocytoma)
3. Mesenchymal tumors (fibroma, lipoma, myxoma)
4. Vascular tumors (hemangioma, aneurysmal bone cyst, hemangiopericytoma)
5. Odontogenic tumors
6. Fibroosseous lesions (osteoma, ossifying fibroma, fibrous dysplasia, osteoblastoma)
7. Granulomatous deposits in sarcoidosis and Wegener granulomatosis

19.4.3 Foreign Bodies

1. Remaining roots

   This is the most common foreign bodies to be found in the sinus. A tooth root or, more commonly, an apex of a tooth may be introduced into the sinus during the surgical removal of a fractured tooth. The remaining root my elicit an inflammatory condition in the sinus. Sometimes, in the absence of infection, the remaining root will remain symptomless for many years until it is discovered accidentally.

2. Surgical dressing of the tooth sockets

   Sometimes, the oroantral fistula passes unnoticed by the dental surgeon with subsequent packing the socket with a packing dressing, e.g., Alvogyl. As a result, the dressing will be introduced into the sinus with the subsequent inflammation.

3. Endodontic materials in the sinus

   Sometimes, during aggressive endodontic filing, pieces of endodontic fillers e.g. gutta percha, zinc oxide or calcium hydroxide may be pushed into the sinus. Also, during retrograde filling of root canals, dental amalgam or other dental filling materials may be introduced into the sinus cavity.

19.4.4 Cysts

Refer to the section of (Cysts of the Maxillary Antrum) on page (200)

19.4.5 Miscellaneous Conditions

Oroantral Fistula

Oroantral fistula is a common complication during dental extraction of the upper maxillary teeth, particularly the first maxillary molar. It requires surgical repair to avoid infection of the sinus and to ameliorates the unpleasant regurgitation of fluids from the nasal cavity when the patient drinks water or fluids. Signs of the oroantral fistula are foul or salty taste, alteration in voice resonance, inability to blow out the cheeks, air shooting from the fistula into the mouth when blowing the nose, and escape of liquids from the mouth through the nose.

Antral Polyps

- Antral polyps are similar to nasal polyps, they are soft outgrowths from the lining mucous membrane
- The exact etiology is unknown, however, most cases are related to chronic rhinosinusitis
- Symptoms include:
    - Nasal obstruction
    - Running nose
    - Constant need to swallow due to post-nasal drip

- ★ Reduced sense of smell or taste
- ★ Nasal bleeding
- ★ Snoring
• Treated by
    - ★ Antihistamines with or without steroids spray
    - ★ Surgical removal is often required
    - ★ Antibiotics are required if there is an associated infection
• Recurrence rate is high

Chapter 20
Oral Manifestations of Skin Diseases

Some skin diseases show oral manifestations, These manifestations my precede the skin lesions by several weeks or months. This makes their recognition by oral health care personnel is important.

20.1 Back to Basics

20.1.1 Skin Structure

The skin is the largest human organ. It covers between 1.5 and 2 m^2, comprising about one sixth of total body weight.

The skin consists of three functional layers, the epidermis, the dermis and the hypodermis (subcutis):

1. Epidermis
   - The epidermis is highly cellular, avascular. Lacks nerves, it produces a proteins termed keratin.
   - There is site to site variation in thickness of the epidermis.
   - The epidermis consists mostly of epithelial cells.
   - But there are other non-epithelial cells present (non-keratinocytes) e.g.:

- ★ Langerhans cells. They contain a sub-cellular organelle found in no other cell, the **Birbeck granules**. They are of hematopoietic origin.
- ★ Melanocytes of neural crest origin and their function is to synthesize melanin.
- ★ Merkel cells which are of neural crest origin and their functions are mechanoreceptors and neuroendocrine function.

2. Dermis or corium
   - The dermis is divided into two zones: The outer zone comprises extensions of the dermis between the downward projection rete pegs of the epidermis and is called the papillary dermis, beneath this zone is the reticular dermis.
   - The connective tissue consists of collagen and elastin together with various glycosaminoglycans which are secreted by the fibroblasts.
   - Collagen fibers are arranged in a specific pattern called Langer's lines. If incision in skin is made along the long axis of the collagen fiber, then little permanent scarring will occur.
   - Scattered within the dermis and often clustered about blood vessels are the mast cells.
   - The nerves of the dermis approach close to the epidermis and often end in specialized sensory structures such as **Pacinian corpuscles**.
   - Dermal blood vessels are organized into 2 structures, the superficial and deep vascular plexuses.
   - At the dermo-epidermal junction are pigmented dendritic cells, the melanocytes.
   - Muscles associated with hair follicles are called **arrector pili**.
   - There are natural holes in this barrier such as the sweat glands and hair ducts.

3. Subcutis (hypodermis)

20.2 Lichen Planus

Definition

Lichen Planus is a chronic skin disease which frequently involves oral mucosa.

Etiology

- Unknown, but T-cell (CD4 and CD8) mediated immune response against basal cells is suspected.
- Upregulation of intercellular adhesion molecule-1 (ICAM-1) and cytokines associated with T-helper type 1 immune response may also play a role.
- Trauma may play a role in the genesis of lichen planus. The occurrence of new lesions at the site of trauma is termed *Koebner's* phenomenon.

Clinically

- Skin lesions appear as flat toped papules which may coalesce into plaques often transversed by white lines called Wickham's stria. Skin lesions are self limiting within 1–2 years leaving areas of hyperpigmentation.
- Skin manifestations affect face, dorsal hands, arms, neck, palms, soles and nails (irregular longitudinal grooving and ridging of the nail plate, thinning of the nail plate).
- Oral lesions may be one of main 5 types:
    1. Reticular form: appears as white patches which can not be wiped off and are usually reticulated or lace like (Wickham's stria). The

most common site is the buccal mucosa. Oral lesions may persist longer than skin lesions. Burning sensation may be felt by some patients although this lesion shows the minimal clinical symptoms.

2. Plaque form: Tends to resemble leukoplakia clinically but has a multifocal distribution. The usual site for this form is the dorsum of the tongue and the buccal mucosa.

3. Erythematous or atrophic form: appears as red patches with very fine white stria. It may be found associated with reticular or erosive forms. The proportion of keratinized areas to atrophic areas varies form one area to another. The attached gingiva is mostly affected in this form. Patients may complain of burning sensation and generalized discomfort.

4. Erosive form: The central area of the lesion is ulcerated. A pseudomembrane usually covers the ulcer. Careful examination usually reveals keratotic stria, peripheral to the ulcer. A significant number of cases present with a picture of desquamative gingivitis. Desquamative gingivitis is not a disease entity but a sign of disease that can be caused by erosive lichen planus, pemphigus vulgaris, or cicatricial pemphigoid. Desquamative gingivitis caused by lichen planus may be accompanied by characteristic Wickham's striae, simplifying the diagnosis, or they may be present without other lesions.

5. Bullous form: This is the rarest form. The bullae range from few millimeters to centimeters in diameter. Such bullae are usually short lived and may rupture leaving a painful ulcer. Lesions are usually seen on the buccal mucosa particularly opposite to the second and third molars. Reticular or striated keratotic areas should be seen with this form of lichen planus. Atrophic, erosive and bullous forms are variations of the same process and should be considered together.

Histologically

1. Hyperkeratosis.
2. Irregular acanthosis.
3. Rete pegs are saw tooth like appearance.
4. In atrophic forms there is severe thinning and flattening of the epithelium
5. Degeneration, apoptosis and necrosis of basal cell layer with production of cleft like spaces.
6. The necrotic basal cells are sometimes called colloid bodies or Civatte bodies.
7. A band of lymphocytic infiltration is found at the dermo-epidermal junction.

For the Diagnostic criteria of lichen planus, see figure (20.1).

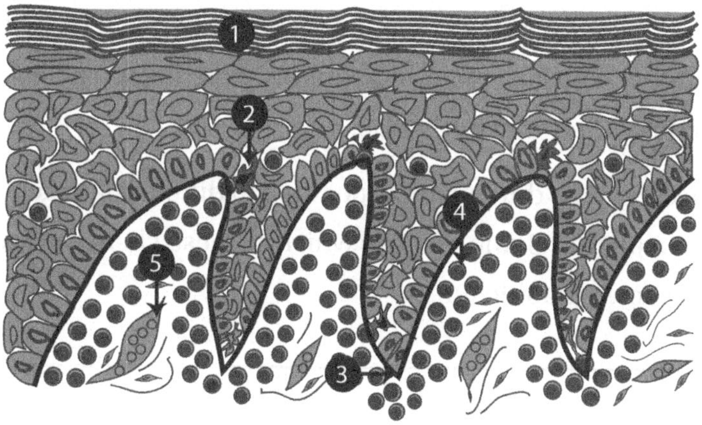

Figure 20.1: Diagnostic criteria of lichen planus. 1: Hyperkeratosis, 2: Apoptotic basal cells (Civatte bodies), 3: Saw-like rete pegs, 4: Lymphocytic band, 5: Blood vessels. Note that most of the apoptotic basal cells are usually surrounded by lymphocytes.

Treatment

- There is no cure for lichen planus.
- First-line of treatment typically involves topical and systemic corticosteroids.
- Removal of any triggers.

20.3 Lichenoid Reactions

This term is given to lichen planus-like lesions caused by specific causes such as systemic drug treatment or graft versus host reaction.

A very wide range of drugs can cause lichenoid reactions of the skin, mucous membranes or both (table 20.1). Graft versus host disease may be associated with lichenoid reaction. Graft versus host reaction is an immunological reaction of the donor graft against the recipient tissue. The clinical features of lichenoid reactions are often indistinguishable from true lichen planus and usually consist only of white striae.

In practice it can be difficult or impossible to differentiate lichenoid reactions from lichen planus. Some features which suggest a lichenoid reaction against drugs are shown in table (20.2).

20.4 Pemphigus

Definition

Pemphigus is an auto-immune vesiculobullous disease which usually shows oral manifestations. For classification of vesiculobullous lesions see "Ulcers & Vesiculobullous Lesions of the Oral Cavity", page (611).

Table 20.1: Examples of drugs capable of causing lichenoid reactions

> **Always Remember**
>
> - Colloidal gold
> - All Beta-blockers
> - Oral hypoglycemics
> - Non-steroidal anti-inflammatory drugs
> - Antimalarials
> - Tricyclic antidepressants
> - Some dental restorative materials

Table 20.2: Features suggesting a lichenoid reaction

> **Always Remember**
>
> - Onset associated with the start of the drug
> - Unilateral lesion or unusual distribution
> - Unusual severity
> - Widespread skin lesions
> - Localized lesion in contact with restoration

The disease is an autoimmune in which there are circulating antibodies against the epithelial inter-cellular cementing substance leading to acantholysis of epithelial cells. By immuno-fluorescence techniques, the antibodies could be detected around epithelial cells.

Historically, the disease was refereed to as true pemphigus to distinguish it form pemphigoid (see later).

In pemphigus the vesicles are intra-epithelial while in pemphigoid the vesicles are subepithelial.

Classification

The disease is classified histologically according to the location of the vesicles into:

1. Pemphigus vulgaris
2. Pemphigus vegetans
3. Pemphigus foliaceous
4. Pemphigus erythematosus

Only pemphigus vulgaris and pemphigus vegetans affect the oral mucosa. In pemphigus vulgaris and pemphigus vegetans the vesicles are supra-basilar i.e. affecting the lower part of the epithelium, while pemphigus foliaceous and pemphigus erythematosus the vesicles are in the superficial part of the prickle cell layer (see also tables 20.3 and figure 20.2). Another form of pemphigus known as familial benign pemphigus (Hailey-Hailey disease) was described by Hailey brothers differs etiologically from other forms of pemphigus as being hereditary and lack an autoimmune background.

Other rare type of pemphigus is the ***paraneoplastic pemphigus (PNP)***. This disorder is a complication of some malignant tumors, usually lymphoma. It may precede the diagnosis of the tumors. Painful ulcers appear on the mouth, lips, and the esophagus. In this variety of pemphigus, the disease process often involves the lungs, causing bronchiolitis obliterans (constrictive bronchiolitis). The disease shows racial predilection in Ashkenazi Jewish population. Complete removal of and/or cure of the tumor may improve the skin disease, but lung damage is generally irreversible.

20.4.1 Pemphigus Vulgaris

- Is the most common type.
- It affects oral mucosa and skin.
- It appears as vesicles or bullae which rupture forming shallow ulcers covered by dry crust.
- If untreated, the disease is almost fatal due to loss of plasma and electrolytes.
- Nikolsky's sign is always positive in pemphigus group. The examiner's finger is firmly pressed against the patient's skin and traction applied, skin separates at the junction of the epidermis and dermis or between layers of the epidermis leaving a red bleeding area.
- Histologically: The disease is characterized by the presence of many *acantholytic cells*. Acantholytic cells are epithelial cells showing loss of intercellular bridges and thus become rounded with pyknotic nuclei. Some of the acantholytic cells appear free floating the in the clefts and is known as *Tzanck cells*. Acantholytic cells will result in the formation of suprabasilar clefts (vesicles). The basal cells remain attached to the basement membrane.

20.4.2 Pemphigus Vegetans

A rare form which appears as a large verrucous plaques. The clefts or vesicles are also suprabasilar.

20.4.3 Familial Benign Pemphigus

(Hailey-Hailey Disease)

- Was described by Hailey brothers in 1939.
- It is a chronic autosomal dominant disorder with incomplete penetrance.
- A history of multiple relapses and remissions is characteristic.
- Decreased numbers of desmosomes have been implicated in the pathogenesis.
- It should be noted that Hailey-Hailey is a genetic form of pemphigus and is not an autoimmune disease.
- Usually appears in the third or fourth decade, although it can occur at any age.
- It typically begins as painful erosive lesions in the skin folds. Common sites include the armpits, groins, and neck, under the breasts and between the buttocks. The lesions tend to come and go and leave no scars.
- Doxycycline is a promising drug for the control of Hailey-Hailey Disease, see page (75).

20.5 Pemphigoid

In pemphigoid, the vesicles are sub-epithelial. Pemphigoid is further classified into the two types:

1. Bullous pemphigoid
2. Benign mucous membrane pemphigoid

20.5.1 Bullous Pemphigoid

Definition

An autoimmune vesiculobullous lesion of skin and oral mucosa.

Etiology

Circulating antibodies against basement membrane (lamina lucida).

Clinically

Large tense bullae containing clear fluid. The bullae do not rupture as easily as those in pemphigus. If uninfected, heal without scarring.

Histologically

Subepidermal non-acantholytic vesicles with lymphocytic infiltration.

20.5.2 Benign Mucous Membrane Pemphigoid

(Cicatricial pemphigoid, mucosal pemphigoid, ocular pemphigoid)

Definition

An autoimmune vesiculobullous lesion of conjunctiva and oral mucosa.

Etiology

Circulating antibodies against basement membrane (lamina lucida). Deposits of immunoglobulins and complement components along the basement membrane zone are characteristic. The antigenic targets are laminin 5 (epiligrin) and a 180 kd protein known as bullous pemphigoid antigen 180 (BPI 180).

Clinically

Large tense bullae containing clear fluid. The bullae do not rupture as easily as those in pemphigus. The disease results in excessive scarring and loss of vision.

Histologically

Subepidermal non-acantholytic vesicles with lymphocytic infiltration.

20.6   Erythema Multiforme

Definition

A hypersensitivity reaction against certain drugs, infections or systemic disorders.

Etiology

The exact etiology is unknown. The reaction is thought to be a cell mediated immune response. In 50% of patients, the disease is precipitated by some events such as:

1. Infections e.g. herpes simplex or histoplasmosis.
2. Drugs e.g. sulfonamides or penicillins.
3. Malignancy e.g. carcinoma or lymphoma.
4. Collagen diseases e.g. lupus erythematosus.

Clinically

The lesions are "**multiform**" and include macules, papules, vesicles and bullae as well as the characteristic "**targets**" or "**iris**" like lesions which consists of red macule or papule with central erosion. A severe form occurs in children known as Steven-Johnson syndrome characterized by ulcerations and blood crusting appearance of lips, oral mucosa and conjunctiva.

Histologically

- Edema of connective tissue.
- Lymphocytic infiltration at the dermoepidermal junction and around blood vessels.
- Degeneration and necrosis of epithelial cells.

20.7 Lupus Erythematosus

Definition

Lupus erythematosus is thought to be an autoimmune disease.

There are two forms:

1. Systemic lupus erythematosus: Which is a serious multisystem disease.
2. Discoid lupus erythematosus: Which is a localized skin lesion.

20.7.1 Systemic Lupus Erythematosus

Etiology

- The etiology is unknown and it is thought that the disease is autoimmune in which both the humoral and the cell-mediated arms of the immune system share in its pathogenesis.
- There is genetic predisposition.
- Ultra-violet rays and female sex hormones may play a role in the pathogenesis.

Clinically

- Is more common in females more than males 9:1
- The most common age is 20–40
- The lesions are widespread with involvement of skin, joints, kidney and serious sacs (commonly the pericardium).
- The onset may be acute with fever, malaise, weight loss, leucopenia, elevated ESR, lymphadenopathy and skin rash. Sometimes the onset of the disease is insidious with development of the rash on the skin followed by other organ involvement.
- Erythema and edema occur on the sun exposed areas of the skin giving the classic butterfly rash.

Histologically

1. Degeneration of basal cell layer.
2. Deposition of IgG and C3 (complement complex) in the basement membrane which could be detected by immunofluorscence. This deposition will result in thickening of the basement membrane.

3. Fibrinoid changes around blood vessels.
4. Edema
5. Inflammatory cell infiltration particularly lymphocytes under the epithelium and around skin appendages (periadnexal).

20.7.2 Discoid Lupus Erythematosus

- Is a skin condition which occurs in the exposed parts of the skin and is made worse by exposure to sunlight. Face and scalp are the most commonly affected sits
- The lesion consists of erythematous scaly macules which show the typical butterfly distribution
- When the scalp is affected, hair loss (scarring alopecia) may occur
- Healing may occur leaving scars and post-inflammatory pigmentation
- Oral manifestations occur in about 20% of cases and consist of erythematous macules without keratosis. Later on the atrophic macules become surrounded by margins or covered by white keratotic spots. Sometimes, alternating red and white zones occur
- These lesions may predispose to squamous cell carcinoma
- Treatment is by topical steroids

20.8 Psoriasis

Definition

Chronic skin disease characterized by increased rate of keratinocyte turnover rate (around 8 times greater than normal).

Etiology

- Unknown
- The disease appears to be an immunoregulartory disorder in which epidermal changes are related to a defect in the control of keratinocyte proliferation.
- Hereditary background is detected in many cases
- Triggering factors include systemic infection, stresses and certain drugs.

Clinically

- Skin lesions: Appears as silvery scaly papules or macules on an erythematous base.
- When the scales are removed, small pinpoint bleeding occurs due to presence of vascular high dermal papillae. This phenomenon is known as *Auspitz sign*.
- The development of new lesions on previously normal skin after trauma is known as Koebner's phenomenon.
- Lesions usually affect extremities at the extensor surfaces such as the elbows and knees.
- Periods of exacerbation and remissions occur. Lesions usually worsen in winter and partially resolve in summer due to the effect of ultraviolet rays of sun.
- Nail changes occur in 30% of cases and consist of yellow-brown discoloration with separation of the nail plate from the underlying bed.
- In the rare variant called pustular psoriasis, multiple small pustules form on erythematous plaques.
- Oral manifestations: are rare and consists of white scaly lesions or erythematous patches with white raised margins.

- Geographic tongue is considered by some authors to be a manifestation of psoriasis.

Histologically

- Hyperparakeratosis
- High connective tissue papillae with thinned overlying epithelium (2-3 cells thick)
- Increased vascularity and lymphocytic infiltration
- Aggregates of PNL between epithelial cells producing sterile micro abscesses that are called ***Munro abscesses***
- See (figure (20.3)) to see how normal skin can progress to psoriasis.

Treatment

- Topical corticosteroids
- Methotrexate
- Retinoids

20.9   Progressive systemic sclerosis

(Systemic scleroderma)

Definition

An autoimmune generalized disorder of connective tissue in which there is thickening of dermal collagen bundles, and fibrosis and vascular abnormalities in internal organs.

Histopathology

1. Hyperkeratosis
2. Atrophy of the epithelium with loss of rete pegs
3. Atrophy of sweat, sebaceous and minor salivary glands
4. Excessive deposition of collagen bundles in the connective tissue with hyalinization
5. Presence of chronic inflammatory cells
6. Vasculitis in the internal organs

20.10 Rheumatoid Arthritis

Definition

- Chronic systemic inflammatory disorder affecting synovial membrane lining of joints, bursae and tendon sheaths
- Also skin, blood vessels, heart, lungs, muscles
- Produces non-suppurative proliferative synovitis, which may progress to destruction of articular cartilage and joint ankylosis

Histopathology

Joints

- Dense perivascular inflammatory infiltrate of T lymphocytes, plasma cells (often with eosinophilic cytoplasmic inclusions called Russell bodies), macrophages; inflammation extends to subchondral bone (relatively specific for rheumatoid arthritis)
- Proliferative synovitis with synovial cell hyperplasia and hypertrophy

- Lymphoplasmacytic infiltrate with variable germinal centers and fibrosis
- Increased vascularity with hemosiderin deposition
- Organizing fibrin floating in joint space as rice bodies
- Neutrophils present on synovial surface; osteoclasts present in bone forming cysts
- Erosions, osteoporosis; pannus[1] formation (synovium, synovial stroma with inflammatory cells, granulomatous tissue, fibroblasts), progressing to fibrous ankylosis (bridges joints), then ossifying to form bony ankylosis
- Minimal evidence of repair (proliferative cartilage, sclerotic bone or osteophytes[2])
- Weichselbaum's lacunae: enlarged chondrocyte lacunae within articular cartilage due to dead chondrocytes

Skin

- Rheumatoid nodules in 25%, usually those with severe disease in skin subject to pressure (ulnar forearm, elbows, occiput, lumbosacral area); also present in viscera; firm, nontender, with central fibrinoid necrosis surrounded by palisading epithelioid histiocytes, lymphocytes, plasma cells; obliterative endarteritis in vasa nervorum and digital arteries causes ulcers, neuropathy, gangrene
- Blood vessels: small to medium size vessels in vital organs (not kidney) affected by severe erosive disease; rheumatoid nodules present, high titers of rheumatoid factor

---

[1] Pannus is an abnormal layer of fibrovascular tissue or granulation tissue. Common sites for pannus formation include over the cornea, over a joint surface (as seen in rheumatoid arthritis), or on a prosthetic heart valve.[1] Pannus may grow in a tumor-like fashion, as in joints where it may erode articular cartilage and bone.

[2] Osteophytes are exostoses (bony projections) that form along joint margins.

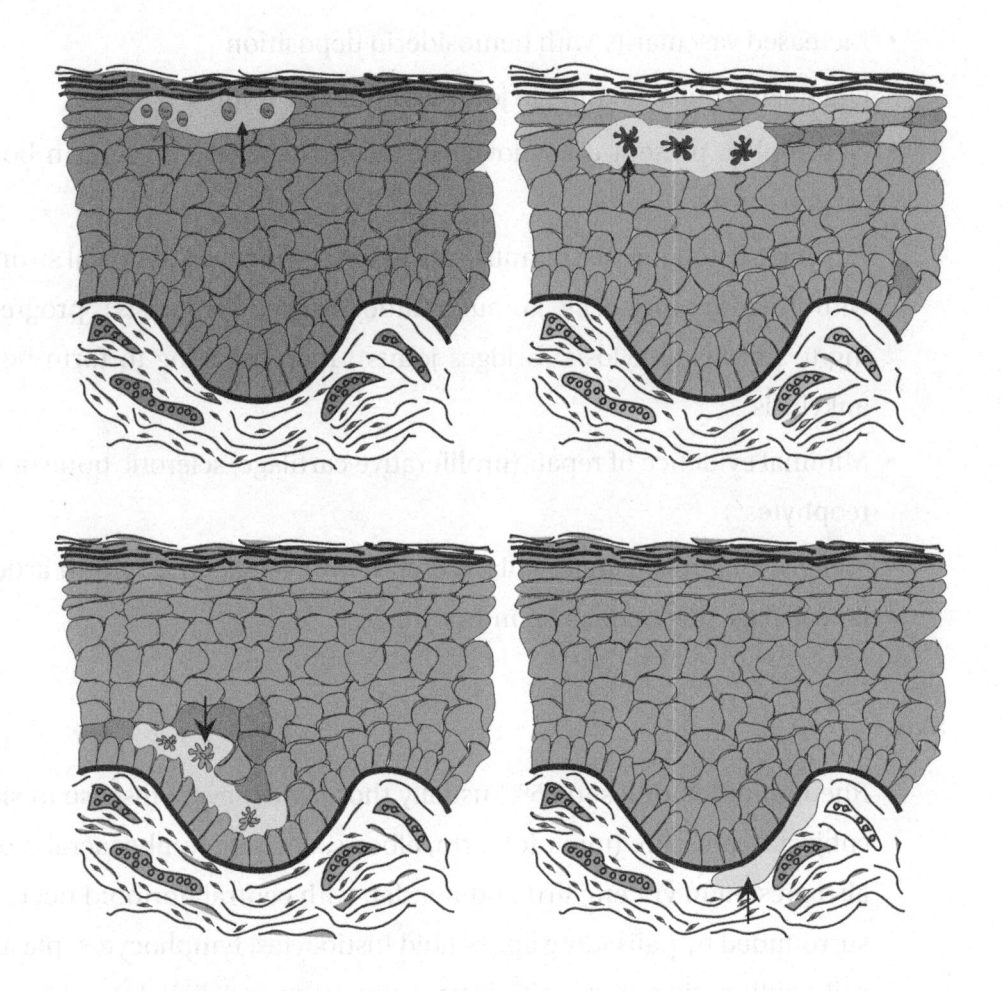

Chapter 20. Oral Manifestations of Skin Diseases

Figure 20.2: Blistering conditions: 1: Subcorneal vesicles as in impetigo (pyogenic infection of the skin), the fluid is rich in PNL. 2: High intra-epithelial vesicles as in pemphigus foliaceus and pemphigus erythematosus, the fluid is rich in acantholytic cells (A). 3: Low intra-epithelial vesicles (supra-basilar clefts) as in pemphigus vulgaris, pemphigus vegetans and Darier's disease. 4: Sub-epithelial vesicles as in pemphigoid and epidermolysis bulosa.

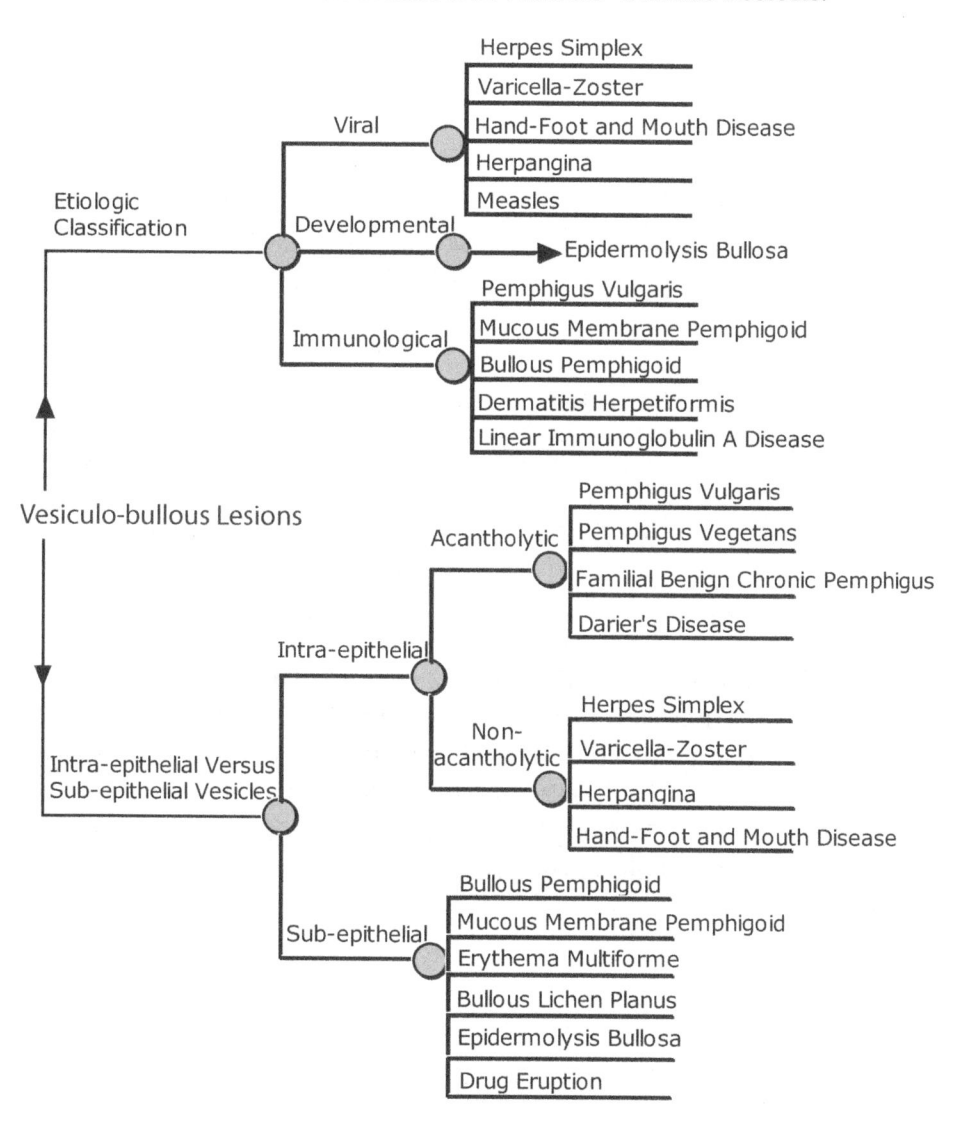

Table 20.3: Classification of Vesiculo-bullous Lesions.

- **Vesiculo-bullous Lesions**
  - **Etiologic Classification**
    - **Viral**
      - Herpes Simplex
      - Varicella-Zoster
      - Hand-Foot and Mouth Disease
      - Herpangina
      - Measles
    - **Developmental**
      - Epidermolysis Bullosa
    - **Immunological**
      - Pemphigus Vulgaris
      - Mucous Membrane Pemphigoid
      - Bullous Pemphigoid
      - Dermatitis Herpetiformis
      - Linear Immunoglobulin A Disease
  - **Intra-epithelial Versus Sub-epithelial Vesicles**
    - **Intra-epithelial**
      - **Acantholytic**
        - Pemphigus Vulgaris
        - Pemphigus Vegetans
        - Familial Benign Chronic Pemphigus
        - Darier's Disease
      - **Non-acantholytic**
        - Herpes Simplex
        - Varicella-Zoster
        - Herpangina
        - Hand-Foot and Mouth Disease
    - **Sub-epithelial**
      - Bullous Pemphigoid
      - Mucous Membrane Pemphigoid
      - Erythema Multiforme
      - Bullous Lichen Planus
      - Epidermolysis Bullosa
      - Drug Eruption

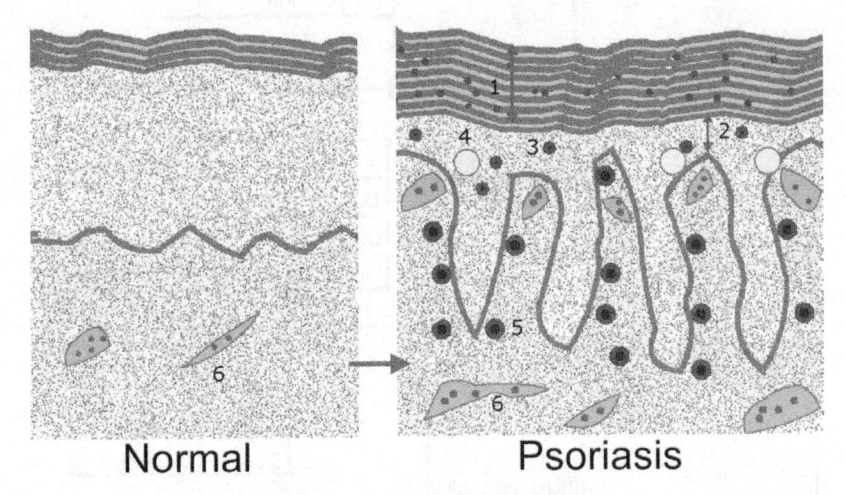

Chapter 20. Oral Manifestations of Skin Diseases

Figure 20.3: The progress of the lesions from normal skin to psoriasis. 1: Hyperparakeratosis, 2: Thinning of the epithelium over the high connective tissue papillae resulting in the Auspitz phenomenon, 3: PNL infiltrating the epithelium, 4: Microabscess (Munro abscess), 5: Lymphocytic infiltration of the connective tissue, 6: Dilated blood vessels.

Chapter 21
WHITE AND RED LESIONS OF THE ORAL CAVITY

Most of the lesions to be mentioned herein have been discussed in their relevant chapters and the reader is advised to refer to these chapters for further details.

The normal pink color of oral mucosa results from reflection of light on the capillary bed of the connective tissue. This normal color requires that the epithelium should be of certain thickness and of definite optical transparency.

21.1 Introduction

White lesions of the oral mucosa occur as a result of (see also figure (21.1)):

1. Increased thickness of epithelium which may result from:
   (a) Hyperkeratosis
   (b) Acanthosis
   (c) Spongiosis resulting form intra and/or inter-cellular edema
2. Alteration of the color of the connective tissue such as decreased vascularity and increased fibrosis

Red lesions of the oral mucosa occur as a result of:

1. Decreased thickness of epithelium due to atrophy, this may be associated with disorganization of the epithelium with formation of high connective tissue papillae.

2. Alteration of the color of the connective tissue due to increased vascularity

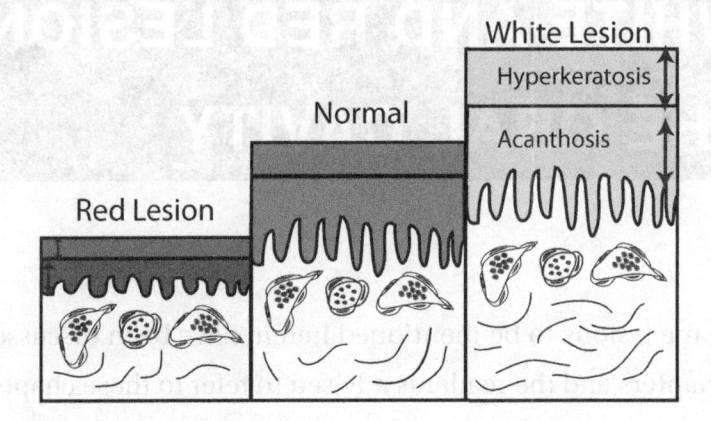

Figure 21.1: White vs red lesions. Left panel, illustrates red lesions resulting from atrophy of the epithelium, middle panel illustrates normal color of oral mucosa while, the right panel illustrates the white lesions resulting from acanthosis and hyperkeratosis.

21.2 White Lesions

21.2.1 Definition

A white lesion is an abnormal area of the oral mucosa which appear whiter than the adjacent normal mucosa.

21.2.2 Classification of white lesions

No satisfactory classification exists and white lesions can be classified according to many criteria. The etiologic classification is the most appropriate.

Classification according to the etiology:

1. Physical agents (Reactive lesions)

- Chemical burns e.g. aspirin burn
- Thermal e.g. thermal burns
- Traumatic e.g. chronic cheek and lip biting

2. Hyperplastic
   - Oral keratosis

3. Preneoplastic (premalignant) and neoplastic lesions

   Leukoplakia, carcinoma in situ, oral submucous fibrosis, verrucous carcinoma and squamous cell carcinoma

4. Developmental disturbances

   Such as leukodema, white spongy nevus, hereditary benign intraepithelial dyskeratosis, Fordyce's spots, pachyonychia congenita, dyskeratosis congenita, and Darier's disease

5. Skin diseases

   Lichen planus, lupus erythematosus and psoriasis

6. Infection

   Candidosis, syphilitic patches, diphtheria and Koplik's spots of measles

7. Miscellaneous

   Linea alba buccalis and skin grafts used to line surgical defects of oral mucosa

Other useful classifications of white lesions

Other classifications of white lesions are mainly clinical and are useful for their differential diagnosis. Some of the most popular classifications are mentioned below:

1. Classification according to whether the lesion can be wiped or not be wiped off:
   (a) Lesions which can be wiped off:

i. Burns such as aspirin burn

ii. Acute pseudomembranous candidosis

(b) Lesions which can not be wiped off:

All other lesions

2. Classification according to whether the lesion is unilateral or bilateral

 (a) Lesions which are usually bilateral:

i. Fordyce's spots

ii. Lichen planus

iii. Leukodema

iv. White spongy nevus

v. Hereditary benign intra-epithelial dyskeratosis

vi. Dyskeratosis congenita

vii. Pachyonychia congenita

viii. Candidosis

 (b) Lesions which are usually Unilateral:

All other lesions

3. Classification according to whether the lesion is purely white or intermingled with red areas

 (a) Lesions which are usually white intermingled with red areas:

i. Speckled leukoplakia

ii. Acute antibiotic stomatitis

iii. Geographic tongue (red patches with white rim)

iv. Atrophic lichen planus

v. Oral submucous fibrosis

vi. Smoker's keratosis (stomatitis nicotina)

 (b) Lesions which are usually purely white:

All other lesions

4. Classification according to whether the lesions show definite malignant potentiality

    (a) Lesions with definite malignant potentiality:
        i. Leukoplakia
        ii. Oral submucous fibrosis
        iii. Actinic keratosis
        iv. Lichen planus
        v. Dyskeratosis congenita
    (b) Lesions with no extra-ordinary risk of malignant potentiality:
        All other lesions

21.2.3 Oral Keratosis

Keratosis by definition is the increased thickness of keratin layer. Most of the oral keratotic lesions are white lesions. The etiology of oral keratosis may be:

1. Frictional (traumatic) keratosis
2. Smoker's keratosis (stomatitis nicotina)
3. Sublingual keratosis
4. Smokeless tobacco keratosis (Betel nut, tobacco chewer's and oral snuff keratosis)
5. Syphilitic keratosis
6. Actinic keratosis (actinic cheilitis)

Frictional (traumatic) keratosis and cheek biting

Definition

White patches caused by prolonged mild abrasion of the oral mucosa by irritants such as sharp tooth, denture clasps, ill fitting dentures and cheek biting. This results in a presumably protective hyperkeratotic white lesion that is analogous to a callus on the skin. Glass blower's keratosis is a variant of frictional keratosis affecting the cheeks and lips in workers of glass factories.

Clinically

At first pale and translucent patches which then become dense and white with rough surface

Histologically

- Hyperkeratosis, acanthosis with prominent granular cell layer
- No dysplasia
- Chronic inflammatory cell infiltration of the connective tissue

Treatment

Removal of the cause

Smoker's keratosis (stomatitis nicotina)

Definition

Smoker's keratosis is seen among heavy, long-term pipe smokers and some cigar smokers.

Clinically

- The lesion usually affects the palate, any part protected by a denture is spared.

- The lesion has two components: Hyperkeratosis and inflammatory reaction of minor salivary glands
- Hence the lesion appears as a white patch with many red spots or umbilicated swellings representing the orifices of minor salivary glands.

Histologically

- The white areas show hyperkeratosis, acanthosis with inflammatory cell infiltration of the underlying connective tissue.
- The diagnostic feature is the swollen, inflamed mucous glands with hyperkeratosis extending to the duct orifices.

Treatment

The patient should be persuaded to stop smoking and the lesion will resolve withing weeks.

Sublingual Keratosis

Definition

The term sublingual keratosis is applied to white lesions on the floor of mouth and ventral tongue. Whether this lesion is a different entity from other leukoplakias is unclear. Malignant change was reported in an unusually high proportion of cases (30%) in one series but this has not been widely confirmed. Probably the risk of malignant transformation is less than 10% and possibly much lower.

Clinically

Sublingual keratosis is a white, soft plaque, usually with a wrinkled surface, an irregular but well-defined outline and sometimes bilateral with a butterfly shape. The plaque typically extends from the anterior floor of the mouth to the undersurface of the tongue. There is usually no associated inflammation.

Histologically

Sublingual keratosis is not distinctive histologically and the appearances are those described for leukoplakia.

Smokeless tobacco keratosis

Definition

The term smokeless tobacco keratosis is applied to white keratotic lesions resulting form the topical use of all forms of tobacco. The tobacco preparations are generally of a higher (alkaline) pH and are often mixed with other ingredients, including shredded areca (betel nut), lime, camphor and spices. Oral mucosa responds to the topically induced effects of tobacco with inflammation and keratosis. Dysplastic changes may follow with a low potential risk of malignant change. Snuff and finely divided or shredded tobacco is more likely to cause oral lesions than coarsely ground tobacco. The dysplastic effect of chewing tobacco may be due to:

- Presence of carcinogenic agents such as nitrosonornicotine.
- Presence of irritants in the tobacco flavoring agents.
- The high alkaline pH of chewing tobacco resulting from the addition of lime (calcium oxide).

Clinically

- White lesions of smokeless tobacco occur in the area where the tobacco is habitually placed.
- The most common area is the mucobuccal fold in the mandibular molar or incisor areas.
- The mucosa develops a granular or wrinkled appearance. Less often, red areas may be admixed with the white plaques.
- The lesions are generally painless and asymptomatic.

Histologically

- Hyperparakeratosis
- Edema
- Chronic inflammatory cell infiltration of the connective tissue.
- Epithelial dysplasia may occasionally develop in these lesions.

Actinic keratosis

(Solar keratosis, Actinic cheilitis, Senile keratosis)

For details see chapter "Premalignant Lesions of the Oral Cavity", page (306).

21.3   Red Lesions

21.3.1   Definition

A red lesion is an abnormal area of the oral mucosa which appear red compared to the surrounding normal mucosa.

21.3.2 Classification of red lesions

The etiologic classification is the most appropriate

1- Physical

Radiation Mucositis

- Radiation mucositis is one of the most painful and distressing inflammatory reaction of the oral mucosa to radiation therapy.
- The degree of injury varies, depending on the dose, portal of the beam, age, and general health of the patient.
- The first reaction is usually noted during the second week after the duration of 5–6 weeks of treatment
- The lesion consists of diffuse erythema, followed by desquamation and ulceration.
- Xerostomia adds to the discomfort and usually persists indefinitely to some degree. Xerostomia also increase the possibility of candidal infection.
- An alteration in taste often precedes the mucosal reaction and may persist, depending on the dose.
- Hydrogen peroxide and water (4:1 solution) and sodium bicarbonate solutions may improve symptoms. Numerous anesthetic mucosal coating agents are available, including combinations of benadryl, viscous lidocaine, and Dyclone.

2- Developmental

- Lingual varices
- Median rhomboid glossitis

- Geographic tongue
- Hereditary hemorrhagic telangiectasia (Rendu-Osler-Weber Syndrome)
- Sturge-Weber Syndrome

3- Benign tumors

- Hemangiomas
- Pyogenic granulomas
- Pregnancy tumors
- Juvenile melanoma (Spitz nevus) (some cases)

4- Premalignant lesions

- Erythroplakia

5- Malignant tumors

- Amelanotic melanomas
- Kaposi's sarcoma
- Hemangioendothelioma
- Hemangiopericytoma
- Angiosarcoma

6- Infections

- Erythematous candidosis
- Antibiotic stomatitis
- Bacillary angiomatosis, see page (261)

7- Blood diseases

- Purpura (hemorrhage into the skin and mucosa)
- Pernicious anemia
- Iron deficiency anemia

8- Miscellaneous causes

- Porphyria
- Vitamin B deficiency
- Petechia and ecchymosis

Chapter 22
Ulcers and Vesiculobullous Lesions of the Oral Cavity

Ulcer by definition is the loss of the epithelium, while erosion is the partial loss of (the superficial layers) of the epithelium. Although it is strictly inaccurate, the two terms (ulcers and erosions) are used synonymously in the medical literature. Vesiculobullous lesions are lesions which start as vesicles or bullae and usually progress into ulcers. Hence both groups of lesions are collected in one entity. Vesicles are small blisters usually (< 1.0 cm) while bullae are larger (> 1.0 cm) in diameter.

22.1 Definitions

Blisters, vesicles, and bullae are fluid-filled spaces due to the separation of two layers of tissues and the leakage of plasma into the space. The most common blister is the frictional blister, commonly found on the heel due to shearing forces set up within the skin as a result of ill-fitting footwear. Such blisters form at the dermo-epidermal junction but other blisters may form at any level within the skin or mucosa and the precise site of blisters gives a very good clue as to their nature.

There are several mechanisms of blister formation:

1. Destruction of the bonds (attachment) between epithelial cells as in pemphigus. Keratinocytes become loose and fall within the blister cavity. These keratinocytes are no longer held in shape by the surrounding cells and become round-up (acanthocytes); the whole process is known as *acantholysis*.
2. The cells may be forced apart by edema fluid as happens in eczema.
3. The cells themselves may be destroyed, leaving gaps, as happens in herpes simplex.
4. The basement membrane or its attachments to the epidermis or dermis may be destroyed as in pemphigoid and epidermolysis Bullosa.

22.2 Classification

22.2.1 Primary versus secondary ulcers

Ulcers can be classified according to whether they start as primary or as secondary, secondary ulcers are ulcers preceded by vesiculobullous lesions.

1. Primary ulcers:

    Are not preceded by vesiculobullous lesions. Examples are:
    - Traumatic ulcers
    - Infective ulcers: e.g. bacterial and fungal infections
    - Neoplastic ulcers
    - Ulcers of systemic diseases such as GIT and blood disorders
    - Aphthous ulcers
    - Behcet's syndrome
    - Reiter's syndrome

2. Secondary ulcers (vesiculobullous lesions):

    Secondary ulcers are preceded by vesiculobullous lesions (see also table 20.3 & figure 20.2). They are further classified into ulcers resulting form intra-epithelial vesicles and ulcers resulting form sub-epithelial vesicles:

    (a) Ulcers resulting from intra-epithelial vesicles

    Are further classified according whether vesicles result form acantholysis (separation of individual keratinocytes from their neighbor due to destruction of the intercellular attachment) or not:

    i. Acantholytic lesions
    - Pemphigus vulgaris
    - Pemphigus vegetans
    - Familial benign chronic pemphigus
    - Darier's disease

    ii. Non-acantholytic lesions (results from hydropic degeneration of a group of keratinocytes)
    - Herpes simplex
    - Herpes zoster
    - Herpangina
    - Hand, foot and mouth disease

    (b) Ulcers resulting from sub-epithelial vesicles
    i. Bullous pemphigoid
    ii. Mucous membrane pemphigoid
    iii. Erythema multiforme
    iv. Bullous lichen planus
    v. Epidermolysis bullosa
    vi. Drug eruptions

22.2.2 Etiologic classification of ulcers

Ulcers and erosions can be the final common manifestation of many conditions ranging from epithelial damage resulting from an immunological attack – as in pemphigus, pemphigoid, lichen planus – to damage because of an immune defect as in HIV disease and leukemia, infections as in herpes viruses, tuberculosis and syphilis, or nutritional defects such as in vitamin deficiencies and some intestinal disease.

Main causes of mouth ulcers

1. Physical causes (reactive ulcers):
   - Trauma:
     * Sharp teeth or restorations
     * Appliances
     * Non-accidental injury
     * Self-inflicted
   - Burns:
     * Heat
     * Cold
   - Chemical
   - Radiation
   - Electric
2. Microbial disease:
   (a) Viral
   - Herpes simplex infection
   - Varicella-Zoster infection
   - Hand, foot and mouth disease
   - Herpangina

- Measles
- Infectious mononucleosis
- HIV

(b) Bacterial
- Acute necrotizing gingivitis
- Noma
- Tuberculosis
- Leprosy
- Syphilis

(c) Fungal
- Histoplasmosis
- Cryptococcosis
- Blastomycosis
- Paracoccidioidomycosis

(d) Parasitic
- Leishmaniasis

3. Neoplasms:
   - Squamous cell carcinoma
   - Basal cell carcinoma

4. Drugs:
   - Cytotoxic drugs
   - NSAIDs

5. Immunological disorders:
   - Recurrent aphthae
   - Beh'et syndrome
   - Reiter syndrome
   - Lichen planus

- Pemphigus vulgaris
- Pemphigoid and variants
- Erythema multiforme
- Epidermolysis bullosa
- Lupus erythematosus

6. Genodermatosis:
   - Epidermolysis bullosa
7. Blood disorders:
   - Anemia
   - Leukemia
   - Neutropenia
8. Gastrointestinal disease:
   - Celiac disease
   - Crohn's disease
   - Ulcerative colitis
9. Disorders of uncertain pathogenesis:
   - Eosinophilic ulcer
   - Wegener's granulomatosis
   - Nasopharyngeal T-cell lymphoma
   - Necrotizing sialometaplasia

22.3 Ulcers due to Physical Injury

Traumatic Ulcers

- Trauma from bites or from dentures and orthodontic appliances is common.

- Self-induced lesions due to lip-biting after a local anesthetic injection.
- Cheek-biting (a neurotic habit).
- Rarer causes include ulceration of the lingual frenum caused by repeated coughing.
- Other local causes include burns from heat or cold, chemicals, electrical injury or irradiation.

Clinical Features

- Usually a single ulcer is seen, with an obvious cause (e.g. a denture flange).
- The patient is otherwise healthy.
- There may be a small degree of ipsilateral cervical lymph node enlargement.
- Chronic irritation may cause hyperplasia or hyperkeratosis of the adjacent mucosa, but induration should raise the suspicion of malignancy.

Management

- Remove etiological factors and prescribe a chlorhexidine 0.2% mouthwash.
- Maintenance of good oral hygiene and the use of benzydamine or hot saline mouth wash may help.
- Most ulcers of local cause heal spontaneously in about 1 week if the cause is removed and such supportive care given.
- Biopsy is needed if there is any suspicion of malignancy (see below) or if the ulcer does not heal within 3 weeks after removal of the cause.

22.4 Ulcers due to Infectious Agents

Infective causes of mouth ulcers include mainly viral infections, especially the herpes viruses. Other viruses that may cause mouth ulcers include Coxsackie and HIV viruses. Bacterial causes of mouth ulcers are less common, apart from acute necrotizing (ulcerative) gingivitis. Syphilis, either the primary or secondary stages, or tuberculosis are uncommon in the developed world at present but are increasing, especially in HIV/AIDS. Fungal causes of ulcers are increasingly seen in immunocompromised persons and travelers. Protozoal causes of ulcers, such as leishmaniasis, are seen in some geographic areas and in HIV/AIDS.

22.5 Ulcers of Neoplastic Lesions

A range of neoplasms may present with ulcers, most commonly these are carcinomas but Kaposi sarcoma, lymphomas and other neoplasms may be seen (see Chapter "Malignant Non-Odontogenic Tumors", page (311).

22.6 Ulcers due to Drugs

(stomatitis medicamentosa)

A wide spectrum of drugs can occasionally cause mouth lesions, by various mechanisms. Ulcers are common in those treated with cytotoxic drugs. The more common examples of drug reactions include:

- Cytotoxic agents, particularly methotrexate.
- Agents producing lichen-planus-like (lichenoid) lesions, such as non-steroidal anti-inflammatory agents, some antihypertensives, antidiabetics, gold salts, antimalarials and other drugs.

- Agents causing local chemical burns (especially aspirin held in the mouth).
- Agents causing erythema multiforme (especially sulfonamides and barbiturates).
- Other drug reactions are uncommon or rare.

22.7 Ulcers of Immunological disorders:

22.7.1 Recurrent Aphthous Stomatitis

(RAS, aphthous ulcer, canker sore)

Definition

- The term aphtha means ulcer. Aphthous ulcers are recurrent ulcers which typically start in young age and are unassociated with systemic disease.
- Recurrent aphthous stomatitis is one of the most common oral mucosal diseases.
- **Prevalence:** Are the most common oral ulcers affecting 5–60% of the population.
- **Age:** Children and young adults.
- **Gender:** Females are affected more than males.

Classification

1. Minor aphthous ulcers (Mikulicz's aphthae)
   Minor aphthous ulcers indicate that the lesion size is between 3–10 mm
2. Major aphthous ulcers

Major aphthous ulcers have the same appearance as minor ulcerations, but are greater than 10 mm in diameter and are extremely painful

3. Herptiform ulcers

Characterized by small, numerous, 1–3 mm lesions that form clusters similar to that of herpes infection.

Etiology

The exact etiology is unknown, however, the following points have been proposed:

- Familial and genetic basis: Approximately 40% of patients with RAS have a familial history, but inheritance may be polygenic with penetrance dependent on other factors.
- Immunological dysregulation with immunological reactivity to unidentified antigens, possibly microbial, such as cross-reacting antigens between the oral mucosa and Streptococcus sanguis or its L form, or heat-shock protein. Cell-mediated immune mechanisms appear to be involved in the pathogenesis: helper T-cells predominate early on, with some natural killer cells. Cytotoxic cells then appear and there is evidence for an antibody-dependent cellular cytotoxicity.
- Hematinic deficiencies (e.g. iron, folic acid, vitamin B-12) in 20% of patients.
- Various microorganisms have been examined for a causal association. ***Helicobacter pylori*** has been detected in lesional tissue of ill-defined oral ulcers, but the frequency of serum immunoglobin G (IgG) antibodies to H pylori is not increased in RAS.
- Little evidence suggests an etiologic association between viruses and RAS. Human herpesviruses (HHV)-6 and HHV-7 DNA have not been

demonstrated in RAS, but HHV-8 DNA is present in HIV-related oral ulcers.

- Dietary deficiency e.g. zinc was also proposed.
- Stress, trauma, various foods (nuts, chocolate, potato crisps) and cessation of tobacco smoking.
- Some women have RAS clearly related to the late phase of the menstrual cycle, and regress in pregnancy.
- Ulcers similar to aphthae (aphthous-like ulcers) are also seen in other conditions.
- An increased incidence of aphthous-like ulcerations has been reported in a variety of systemic disorders. These are:
  - ★ Behçet syndrome
  - ★ Celiac disease
  - ★ Cyclic neutropenia
  - ★ Nutritional deficiencies (iron, folate, zinc, B 1 , B 2 , B 6 , and B 12)
  - ★ Immunoglobulin A (IgA) deficiency
  - ★ Immunocompromised conditions, including human immunodeficiency virus (HIV) disease
  - ★ Inflammatory bowel disease

Clinical Features

Their clinical features differ according to types, (see table 22.1 for the clinical criteria of aphthous ulcers).

Minor Aphthae (Mikulicz's aphthae) are:

- Small, 2–4 mm in diameter
- Ovoid or rounded

Table 22.1: Key Features of Aphthae (Recurrent Aphthous Stomatitis (RAS)).

> **Always Remember**
>
> **Etiology**
> - Not well understood
> - Many Factors: autoimmune, viral, bacterial, hormonal, diet, hereditary background
>
> **Clinical Features**
> - Typically early onset with recurrent ulcers usually lasting 1 week to 1 month.
> - Incidence: Up to 20% of population.
> - Three distinct clinical patterns:
>   1. Minor - small ulcers (<4 mm) on mobile mucosae, healing within 14 days, no scarring.
>   2. Major - large ulcers (may be >1 cm), any site including dorsum of tongue and hard palate, healing within 1-3 months, with scarring.
>   3. Herpetiform ulcers-multiple minute ulcers that coalesce to produce ragged ulcers.
>
> **Management**
> - Diagnosed from history and clinical features.
> - No diagnostic test of value.
> - A blood picture is useful to exclude possible deficiencies and coeliac disease.
> - Treat any underlying predisposing factors
> - Treat aphthae with chlorhexidine aqueous mouthwash or topical corticosteroids.

- Have a yellowish depressed floor
- Have a pronounced red inflammatory halo
- The ulcers are typically painful
- Last 7–10 days
- May occur anywhere in the oral cavity and the oropharynx
- Tend *not* to be seen on gingiva, palate or dorsum of tongue
- Heal with no obvious scarring
- Most patients develop not more than six ulcers at any single episode.

Major Aphthae (Sutton's ulcers)

- Are less common, much larger, and more persistent than minor aphthae, and can affect the soft palate and dorsum of tongue as well as other sites. Sometimes termed periadenitis mucosa necrotica recurrens (PMNR),
- Can exceed 1 cm in diameter
- Are most common on the palate, fauces and lips,
- Can take months to heal
- May leave scars on healing
- At any one episode there are usually fewer than six ulcers present.

Herpetiform Ulcers

- Herpetiform ulcers clinically resemble herpetic stomatitis.
- Start as multiple pinpoint aphthae
- Enlarge and fuse to produce irregular ulcers
- Can be seen on any mucosa, but especially on the tongue ventrum.

Investigations

- There is no specific diagnostic test of value.
- Rarely, biopsy may be indicated to establish definitive diagnosis.

Histologically

- Ulcer covered by fibrinous exudate infiltrated by PNL overlying granulation tissue with dilated capillaries and edema.
- When fibroblastic repair reaction starts, scarring become apparent clinically.

Treatment

- Numerous therapies have been tried for recurrent aphthous stomatitis, most with only minimal success.
- The majority of aphthous ulcers heals within 10 to 14 days and requires no treatment;
- However, patients with severe symptoms may require medical intervention.
- Temporary pain relief can be obtained with topical anesthetic agents (e.g. viscous lidocaine).
- Tetracycline oral suspension and antiseptic mouthwashes have also been used, with varying success.
- Topical steroids are the main line of therapy and may shorten the duration of the ulcers if applied during the early phase. These agents may be applied either in a solution (e.g., dexamethasone oral suspension, 0.5 mg/5 ml) or in an ointment (e. g. fluocinolone or clobetasol). Ointments work much better in the oral cavity than creams or gels do.

- Systemic steroids are indicated when the number of ulcers is large or when the outbreak has persisted for a long time.
- Good oral hygiene should be maintained; chlorhexidine or triclosan mouthwashes help achieve this and may help reduce ulcer duration.

Prognosis

The natural history is of spontaneous resolution with age.

22.7.2 Behçet's Syndrome (Behçet's Disease)

- Behcet's Syndrome consists *essentially* of a triad of:
    1. Multiple aphthous ulcers
    2. Genital ulcers
    3. Uveitis
- This rare condition affects mainly young adult males and is most common in people from the Middle East, Japan, China and Korea.

Etiology

- An immunogenetic basis, with a specific association with HLA genetic type HLA-B5101.
- Immunological changes are like those in aphthae.
- The precipitating factor is unknown but may be *Streptococcus sanguis*.
- There appears to be a subset of T cells which react to an immunostimulatory human heat shock protein with cross-reactivity to streptococci, and produce tumor necrosis factor (TNF) and interleukin 8 (IL-8).
- The interleukin leads to the chemo-attraction of neutrophils, which are also hyperactive and release superoxide, leading to vasculitis.

Clinical Features

Behçet's syndrome is a multisystem disease affecting the mouth in most cases and many other sites including, commonly:

- Genitals: Ulcers resembling oral aphthae.
- Eyes: Uveitis is one of the more important ocular lesions and visual acuity is often impaired.
- Skin: Erythema nodosum (painful red lumps on the shins), various rashes may develop as well as pustules at the site of venepuncture[1] (*pathergy*[2]).
- Pathergy is seen with both Behçet's disease and pyoderma gangrenosum[3]. A highly similar phenomenon known as the **Koebner phenomenon** occurs in autoimmune diseases such as psoriasis, (page 591) and systemic lupus erythematosus, (page 589).
- Pathergy may be helpful in the diagnosis of Behçet's disease by attempting to induce a pathergy reaction with a test known as a "Skin Prick Test".
- Joints: large joint arthropathy is not uncommon.
- Neurological system: headache, psychiatric, motor or sensory manifestations.
- Vascular system: thrombosis of large veins may be life-threatening.

Diagnosis

- Behçet's syndrome is a clinical diagnosis, the cardinal features being oral and genital ulceration, uveitis and erythema nodosum.

---

[1] the puncture of a vein as part of a medical procedure, typically to withdraw a blood sample or for an intravenous injection.

[2] Pathergy is a skin condition in which a minor trauma, hapten or antigen leads to the development of skin lesions or ulcers that may be resistant to healing.

[3] Pyoderma gangrenosum is a rare, non-infectious inflammatory skin disease where painful pustules or nodules become ulcers that progressively enlarge.

- Other causes of this group of lesions, such as ulcerative colitis, Crohn's disease, mixed connective tissue disease, lupus erythematosus and Reiter's syndrome, must be excluded.

Diagnostic criteria for Behcet's syndrome are not completely agreed but include:

- Recurrent oral ulcerations, plus two or more of the following:
    1. Recurrent genital ulceration
    2. Eye lesions
    3. Skin lesions
    4. Positive pathergy test (when a needle containing saline is inserted subcutaneously in the skin of the forearm, a positive pathergy test is elicited when an indurated pustule forms within 48–72 hours).

Treatment

- Oral ulcers are treated as for aphthae.
- Systemic manifestations require immunosuppression using, corticosteroids, colchicines or thalidomide.

22.7.3 Reiter's Syndrome

- A disease of unknown etiology characterized by a triad of:
    1. Urethritis (non-gonococcal urethritis, usually due to chlamydial infection)
    2. Arthritis
    3. Conjunctivitis

- Oral lesions consist of red macules with whitish raised borders which may ulcerate to produce aphthous-like ulcers. On the tongue the lesions are similar to that of geographic tongue.
- **Histologically**, the lesions are similar to psoriasis.
- **Mucocutaneous-ocular syndromes** are syndromes characterized by simultaneous involvement of the skin, oral mucosa and the eyes. These include:
    1. Behcet's syndrome
    2. Reiter's syndrome
    3. Steven Johnson's syndrome

22.8 Ulcers of Genodermatosis

22.8.1 Epidermolysis bullosa

Was discussed in the chapter "Developmental Disturbances of Oral & Para-Oral Tissues", page (77)

22.9 Ulcers due to Blood Disorders

- Hematological disease can cause ulcers. Mouth ulcers may be seen in leukemias.
- Oral features may include purpura, gingival bleeding, lymphadenopathy, recurrent herpes labialis and candidiasis.

22.10 Ulcers of Gastrointestinal Tract Diseases

22.10.1 Celiac Disease

A disease occurring in children and adults characterized by sensitivity to wheat gluten, with chronic inflammation and atrophy of the mucosa of the upper small intestine; manifestations include diarrhea, malabsorption, steatorrhea, and nutritional and vitamin deficiencies. Oral manifestations are similar to that of pernicious anemia.

22.10.2 Ulcerative Colitis

A chronic disease of unknown cause characterized by ulceration of the colon and rectum, with rectal bleeding, mucosal crypt abscesses, inflammatory pseudopolyps, abdominal pain, and diarrhea; frequently causes anemia, hypoproteinemia, and electrolyte imbalance, and is less frequently complicated by peritonitis, or carcinoma of the colon.

22.10.3 Crohn's Disease

See orofacial granulomatosis in chapter "Infections of the Oral and Para-Oral Tissues", page (522).

22.11 Ulcers of uncertain pathogenesis

22.11.1 Eosinophilic Ulcer

(atypical or traumatic eosinophilic granuloma)

Definition: This is a tumor-like ulcerative lesion with a microscopic picture similar to that of Langerhans cell histiocytosis.

Etiology: Although, the etiology remains unknown, history of trauma is reported in some cases.

Clinically, appears as an ulcerated mass which could be mistaken for carcinoma but is typically soft. The most common site is the tongue and the gingiva.

Histologically, there is a dense aggregation of *eosinophils* and cells which resemble histiocytes. The histiocytes lack the ultrastructural features and surface markers of Langerhans cells.

Differential diagnosis: From Langerhans cell histiocytosis which can be excluded by the absence of Langerhans cell markers.

Treatment: Lesions usually heal spontaneously within 3–8 weeks.

22.11.2 Lethal midline granuloma syndrome

Lethal midline granuloma syndrome may result from either Wagener's granulomatosis or nasopharyngeal T-cell or NK-cell lymphomas. In their early stages, they are clinically similar. Both conditions produce sever destruction of the middle face and a fatal outcome.

22.11.3 Wegener's granulomatosis

Comprises the triad of granulomatous inflammation of the *nasal* region, *pulmonary* and *renal* involvement. It is associated with production of **antineutrophil cytoplasmic antibodies** (ANCAs) which are useful in diagnosis.

Etiology

Unknown, infection and immune dysfunction were postulated but not proven.

Clinically

- **Sex:** Men appear to be more frequently affected
- **Age:** Between 40 and 55 years. The disease has rarely also been seen in children.
- **Clinical features:**
  * Early features consist of granulomatous inflammation of the nasal cavity.
  * Later, destruction of the nasal septum can lead to a *saddle nose* deformity.
  * An occasional feature is a distinctive and proliferative gingivitis with a granular surface and deep red in color that has been described as "*strawberry gums*".
  * This can form the earliest clinical manifestation of the disease. A few or many teeth may be involved. This form of gingivitis, after confirmation by biopsy, can allow treatment to be started at an unusually early stage.
  * Mucosal ulcers may develop in the later stages and may dominate the picture.
  * Unlike the palatal ulceration that may result from a nasopharyngeal lymphoma, the ulcers of Wegener's granulomatosis can be large, superficial, and widely distributed. Cervical lymphadenopathy may be associated.

Microscopy:

- Inflammation with a mixed cellular picture and, frequently, numerous *eosinophils.*
- An essential feature is necrotizing vasculitis of small arteries, associated with multinucleated giant cells.
- The giant cells are involved in the vasculitis but are as frequently found in the adjacent tissues. They are typically compact with four or five nuclei but may resemble *Langhans giant cells.*
- Although Granulomas are characteristic of this disease, they are inconspicuous, usually difficult to find, and rarely seen in oral biopsies.
- Foci of necrosis and microabscesses.
- Biopsies of gingival lesions typically show only the giant cells and are unlikely to show vasculitis since arteries of sufficient size are unlikely to be included. However, gingival tissues show superficial proliferation throwing the epithelium up into folds which produce the granulomatous appearance seen clinically.

Behavior and management

- Early recognition of Wegener's granulomatosis is essential as it can be rapidly fatal.
- Occasionally, it can be recognized early by the gingival lesions which precede systemic disease and can permit exceptionally early treatment.
- Later manifestations are typically pulmonary cavitation and renal disease, which is the main cause of death.
- Joint pains are common and rashes are sometimes a feature.
- The diagnosis must be established by biopsy at the earliest possible moment and detection of ANCAs is helpful.

- ANCAs show fine granular cytoplasmic fluorescence and are present in approximately 85%.
- Staining for classical antineutrophil cytoplasmic antibodies (cANCA) is more strongly positive in Wegener's granulomatosis.
- Staining for perinuclear antineutrophil cytoplasmic antibodies (pANCA) is positive in all of these, apart from classical polyarteritis nodosa where it is weak. They are valuable for distinguishing Wegener's granulomatosis from nasopharyngeal lymphoma when it presents a similar clinical picture.
- Though ANCAs are not specific to Wegener's granulomatosis, its clinical picture is quite different from that of other types of vasculitis.
- Examination of the nasopharynx, chest radiographs, and renal function tests should also be carried out.
- Hematuria is likely to indicate glomerulonephritis and a poor prognosis.
- Early treatment is usually with *prednisolone* plus *cytotoxic* drugs such as cyclophosphamide or azathioprine.
- Arrest of the disease with co-trimoxazole has been reported on several occasions but remains a controversial.

22.11.4 Nasopharyngeal T-cell lymphomas

Nasopharyngeal (T-cell and NK-cell) lymphomas

- These are rare cause of midline granuloma syndrome. In their early stages they can be indistinguishable clinically from Wagner's granulomatosis.
- Constant association with **Epstein-Barr virus** have been reported.
- Extension of the disease through the palate can cause swelling and ulceration as a presenting feature. Small ulcer may extend until the whole

of the palate becomes necrotic. A deep biopsy is necessary to obtain lesional tissue not obscured by necrosis.

- Histological diagnosis is difficult as these lymphomas are cellularly pleomorphic. They attack blood vessels and thus simulate vasculitis. Secondary inflammation may also obscure the lymphoma cells, so that several biopsies may be required.
- Death may result from dissemination of lymphoma but this may be delayed by radiotherapy.

22.12   Guide Lines in the Diagnosis of Ulcers

- The most important feature of ulceration is whether the ulcer is persistent, since this may indicate that the ulcer is caused by:
    * Neoplasia such as carcinoma
    * Chronic trauma
    * Chronic skin disease such as pemphigus
    * Chronic infection such as syphilis, tuberculosis or mycosis.
- An important feature is whether one or more than one ulcer is present, since malignant tumors usually cause a single lesion.
- A single ulcer persisting for more than 3 weeks without signs of obvious healing must be taken seriously, as it could be a neoplasm.
- Multiple persistent ulcers are mainly caused by:
    * Skin diseases, such as pemphigus, pemphigoid or lichen planus
    * Gastrointestinal disease
    * Immune defect.
- Multiple non-persistent ulcers can be caused by aphthae, when the ulcers heal spontaneously, usually within 1 week to 1 month. If this is not the case, an alternative diagnosis should be considered.

- Erosions or ulcers on both sides at the commissures of the lips are usually angular stomatitis (cheilitis), but sores are also sometimes caused at the angles by trauma (such as dental treatment) or infection (such as recurrent herpes labialis).
- Making a diagnosis of the cause for oral soreness or ulceration is based mainly on the history and clinical features. The number, persistence, shape, character of the edge of the ulcer and the appearance of the ulcer base should also be noted. Ulcers should always be examined for induration (firmness on palpation), which may be indicative of malignancy. Unless the cause is undoubtedly local, general physical examination is also indicated, looking especially for mucocutaneous lesions, lymphadenopathy or fever.
- Features that might suggest a systemic background to mouth ulcers include:
  - Extra-oral features such as:
    - Skin lesions
    - Ocular lesions
    - Anogenital lesions
    - Purpura
    - Fever
    - Lymphadenopathy
    - Hepatomegaly
    - Splenomegaly
    - chronic cough
    - gastrointestinal complaints (e.g. pain, altered bowel habits, blood in feces)
    - loss of weight or, in children, a failure to thrive
    - weakness

- ★ An atypical history or ulcer behavior such as:
  - ∗ onset of ulcers in later adult life
  - ∗ exacerbation of ulcers
  - ∗ severe aphthae
  - ∗ aphthae unresponsive to topical hydrocortisone or triamcinolone
- ★ Other oral lesions, especially:
  - ∗ candidiasis
  - ∗ herpetic lesions
  - ∗ glossitis
  - ∗ petechiae
  - ∗ gingival bleeding
  - ∗ gingival swelling
  - ∗ necrotizing gingivitis or periodontitis
  - ∗ hairy leukoplakia
  - ∗ Kaposi sarcoma.

22.13   Management of Oral Ulcers

- Treat the underlying cause.
- Remove etiological factors.
- Ensure any possible traumatic element is removed (e.g. a denture flange).
- Prescribe a chlorhexidine 0.2% aqueous mouthwash.
- Maintain good oral hygiene.
- A benzydamine mouthwash or spray may help ease discomfort.

- Topical corticosteroids are useful in the management of many oral ulcerative conditions where there is no systemic involvement, such as recurrent aphthous stomatitis and oral lichen planus.
- Creams, gels and inhalers are better than ointments since the latter adhere poorly to the mucosa. However, creams can be bitter and gels can irritate.
- Patients should not eat or drink for 30 minutes after using the steroid, in order to prolong contact with the lesion.
- Adverse effects are important mainly with systemic steroids. With many topical steroids there is little systemic absorption and thus no significant adrenocortical suppression. In patients using potent topical steroids for more than a month it is prudent to add an antifungal, since candidiasis may arise.

Chapter 23
Brown and Black Pigmented Lesions

Most of the lesions to be mentioned here have been discussed in their relevant chapters and the reader is advised to refer to these chapters for further details. Lesions mentioned for the first time are discussed in more detail.

23.1 Overview

Classification of Brown or Black Pigmented Lesions

1. Physiologic Pigmentation
2. Developmental Pigmentation
3. Neoplastic Pigmentation
4. Hormonal Pigmentation
5. Skin Diseases
6. Miscellaneous conditions

23.2 Physiologic Pigmentation

23.2.1 Racial Pigmentation (Oral Melanosis)

This is brown or black pigmentation occurring in dark skinned people, usually affecting the gingiva but the inner aspect of lips is typically spared.

23.2.2 Melasma (Mask of Pregnancy)

- Melasma is an acquired pigmentation, commonly seen in pregnancy and in women taking contraceptive pills.
- Melasma usually disappears several months after delivery.

23.3 Developmental Pigmentation

23.3.1 Incontinentia pigmenti

(*Bloch-Sulzberger syndrome*)

- An X-linked dominant genetic disorder that affects the skin, hair, teeth, nails and central nervous system. It is named from its appearance under a microscope.
- The name incontinentia pigmenti is derived from the histological characteristics of the disease, that is, melanin incontinence by melanocytes in the basal epidermal layer.
- The disease is usually lethal in males.
- Skin manifestations include blistering, vesicles, bullae and melanin pigmentation.

- Dental manifestations include hypodontia, microdontia and retarded eruption of teeth.

23.3.2 Peutz-Jeghers syndrome

Refer to chapter "Developmental Disturbances of Oral & Para-Oral Tissues", page (on page 70).

23.3.3 Xeroderma Pigmentosa

Refer to the chapter "Developmental Disturbances of Oral & Para-Oral Tissues", page (on page 70).

23.3.4 Polystotic fibrous dysplasia

Refer to the chapter "Bone Diseases", page (446).

23.4 Neoplastic

23.4.1 Pigmented nevi

Refer to the chapter "Benign Non-Odontogenic Tumors & Tumor-Like Lesions" (on page 273).

23.4.2 Multiple neurofibromatosis (Von Recklinghausen disease of skin)

Refer to the chapter "Benign Non-Odontogenic Tumors & Tumor-Like Lesions" (on page 285).

23.4.3 Malignant melanomas

Refer to the chapter "Malignant Non-Odontogenic Tumors" (on page 345).

23.5 Hormonal Pigmentation

23.5.1 Addison's disease (adrenal cortex insufficiency)

- Addison's disease (also chronic adrenal insufficiency, hypocortisolism, and hypoadrenalism) is a rare, chronic endocrine disorder in which the adrenal glands do not produce sufficient steroid hormones (glucocorticoids and often mineralocorticoids).
- It is characterized by a number of relatively nonspecific symptoms, such as abdominal pain and weakness, but under certain circumstances, these may progress to Addisonian crisis, a severe illness which may include very low blood pressure and coma.

23.5.2 Hyperpituitarism

particularly Cushing disease which is usually due to pituitary gland adenoma resulting in increased ACTH that stimulates adrenal cortex.

23.6 Skin Diseases

23.6.1 Lichen Planus

Melanin pigmentation may be associated with some cases of lichen planus.

23.6.2 Freckles (Ephelides)

- Ephelides represent an increase in melanin synthesis by melanocytes, without an increase in their number.
- On the skin, this increased melanogenesis can be attributed to sun ray exposure.
- Ephelides can therefore be encountered on the vermilion border of the lips, with the lower lip being the favored site since it tends to receive more solar exposure than the upper lip.
- The lesion is macular and ranges from being tiny small to over a centimeter in diameter. Some patients report a prior episode of trauma to the area.
- Lip ephelides are asymptomatic and occur equally in men and women. They are rarely seen in children.
- **Microscopically:** The basal cells contain numerous melanin pigment granules without proliferation of melanocytes. Melanin incontinence into the submucosa is commonly seen. Rarely, melanin-containing dendritic cells are seen to extend high into a thickened spinous layer. Lesions of this nature are diagnosed as melanoacanthoma. To differentiate between melanocytes and pigmented basal cells, DOPA staining is performed, melanocytes are DOPA positive while other pigmented cells are DOPA negative.
- No treatment is required. Sun avoidance or use of sun protectors is indicated.
- The intraoral counterpart to the ephelis is the *oral melanotic macule* (see later in this chapter).

23.7 Miscellaneous conditions

23.7.1 Amalgam Tattoo

Fragments of amalgam frequently become embedded in the oral mucosa and forms the most common pigmented lesions which may simulate melanomas. Most of theses amalgam lesions appear radiopaque.

23.7.2 Graphite Tattoo

Graphite tattoos tend to occur on the palate and represent traumatic implantation from a lead pencil. The lesions are usually macular, and gray or black.

23.7.3 Drug-induced pigmentation

- Tetracycline associated pigmentation may be found after treatment with prolonged high doses of minocycline.
- Pigmentation is thought to be due to increased melanin production or as a result of formation of drug complexes in melanocytes.

23.7.4 Heavy metal pigmentation

- Some heavy metals (lead, mercury, arsenic and bismuth) may be responsible for oral pigmentation.
- This phenomenon occurs usually after occupational exposure to vapors of these metals.
- These heavy metals may be deposited in both skin and oral mucosa especially in the gingiva.

- The characteristic color is *grey to black* and the distribution is linear when found along the gingival margins. The intensity of the staining is proportional to the degree of gingival inflammation and appears to be a result of the reaction of the heavy metal with bacterially produced hydrogen sulfide in the inflammatory zones.

23.7.5 Black hairy tongue

Refer to the chapter "Developmental Disturbances of Oral & Para-Oral Tissues" (on page 86).

23.7.6 Acanthosis nigricans

- An eruption of warty growths associated with hyperpigmentation occurring in the skin of the axillae, neck, anogenital area, groin, and around the mouth
- In adults, may be associated with internal malignancy, endocrine disorders, or obesity; a benign (juvenile) type occurs in children.
- The exact etiology is not known, it is speculated that some tumor cells can secrete peptides acting as melanocyte stimulating hormone.

23.7.7 Oral Melanotic Macules

(Focal Melanosis)

Definition

- The term melanotic macule has been used to describe a benign pigmented lesion of the oral cavity, characterized by an increase in melanin

- pigmentation along the basal cell layer of the epithelium and the lamina propria.
- In the literature, the oral melanotic macule has been given various perplexing, such as ephelis and lentigo.
- **Ephelis** (*freckle*) is a circumscribed brown macule over skin that has been exposed to sunlight.
- Histologically, ephelis shows increased melanin pigmentation in the basal-cell layer *without* an increase in the number of melanocytes.
- Ephelides are not found on mucous membranes. Although the histologic appearance of the melanotic macule of the oral mucosa is similar to that of ephelis of the skin.
- It is not at all related to exposure to sun and thus the term ephelis for the intraoral lesion is a misnomer.
- The term *lentigo* has also been suggested for oral melanotic macules. But since melanotic macules of the oral mucosa do not exhibit a significant increase in the number of melanocytes, the term lentigo is not considered appropriate for this type of lesion.

Etiology

- The exact etiology is unknown.
- Postinflammatory or posttraumatic causes was proposed.
- Oral melanotic macules may be associated with HIV infection and may be seen in up to 6% of AIDS patients.
- Also the condition may occurs in some other disorders such as Addison's disease, Peutz-Jeghers syndrome, or Laugier-Hunziker syndrome.

Clinically

- Labial melanotic macules most often are seen in childhood and the 20 to 30 years age.
- The intraoral lesions usually occur in patients older than 40.
- More commonly found in women.
- The melanotic macule is typically a well circumscribed flat area of pigmentation that may be brown, black, blue or grey in color. Most of the lesions are less than 1 cm in diameter, although in occasional cases they may be larger in size.
- The oral melanotic macule is usually located on the vermilion border of the lips and termed as the *labial melanotic macule*.
- Intraorally, it may be found on the gingiva, buccal mucosa or the palate and is termed as the *oral melanotic macule*.

Histopathology

- Histologically there is excess melanin pigmentation in the basal cell layer and in the upper part of the lamina propria.
- Regarding histopathology, the dark color of the lesion is due to increase in melanin pigment of the basal cell layer, not from an increased number of melanocytes.
- Melanin may also be found in the lamina propria.

Treatment

- Surgical excision.
- Biopsy to rule out the possibility of an early malignant melanoma.

REFERENCES

[1] Witkop C. Amelogenesis imperfecta, dentinogenesis imperfecta and dentin dysplasia revisited: problems in classification. Journal of Oral Pathology & Medicine. 1988;17(9-10):547–553.

[2] Neville BW, Damm DD, Allen CM, Chi AC. Oral and maxillofacial pathology. Elsevier Health Sciences; 2015.

[3] Shear M, Speight P. Cysts of the oral and maxillofacial regions. Wiley-Blackwell; 2008.

[4] Argyris PP, Wetzel SL, Pambuccian SE, Gopalakrishnan R, Koutlas IG. Primordial Odontogenic Cyst with Induction Phenomenon (Zonal Fibroblastic Hypercellularity) and Dentinoid Material Versus Archegonous Cystic Odontoma: You Choose! Head and neck pathology. 2016;10(2):237–244.

[5] Levison D, Reid R. Muir's Textbook of Pathology. 14th ed. Levison D, Reid R, Fleming S, Harrison D, Burt A, editors. Hodder Arnold Publication; 2008.

[6] Anneroth G, Batsakis J, Luna M. Review of the literature and a recommended system of malignancy grading in oral squamous cell carcinomas. Scand Dent Res. 1987;7;95:229–249.

[7] DeLong L, Burkhart N. General and oral pathology for the dental hygienist. LWW; 2013.

[8] El-Khoury J, Kibbi AG, Abbas O. Mucocutaneous pseudoepitheliomatous hyperplasia: a review. Am J Dermatopathol. 2012 Apr;34(2):165–175. Available from: http://dx.doi.org/10.1097/DAD.0b013e31821816ab.

[9] Eversole L. Contemporary Oral and Maxillofacial Pathology. St. Louis: Mosby; 2004.

[10] Eversole L. Clinical outline of oral pathology: diagnosis and treatment. Pmph Bc Decker; 2002.

[11] M CD, Fletcher CD. Diagnostic histopathology of tumors. 4th ed. Elsevier, Saunders; 2013.

[12] Langlais R. Color Atlas of Common Oral Diseases. Hagerstwon: Lippincott Williams & Wilkins; 2009.

[13] Langland OE, Langlais RP, Preece JW. Principles of dental imaging. Lippincott Williams & Wilkins; 2002.

[14] López de Blanc S, Sambuelli R, Femopase F, Luna N, Gravotta M, David D, et al. Bacillary angiomatosis affecting the oral cavity. Report of two cases and review. J Oral Pathol Med. 2000 Feb;29(2):91–96.

[15] MacDonald-Jankowski DS. Fibro-osseous lesions of the face and jaws. Clin Radiol. 2004 Jan;59(1):11–25.

[16] Marx RE, Stern D. Oral and Maxillofacial Pathology: A Rationale for Diagnosis and Treatment. Quintessence Publishing Company; 2012. Available from: http://books.google.com.sa/books?id=mCk5ywAACAAJ.

[17] Pogrel A. The diagnosis and management of giant cell lesions of the jaws. Annals of Maxillofacial Surgery. 2012;2(2):102–106. Available from: http://www.amsjournal.com/article.asp?issn=2231-0746;year=2012;volume=2;issue=2;spage=102;epage=106;aulast=Pogrel;t=6.

[18] Regezi J. Oral Pathology. Philadelphia: Saunders; 2007.

[19] Scully C. Oral Medicine and Pathology at a Glance. Wiley-Blackwell; 2010.

[20] Southam JV, Soames JC. Oral Pathology. Oxford shire: Oxford University Press; 2005.

[21] Zayour M, Lazova R. Pseudoepitheliomatous hyperplasia: a review. Am J Dermatopathol. 2011 Apr;33(2):112–22; quiz 123–6. Available from: http://dx.doi.org/10.1097/DAD.0b013e3181fcfb47.

[22] Malik S, Singh V, Singh G, Dahiya N. Central Giant Cell Granuloma of the Mandible: A Rare Presentation. IJHNS, Jaypee. 2014;Available from: http://www.jaypeejournals.com/eJournals/ShowText.aspx?ID=3993&Type=FREE&TYP=TOP&IN=_eJournals/images/JPLOGO.gif&IID=313&isPDF=YES.

[23] Powers-Fletcher M. A review of the biology and the laboratory diagnosis of Treponema pallidum. Journal of Continuing Education Topics & Issues. 2011;13(3). Available from: http://www.freepatentsonline.com/article/Journal-Continuing-Education-Topics-Issues/268477987.html.

References

[24] Shah A, Latoo S, Ahmad I. Multiple Myeloma and Dentistry - An Overview. MULTIPLE MYELOMA–AN OVERVIEW. 2011;p. 207. Available from: http://cdn.intechopen.com/pdfs-wm/26509.pdf.

[25] Sharma NK, Singh AK, Pandey A, Verma V. Solitary plasmacytoma of the mandible: A rare case report. Natl J Maxillofac Surg. 2015;6(1):76–79. Available from: http://dx.doi.org/10.4103/0975-5950.168214.

[26] Southam JV, Soames JC. Oral Pathology. Oxford Oxford shire: Oxford University Press; 2005.

[27] Ibsen O, Phelan JA. Oral Pathology for the Dental Hygienist. Sixth ed. Elsevier Saunders; 2014.

[28] Rosen Y. photos pulmonary pathology; 2019. Available from: https://commons.wikimedia.org/w/index.php?curid=17387675.

[29] Nephron. Own work, CC BY-SA 3.0; 2019. Available from: https://commons.wikimedia.org/w/index.php?curid=7740036.

[30] Shetty SJ, Pereira T, Desai RS. Inflammatory myofibroblastic tumor of the oral cavity: A case report and literature review. Journal of cancer research and therapeutics. 2019;15:725–728. Available from: http://www.cancerjournal.net/text.asp?2019/15/3/725/244198.

[31] AlKindi MG. A rare case of inflammatory myofibroblastic tumor of the mandible mimicking a malignant tumor. The Saudi dental journal. 2017 Jan;29:36–40.

[32] Binmadi NO, Packman H, Papadimitriou JC, Scheper M. Oral inflammatory myofibroblastic tumor: case report and review of literature. The open dentistry journal. 2011 Apr;5:66–70. Available from: https://www.ncbi.nlm.nih.gov/pmc/articles/PMC3091292/.

[33] Balighi K, Azizpour A, Sadeghinia A, Saeidi V. A Case Report of Paraneoplastic Pemphigus Associated With Retroperitoneal Inflammatory Myofibroblastic Tumor. Acta medica Iranica. 2017 May;55:340–343.

[34] Odell EW. Cawson's Essentials of Oral Pathology and Oral Medicine. Elsevier Health Sciences; 2017.

[35] Kim SM. Definition and management of odontogenic maxillary sinusitis. Maxillofacial plastic and reconstructive surgery. 2019 Dec;41:13.

[36] Chiu A, Palmer J, Adappa N. Atlas of Endoscopic Sinus and Skull Base Surgery. Elsevier; 2018.

[37] Abdel-Azim, A M and Abdel-Azim, A A. Oral and Maxillofacial Pathology: Tips and Tricks. theWay; 2020. Available from: `https://dr-adel.site/`.

[38] Abdel-Azim, A M and Abdel-Azim, A A. Oral and Maxillofacial Pathology: A Study Guide. theWay; 2019. Available from: `https://dr-adel.site/`.

[39] National Academies of Sciences, Engineering, and Medicine. Temporomandibular Disorders: Priorities for Research and Care. The National Academies Press, Washington, DC; 2020. Available from: `https://doi.org/10.17226/25652`.

INDEX

A
aberrancy, 89
abfraction, 207
abrasion, 205
abscess, 223
    acute periapical, 162
    chronic periapical, 167
    periapical, 162
    periodontal, 508
acantholysis, 76, 584
acantholytic, 613
acantholytic cells, 76, 585
Acanthosis, 76
acanthosis nigricans, 645
achondroplasia, 456
acidogenic bacteria, 109
acinic cell adenocarcinoma, 437
acinic cell tumor, 437
acquired
    enamel hypoplasia, 30
    generalized enamel hypoplasia, 30
acquired enamel pellicle, 104, 112
actinic keratosis, 306, 607
actinomycosis, 519
acute necrotizing ulcerative gingivitis, 500
acute streptococcal gingivitis, 503
acute suppurative parotitis, 409
Addison's disease, 642
adenocystic carcinoma, 435
adenoid squamous cell carcinoma, 320
adenomatoid odontogenic tumor, 368
adult osteopetrosis, 453
aerodontalgia, 143
aglossia, 80
agnathia, 64
AIDS, 555
alleles, 2
alveolar osteitis, 464
amastigotes, 536

amelanotic melanoma, 347
ameloblastic carcinoma, 398
ameloblastic fibroma, 390
ameloblastic fibro-odontome, 393
ameloblastic fibrosarcoma, 401
ameloblastic odontome, 393
ameloblastoma, 357
amelodentinal junction, 32
amelogenesis imperfecta, 35
anachoresis, 142
ANCAs, 632
aneuploidy, 239
aneurysmal bone cyst, 196
angina
    Ludwig's, 166, 228, 506
    Vincent, 501
angiogenesis, 235
angiosarcoma, 342
angular cheilitis, 531
anhidrosis, 21
ankyloglossia, 81
ankylosis, 213, 217, 218
    bonny, 595
    fibrous, 595
    joint, 594
    TMJ, 472
    tooth, 218
anodontia
    false, 19
    true, 19

anthrax, 511
antimongoloid, 54
antineutrophil cytoplasmic antibodies, 630
antioncogenes, 242
antral mucocele, 201
antral pseudocyst, 200
ANUG, 500
aphthous
    major, 623
    minor, 621
aphthous stomatitis, 619
aplasia
    of mandible, 64
    salivary gland, 89
apoptosis, 242
apoptotic, 239
arrested caries, 100
Ascher syndrome, 66
aspergillus, 571
Aspergillus niger, 109
astroid bodies, 524
ataxia telangiectasia, 243
atresia, 89
attrition, 203
auriculotemporal syndrome, 412
Auspitz sign, 592
avulsion, 222
azathioprine, 633

Index

B

bacillary angiomatosis, 261
barodontalgia, 143
basal cell carcinoma, 323
basilar hyperplasia, 292
basket weave appearance, 74
beads, 121
Behcet's syndrome, 625
Bence Jones proteins, 338
benign cementoblastoma, 377
benign mucous membrane pemphigoid, 587
bifid tongue, 84
bilateral acoustic neurofibromatosis, 286
biofilm, 111
birthmarks, 281
bisphosphonates bone necrosis, 478
black tongue, 87
blepharochalasis, 66
Bloch-Sulzberger syndrome, 640
Bodansky unit, 462
Bohn's nodule, 181
Bohn's nodules, 91
borellia vincenti, 500
botryoid odontogenic cyst, 180
branchial cleft cyst, 199
BRCA1, 249
BRCA2, 249
Broder's classification, 313

Bruxism, 205
bruxism, 203
bullous pemphigoid, 587
Burkitt's lymphoma, 241, 336

C

Calcific Metamorphosis, 156
calcification
    defective, 33
    dentinogenesis imperfecta, 41
    dystrophic, 155, 156, 472
    pulp, 154
    regional odontodysplasia, 46
calcifying epithelial odontogenic cyst, 191
calcifying odontogenic cyst, 369
calcitriol, 95
calculus, 129
    sub-gingival, 129
    supra-gingival, 129
cANCA, 633
cancrum oris, 502
candida albicans, 296, 496, 526
candidiasis, 526
Cannon's disease, 73
capillary hemangioma, 281
Carabelli cusp, 26
carcinogenesis, 240
carcinoma in situ, 303
caries
    arrested, 100

cemental, 100
   hidden, 100
   pit and fissure, 99
   rampant or chronic, 100
   recurrent, 100
   residual, 100
   secondary, 100
   senile, 100
   smooth surface, 99
   white spot lesion, 100
cavernous hemangioma, 282
Cavernous Sinus Thrombosis, 230
celiac disease, 629
cell
   goblet, 567
cell nests, 292
cellular immortalization, 239
cellulitis, 223
cemental caries, 100
cementifying fibroma, 379
Cementoma
   True, 377
cemento-ossifying fibroma, 379
central giant cell granuloma, 481
central mucoepidermoid carcinoma, 435
central odontogenic fibroma, 374
cervical lymphoepithelial cyst, 199
chancre, 513
cheek biting, 603

cheilitis granulomatosa, 522
cheillits
   glandularis, 67
   granulomatosa, 68, 69
chemical carcinogens, 245
cherubism, 450
chicken pox, 543
chlorhexidine, 33
cholesterol clefts, 161, 174, 175
chondroma, 266
chondrosarcoma, 332
   conventional, 332
chromosomal rearrangement, 241
chronic caries, 100
chronic sialoadenitis, 410
Cicatricial pemphigoid, 587
Civatte bodies, 581
clear cell odontogenic carcinoma, 401
cleft lip, 66
cleft lip and palate, 57
cleft palate, 65
cleft tongue, 84
Cleidocranial Dysplasia, 18
colobomata, 54
complex composite odontome, 392
compound composite odontome, 392
conchoidal bodies, 524
concrescence, 24
concussion, 221
congenita, 601, 602

congenital lip pits, 67
congenital syphilis, 27, 514
corps ronds and grains, 76
co-trimoxazole, 633
Cowdry, 301
Coxsackie, 545
cranio-facial dysostosis, 56
craniosynostosis, 56, 455
crater shape, 501
Crohn's disease, 525, 629
Crouzon syndrome, 56
cyclophosphamide, 633
cyst
    gingival cyst of adult, 91
    gingival cyst of newborn, 91
    latent bone, 90
    thyroglossal tract, 88
cystic primary intraosseous carcinoma, 400
cyst-like lesions, 196
cytotoxic drugs, 28

D
Darier's disease, 75, 291, 613
deafmutism, 54
delayed healing, 468
dens evaginatus, 25
dens in dente, 25
dens invaginatus, 25
dental fluorosis, 31
dental plaque, 111

denticles
    false, 155
    true, 155
dentigerous cyst, 182
dentin
    atubular, 44, 156
    tubular, 101
dentinal dysplasia, 43, 155, 157
dentinal sclerosis, 207
dentinogenesis imperfecta, 39, 155, 157
dentinogenesis imperfecta type I, 39
dentinogenesis imperfecta type II, 41
dentinogenesis imperfecta type III, 42
denture fissuratum, 262
denture papillomatosis, 263
denture-induced granuloma, 262
dermoid cyst, 194
desomosomes, 77
developmental lateral periodontal cyst, 179
dextran, 109
diabetes, 11, 441, 465, 468, 486, 527, 533
differentiation, 235
diffuse syphilitic glossitis, 514
diffuse syphilitic osteitis, 514
dilaceration, 24
dimorphic, 496
diphtheria, 511
disaccharides, 105

distomolar, 16
distraction osteogenesis, 221
DNA of tumor cells, 239
DNA repair genes, 242
double lip, 66
Down's syndrome, 97
doxycycline, 77, 586
dry socket, 464
dyskaryosis, 293
dyskeratosis, 74
dyskeratosis congenita, 79, 291, 603
dyskeratotic cells, 76
dysphagia, 80
dystropy of nails, 79

E

early onset idiopathic hypoparathyroidism, 96
EBV, 322
EBV virus, 552
ectopic, 26
Ehlers-Danlos syndrome, 93, 155
enamel hypoplasia, 28, 514
enamel pearl, 26
enameloma, 372
endogenous pigments, 33
eosinophilic granuloma, 485
eosinophilic ulcer, 629
ephelides, 643
epidermolysis bullosa, 77, 628
epimyoepithelial islands, 420

epithelial dysplasia, 291
Epstein-Barr virus, 296, 337, 633
Epstein's pearls, 92
epulis fissuratum, 262
epulis granulomatosa, 262
erosion, 206
eruption
    delayed, 47
    early, 46
eruption cyst, 181
eruption hematoma, 181
erythema multiforme, 588
erythroblastosis fetalis, 33, 34
erythromycin, 504
erythroplakia, 303
eubacteria, 497
Ewing's sarcoma, 333
exanthematous fevers, 29
expressivity, 3, 285, 389
external resorption, 211
extramedullary plasmacytoma, 341

F

facial hemihypertrophy, 62
facial hemihypoplasia, 63
facial paresis, 69
familial benign pemphigus, 586
familial gigantiform cementoma, 388
Fanconi's syndrome, 79, 243
fibrinolytic enzymes, 465
fibroepithelial polyp, 262

Index

fibroma, 257
fibromatosis gingivae, 90
fibrosarcoma, 326
fibrous dysplasia, 446
fibrous epulis, 262
filamentous bacteria, 497
fissural cysts, 191
fissured tongue, 69, 84
florid cemental dysplasia, 386
florid cemento-osseous dysplasia, 386
fluorides, 29
focal cemento-osseous dysplasia, 382
focal epithelial hyperplasia, 253
focal melanosis, 645
focal reversible pulpitis, 146
Forchheimer's sign, 551
Fordyce's granules, 72
Fordyce's spots, 72
Franceschetti's, 53
freckles, 643
frenal tag, 259
Frey's syndrome, 412
frictional keratosis, 603
frontonasal, 54
fungal ball, 571
furred tongue, 87
fusiform bacilli, 500
fusion, 23
fusispirochetal infection, 500

G

Gardener syndrome, 249
Gardener's syndrome, 93
gemination, 23
gene
    ameloblastin, 36
    amplification, 241
    APC, 93, 249
    ATP2A2, 75
    BRAF, 274
    CBFA1, 18
    COL1A1, 39, 458
    COL1A2, 39, 458
    DSPP, 41
    EB, 77
    enamelin, 36
    FGF23, 95
    FGFR-2, 56
    GNAS1, 447
    MDM2, 329
    NF-1, 249
    NF-2, 249
    OFD1, 97
    PHEX, 95
    RB1, 329
    SOX9, 55
    SRY, 6
    STK11, 71
    TP53 (p53), 329
    treacle, 54

tuftelin, 36
geographic tongue, 85
German measles, 550
germ-free, 107
ghost cell odontogenic carcinoma, 400
ghost teeth, 45
giant cell tumor of bone, 483
gingival cyst of adult, 91, 182
gingival cyst of newborn, 181
gingival cysts of newborn, 91
gingivitis
    acute necrotizing ulcerative, 500
    acute streptococcal, 503
glandular fever, 552
glandular odontogenic cyst, 180
globulomaxillary cyst, 193
glossitis areata exofoliativa, 85
glossoptosis, 54
gnotobiote rats, 108
Gorlin cyst, 191, 369
Gorlin-Goltz syndrome, 191, 249
granular cell myoblastoma, 271
granular cell tumor, 271
granuloma
    periapical, 159
gum boil, 164, 168
gumma, 514

H

Hailey-Hailey Disease, 586
hairy leukoplakia, 299
hairy tongue, 86
hand-foot and mouth disease, 545
Hand-Schuller-Christian Disease, 486
Hansen's disease, 514
Hashimoto's thyroiditis, 422
Heck's disease, 253
hemangioendothelioma, 343
hemangiomas, 281
hemangiopericytoma, 343
hemifacial atrophy, 63
hemifacial hypertrophy, 62
hereditary benign intraepithelial dyskeratosis, 74
hereditary ectodermal dysplasia, 20
hereditary gingival fibromatosis, 90
hereditary hemorrhagic telangiectasia, 78
hereditary hypophosphatemia, 94
hereditary retinoblastoma, 329
herpangina, 546
herpes simplex, 539
herpes simplex virus, 295
herpetiform ulcers, 623
heterozygote, 2, 3
hiatus semilunaris, 566
Higmore antrum, 565
Histocytosis X, 484
Holandric inheritance, 6
homozygote, 2, 3
HPV, 295

human papilloma virus, 295
Hutchinson's teeth, 28
hyalinization, 305, 359, 438
Hypercementosis, 168
hypercementosis, 217
Hyperkeratosis, 76
hyperkeratosis, 70, 74
hyperparathyroidism, 488
hyperpituitarism, 642
hyperplasia, 234
hypertrichosis, 90
hypocalcified amelogenesis imperfecta, 37
hypocementosis, 218
hypomaturation amelogenesis imperfecta, 38
hypophosphatasia, 93, 218
hypophosphatemia, 95
hypoplastic amelogenesis imperfecta, 36
hypotrichosis, 21

I

IgG4-related disease, 418
immunology of dental caries, 122
immunosuppression, 248
immunosurveillance, 247
incisive canal cyst, 195
inclusion bodies, 301
incontinentia pigmenti, 640
infantile osteopetrosis, 453

infectious mononucleosis, 552
inflammatory lateral periodontal cyst, 178
inflammatory periapical cyst, 173
insulin-resistant diabetes, 22
interferon alpha, 483
interglobular spaces, 41
internal resorption, 214
interprismatic substance, 33
irradiation, 246
irradiation necrosis, 479
ischemia, 150
isotretinoin, 76

J

Jaffe-Lichtenstein syndrome, 446
juvenile melanoma, 277

K

Kaposi's sarcoma, 334
keratin pearls, 292
keratoacanthoma, 254, 291
keratoconguctivitis sicca, 419
keratocystic odontogenic tumor, 187
keratosis
    actinic, 297, 306, 607
    follicularis, 75
    frictional, 603
    oral, 603
    senile, 306
    smokeless, 606

smokers, 604
sublingual, 605
King Armstrong unit, 462
Koebner's phenomenon, 579, 592
Koplik's spots, 547
Kveim antigen, 523

L

lactoferrin, 105
Langerhans histiocytes, 484
Langhans giant cells, 69, 632
latent bone cyst, 90, 198
Laugier-Hunziker syndrome, 646
leiomyoma, 270
Leishman-Donovan, 536
Leishmaniasis, 535
leprosy, 514
lethal midline granuloma syndrome, 630
Letterer-Swie disease, 487
leukoedema, 72
leukoplakia, 297
levan, 110
lichen planus, 305, 579, 603, 642
lichenoid reactions, 582
Li-Fraumeni syndrome, 329
Li-Fraumni syndrome, 248
lingual pelicata, 84
lingual thyroid nodule, 88
lingual tonsils, 83
lingual varicosities, 82

lipoma, 266
liquefaction foci, 121
lobular capillary hemangioma, 259
loss of polarity, 291
Ludwig's angina, 228
lupus erythematosus, 589
luxation, 221
lymphangioma, 283
lymphoepithelial cysts, 198
lymphoepithelioma, 322
lymphomas, 336
Lyon effect, 37
Lyon hypothesis, 37
lyonization, 21
lyphoepithelial lesion, 420
lysozymes, 105

M

Maccune-Albright syndrome, 446, 447
macrodontia, 21
macroglossia, 81
macrognathia, 65
macrostomia, 62
major aphthae, 623
Malassez epithelial rests, 174, 179, 182
malignant ameloblastoma, 397
malignant melanoma, 345
malignant pleomorphic adenoma, 433
Mallassez, epithelial rests, 161
MAPK, 274
Marble bone disease, 452

Index

marsupialization, 178
maxillofacial gangrene, 502
Mazabraud syndrome, 447
measles, 546
median alveolar cyst, 192
median mandibular cyst, 193
median palatal cyst, 192
median rhomboid glossitis, 531
median rhomboidal glossitis, 85
medication-related osteonecrosis, 476
melanoma
    cutaneous, 345
    juvenile, 277
    mucosal, 350
melasma, 640
Melkersson - Rosenthal syndrome, 69
Melkersson Rosenthal syndrome, 522
mesiodens, 16
metastatic tumors of the jaws, 352
metazoa, 495
Metronidazol, 501
microdontia, 22
microglossia, 81
micrognathia, 64
microstomia, 62
Mikulicz syndrome, 422
Miller, 107
Miller experiment, 107
Miller's theory, 115
minocylcline, 644

minor aphthae, 621
mitogen-activated protein kinase, 274
Mitotic, 239
MMR, 550
molluscum contagiosum, 291
Mongolian spots, 278
Mongolism, 97
moniliasis, 526
monosaccharides, 105
Moon's molar, 28
Moon's molar molar, 514
mosaic appearance, 463
moth-eaten, 352
mottled enamel, 31
moulds, 496
mucicarmine stain, 434
mucoceles, 416
mucous extravasation cyst, 416
mucous patches, 513
mucous retention cyst, 416
Mulberry molar, 514
mulberry molar, 28
multicellular, 496
multiple neurofibromatosis, 285
mumps, 412
Munro, 593
mycetoma, 571
myeloma
    plasma cell, 338
    solitary plasma cell, 341

myoepithelioma, 426
myxoma, 265
myxomatous, 426

N

nasolabial cyst, 193
nasopalatine duct cysts, 195
nasopharyngeal carcinoma, 322
nasopharyngeal lymphoma, 633
nasopharyngeal T-cell lymphomas, 633
natal teeth, 17
necrotizing sialometaplasia, 440
neonatal teeth, 17
neoplasm, 233
neurofibroma, 284
neurofibromatosis, 249
neurolemmoma, 286
nevi, 272
nevoid basal cell carcinoma syndrome, 191
nevus
   blue, 278
   compound, 277
   halo, 280
   intradermal, 276
   junctional, 275
   melanocytic, 273
   of Ota, 280
   pigmented, 273
   Sutton, 280
   vascular, 281
   white spongy, 73
nevus flammeus, 282
Nikolsky's sign, 585
noma, 501, 502
Non-acantholytic, 613
nuclear rows of Verocay, 287

O

oblique facial cleft, 61
odonto-ameloblastoma, 393
odontogenic carcinoma, 399
odontogenic keratocyst, 187
odontogenic myxoma, 375
oligohydramnios, 55
oncocytes, 428
oncocytoma, 428
oncocytosis, 429
oncogenes, 240
oncogenic viruses, 243
onion skin appearance, 334
oral facial digital syndrome, 96
oral keratosis, 603
oral lymphoepithelial cyst, 199
oral melanotic macule, 645
oral submucous fibrosis, 304
Orland experiment, 107
oroantral fistula, 568, 574
orofacial granulomatosis, 522
Osler Weber-Rendu disease, 282
ossifying fibroma, 379, 481
osteitis deformans, 459

Osteitis fibrosa cystica, 488
Osteodentin, 158
osteodentin, 209
osteogenesis imperfecta, 39, 457
osteoid osteoma, 269, 481
osteoma, 268, 481
osteomalacia, 491
osteomyelitis
    acute pyogenic, 468
    chronic non-pyogenic, 473
    chronic pyogenic, 472
    chronic with proliferative periostitis, 473
    diffuse sclerosing, 474
    focal sclerosing, 475
    Garre's, 473
osteopetrosis, 452
osteoporosis, 492
osteoradionecrosis, 479
osteosarcoma, 327
ostium maxillare, 566
otodental syndrome, 22
oxyphilic adenoma, 428

P

p53, 295
pachonychia congenita, 291
pachyonychia congenita, 79
Paget's disease, 218
Paget's disease of bone, 65, 329, 459
palatine papilla cyst, 196
palpebral fissure, 54
pANCA, 633
papillary cystadenoma lymphomatosum, 430
papillary hyperplasia of the palate, 263
papilloma, 251
paradental cyst, 178, 182
paramolar, 16
paramyxovirus, 412
paraneoplastic pemphigus, 584
parulis, 164, 168
Paterson-Kelly syndrome, 80
pathergy, 626
pemphigoid, 586
pemphigus, 582
pemphigus vegetans, 585
pemphigus vulgaris, 585
penetrance, 4, 54, 389, 451, 586, 620
penicillin, 504
pentostam, 536
periapical abscess, 162
periapical cemental dysplasia, 384
periapical cemento-osseous dysplasia, 384
periapical granuloma, 159
pericoronitis, 504
pericyte, 343
periostitis ossificans, 473
peripheral giant cell granuloma, 264
peripheral odontogenic fibroma, 373

perleche, 529
peroxidases, 105
Peutz - Jeghers syndrome, 70
picornaviruses, 545
Pierre Robin syndrome, 54
pigmentation
    black hairy tongue, 86, 645
    black tongue, 87
    drug-induced, 644
    heavy metal, 644
Pindborg tumor, 366
pink spot, 214, 216
pit and fissure caries, 99
plasma cell myeloma, 338
plasmacytoma, 338
pleomorphic adenoma, 424
Plumer-Vinson syndrome, 80
pneumatization, 566
point mutation, 241
polyarteritis nodusa, 419
polyploidy, 239
polyposis coli, 93
polysaccharides, 106
porphyria, 34
Porphyries, 33
port-wine nevus, 282
post-permanent Dentition, 17
Pott's disease, 519
precancerous conditions, 289
pre-deciduous dentition, 17

prednisolone, 633
prednisone, 341
pregnancy tumor, 262
premalignant lesions, 289
primary intraosseous carcinoma of jaw, 399
primordial cyst, 186
progressive systemic sclerosis, 593
prokaryotes, 497
prolabium, 60
prominent circumvallate papillae, 82
prominent foliate papillae, 83
prostate cancer, 353
proteolosis-chelation theory, 116
proteolytic theory, 115
protooncogenes, 240
protozoa, 495
psammoma-like bodies, 438
pseudocyst
    of the maxillary antrum, 200
    salivary gland, 416
pseudoepitheliomatous, 272
pseudoepitheliomatous hyperplasia, 255
pseudomembrane, 513
psoriasis, 591
PTCH gene, 249
ptyalism, 407
pulp
    calcification, 154
    polyp, 152

pulp hyperemia, 146
pulp necrosis, 150
pulp stones, 154
pulpitis
    acute, 149
    chronic, 151
    chronic hyperplastic, 152
    focal reversible, 146
pyogenic granuloma, 259
pyronine bodies, 161

R

racial pigmentation, 640
radiation mucositis, 608
radicular cyst, 173
rampant caries, 100
Ramsay-Hunt syndrome, 544
ranula, 417
recurrent caries, 100
recurrent parotitis, 411
refinement of carbohydrates, 106
regional odontodysplasia, 45
Reiter's syndrome, 612, 627
Rendu-Osler-Weber disease, 78
residual caries, 100
residual cyst, 178
resorption of teeth, 209
retention cyst of the maxillary sinus, 202
retrocuspid papilla, 259
Retzus brown stria, 118

rhabdomyoma, 270
rhagedes, 514
rheumatoid arthritis, 594
rickets, 490
rodent ulcer, 323
rootless teeth, 43
Rothmund-Thomson syndrome, 329
rubella, 550
rubeola, 546
Rushton bodies, 175
Russell bodies, 161, 175

S

saddle nose, 631
salivary antibodies, 104
salivary calculus, 414
salivary duct stenosis, 415
sarcoidosis, 522
scarlet fever, 510
Schaumann bodies, 524
schizodontia, 23
Schwannoma, 286
secondary dentin, 208
secondary tumors, 352
sequelae of caries, 101
sex limited traits, 4
shell tooth, 42
shingles, 543
shovel-shaped, 25
sialoadenosis, 441
sialolithiasis, 414

sialo-odontogenic cyst, 180
sialoprotein, 41
sialorrhoea, 407
sialosis, 441
Sjogren's syndrome, 418
smokeless tobacco keratosis, 606
smoker's keratosis, 604
smooth surface caries, 99
solid primary intraosseous carcinoma, 400
solitary bone cyst, 197
solitary plasma cell myeloma, 341
spindle cell carcinoma, 318
spirochete, 500
squamous cell carcinoma, 313
squamous odontogenic tumor, 371
Stafne bone cyst, 90
Stephan curve, 113
stomatitis medicamentosa, 618
stomatitis nicotina, 604
strawberry gums, 631
strawberry tongue, 510
Streeter's syndrome, 20
Streptococcus mutans, 109
stroma, 235
Sturge-Weber syndrome, 282, 609
sublingual keratosis, 605
submucous cleft palate, 61
sucrose, 105
sulfasalazine, 525

sulfur granules, 521
supernumerary Cusps, 26
supernumerary roots, 26
supernumerary teeth, 16
supplemental teeth, 16
suprabasilar clefts, 76
surgical ciliated cyst, 201
syphilis, 512
    acquired, 513
    congenital, 28
    postnatal, 512
    prenatal, 512
systemic lupus erythematosus, 590
systemic mycoses, 534

T

Talon cusp, 26
tartar, 129
tattoo
    amalgam, 644
    graphite, 644
taurodontism, 24
teething problems, 48
telangiectasia, 79, 609
telangiectasias, 307
Teratogens, 10
tertiary dentin, 208
Tetracycline, 33, 78, 624, 644
tetracycline, 29
thrush, 528
thymoma, 533

thyroglossal tract cyst, 88, 196
torus
    mandibularis, 66
    palatinus, 65
Touton giant cells, 276
transverse clefts, 121
transverse facial cleft, 61
traumatic bone cyst, 197
traumatic neuroma, 287
traumatic ulcers, 616
Treacher Collins syndrome, 53
treponema pallidium, 512
triamcinolone acetonide, 482
trisomy 21, 97
tuberculosis, 517
    lymph node, 518
tuberculous lymphadenitis, 518
Tzanck cells, 585

U
ulcerative colitis, 629
ulcers, 612
unicellular, 496
unicystic ameloblastoma, 363

V
Van der Woude syndrome, 57, 58
varicella, 543
Verocay bodies, 287
verruca vulgaris, 252
verrucous carcinoma, 320

vesiculobullous, 611
vesiculobullous lesions, 582
Vincent angina, 501
Vincent organisms, 500
viral insertion, 241
viral structure, 537
visceral Leishmaniasis, 537
vitamin D-resistant rickets, 94
Von Recklinghausen disease of skin, 285
von-Hippel Lindau disease, 282
Von-Recklinghausen's disease of bone, 488

W
wart
    common, 252
    flat, 252
    palmoplantar, 252
Warthin-Finkeldey, 549
Warthin's tumor, 430
Warthin-Starry silver staining, 261
Wegener's granulomatosis, 630
white spongy nevus, 73
Wickham's stria, 579
Witkop classification, 36
Witkop's disease, 74

X
xeroderma pigmentosa, 70, 346
xerostomia, 405, 608

Y
yeasts, 496

Z
zoster Virus, 543

Index